Praise for

ODD GIRL OUT

"This is the book we have been waiting for. It's a wake-up call to all of us who care deeply about girls' development. Simmons has given voice to the girls who struggle everyday with friendships. She has uncovered a hidden world of aggression that unfolds behind adults' backs."
— Susan Wellman, President of The Ophelia Project

"Passionate and beautifully written. A significant contribution to our understanding of the psychology of girls."
— Michael Thompson, coauthor of *Raising Cain*

"Required reading for young girls and their mothers."
— *Boston Globe*

"A bold and myth-shattering work." — *Seattle Weekly*

"Peels away the smiley surfaces of adolescent female society to expose one of girlhood's dark secrets: the vicious psychological warfare waged every day in the halls of our middle schools and high schools."
— *San Francisco Chronicle*

"There has not been so much interest in young females since psychologist Mary Pipher chronicled anorexics and suicide victims in her 1994 bestseller, *Reviving Ophelia*." — *Washington Post*

ODD *girl* OUT

ODD *girl* OUT

the
hidden
culture of
aggression
in girls

COMPLETELY REVISED AND UPDATED

RACHEL SIMMONS

MARINER BOOKS
HOUGHTON MIFFLIN HARCOURT
boston new york

First Mariner Books edition 2011

www.hmhco.com

The Library of Congress Cataloging has cataloged the hardcover edition as follows:
Simmons, Rachel, 1974–
Odd girl out: the hidden culture of aggression in girls/
Rachel Simmons. — 1st ed.
p.   cm.
ISBN 978-0-15-100604-5   ISBN 978-0-15-602734-2 (pbk.)
ISBN 978-0-547-52019-3 (rev. ed.)
1. Aggressiveness in children. 2. Girls — Psychology.   I. Title.
BF723.A35 .S56 2002
302.5'4'08342 — dc21   2001006864

Text set in Galliard
Book design by Kaelin Chappell

Printed in the United States of America

DOC 10 9 8

To my parents,
Claire and Luiz Simmons,
whose constant faith, love,
and support made this book possible
and
To Jane Isay:
heroine, world changer, and friend,
who believed, and believed, and believed.

contents

ODD *girl* OUT

When it was first published, *Odd Girl Out* lit a fuse in the culture, setting off a passionate public dialogue about girls and bullying. Parents and girls who had struggled without recognition suddenly gained a platform, language, and community. Now, this thing that had lived in the shadows had come to light.

Although I wrote the book as a journalist telling a story, I ended up becoming part of the story itself. *Odd Girl Out*'s publication launched me on a book tour that never quite came to an end. I began working with schools, families, and youth professionals to fight the bullying epidemic. I became a classroom teacher and co-founded the Girls Leadership Institute, a nonprofit organization that teaches girls, schools, and families skills for healthy relationships. I wrote two more books: *Odd Girl Speaks Out,* a collection of girls' writing about bullying and friendship, and *The Curse of the Good Girl: Raising Authentic Girls with Courage and Confidence.*

This is why I had to revise the book. I wrote it as an observer, but I have revised it as a practitioner. The new edition contains a decade of strategies, insights, and wisdom I have gathered while teaching and living with girls, interviewing administrators, coaching parents, and talking with school counselors. In four new chapters, readers will get down-to-earth tools to help a girl survive one of the most painful events of her life. I share the lessons I learned the hard way and the best practices I collected from extraordinary colleagues.

When I first wrote *Odd Girl Out,* there was no texting, no Facebook, no cell phone cameras, no video chats. Today, girl bullying has gone digital. Cell phones and computers have become a new kind of bathroom wall, giving users the ability to destroy relationships and reputations with a few clicks. Social media has been a game changer, transforming the landscape of girl bullying.

Technology has also altered girls' everyday relationships, indeed girls' very sense of self. It is not uncommon for a girl to say, "I don't exist if I'm not on Facebook." Many girls sleep with their cell phones on their chests, waiting for them to vibrate with news in the night. They treat their cell phones like extensions of their bodies and are inconsolable if they lose access. In 2010, the average teen texted three thousand times per month.

There is now a seamless integration between girls' virtual and real lives, and this new era of BFF 2.0 has brought both blessing and curse. On the one hand, cell phones and social networking sites like Facebook allow girls to connect in exhilarating new ways. On the other hand, Facebook makes many girls anxious, jealous, and even paranoid about their friendships. Girls have instant access to photographs of parties they were excluded from, or conversations they were not invited to join. Cell phones are posing thorny new questions about friendship, such as: Is my friend mad at me if I text her and she doesn't reply? Why is she texting while I'm talking to her?

This new edition guides readers through the sprawling world girls now inhabit online. In two new chapters, I explain the ins and outs of cyberbullying. I also explore the more common cyberdrama, or day-to-day conflicts and confusion that social media can ignite. I share concrete advice on how to guide girls through the new challenges they are facing.

Still other changes have evolved within the hidden culture of girls' aggression. As the issue of girl bullying has risen to new prominence, it has attracted a more troubling kind of attention. Reality television show producers discovered that mean girls sell, and they churned out scores of programs featuring breathtakingly aggressive females. These programs rewarded their stars with book deals, product lines, and other spoils of celebrity—and gained a rapt teen following. The scramble to commodify the mean girl trickled down to even the youngest consumers: children's television programming began to highlight an array of snarky, sarcastic girl characters. As a result, girls now observe ten times the amount of relational aggression on television that they see in real life. In an analysis of television programs, researchers found that the meanest female characters on television were frequently rewarded for their behavior.

Invariably, these changes in the culture inflect girls' relationships. With more aggression to absorb, there is more to mimic. When aggression is sold as entertainment or an accessory to friendship, it is harder to define the behavior as problematic. Girls perceive an incentive to claim power through aggression. More than ever before, girls face pressure to be and act and look in ways that undermine their healthy development.

In my travels over the last ten years, there is one comment that I hear almost everywhere: girl bullying is not only meaner; it's younger.[1] While three-year-old girls have always used relational aggression (the use of friendship as a weapon) to control their peers, today's girls seem to reach developmental milestones sooner. Name-calling, exclusion, and popularity wars start as early as kindergarten. It is unclear if girls are mimicking behavior they do not really understand, or if we are now noticing what was there all along. Still, the age creep of girl bullying, even if it has yet to be backed up by research, is difficult to ignore. Parents cannot wait until their girls are in elementary school to educate themselves and their daughters about aggression and bullying.

Not all the changes of the last decade are troubling. There has been remarkable social change. The number of researchers studying girls' aggression has skyrocketed. Scores of studies have been completed and published, providing the first critical mass of research on girls' psychological aggression.[2] Today, it is harder to argue that the cruelty of girls is a trivial phase, rite of passage, or "girls being girls." Just a few years ago, the term "relational aggression" was largely unknown. Now, training to understand and intervene in girls' aggression is increasingly common in school districts across the country.

State and federal governments are also taking notice. By early 2011, twenty states had passed legislation requiring schools to create anti-bullying policy (my father, a state legislator, is the primary sponsor of Maryland's Safe Schools Reporting Act). The federal government launched Stop Bullying Now, a wide-ranging, multi-agency initiative to reduce bullying in schools. And news media is also taking notice: after several tormented children and teens committed suicide, the plight of bullied youth and their families became breaking news. National news programs like NBC's *Today* and CNN's *American Morning* led with stories of peer assault, cybercruelty, and bullying among teens. The unwelcome attention this exposure brought to school communities put others on notice: crises that were once private community matters could wind up leading a national newscast. The issue's new prominence has inspired more parent advocacy and increased vigilance among school administrators.

There have also been some surprises along the way. I have noticed increasing numbers of boys and their parents gathering in the audience of my talks. After student assemblies, boys wait in line along with girls to ask me questions. They share stories of being targeted by a class's "mean girls," or admit to "acting like mean girls" themselves. Research confirms a shrinking gender gap in behaviors like relational aggression, especially by the time boys reach middle school. These behaviors are clearly not owned by girls, and adolescent boys are telling researchers that relational and social aggression—actions that damage friendship and reputation—concern them more than physical intimidation.

It is unclear if the incidence of these behaviors is higher today, or if we now have a language to name what is happening. Researchers who once asked boys only about physical violence are now reframing their questions. Although it is true that girls disproportionately engage in some of these behaviors, it is also surely time for boys to have their say. In the meantime, this book may be written about girls, but many of its stories and strategies apply to boys and girls alike.

Despite the extraordinary changes of the last decade, girl bullying looks a lot like it always did, and it is far from over. Every day, girls eat lunch in bathroom stalls because they are too afraid to sit alone in the cafeteria. They sit in class, anxious and panicked, obsessively wondering who will play with them at recess. They open their cell phones to screens blinking with venom. They also struggle to confront toxic friends and speak their truths. As ever, girls need our help and support.

By now, I have spoken to tens of thousands of people. Many enjoy my advice, but most want to hear stories. They are curious about the other parents and girls I have met: How did they feel? What choices did they face? How did they overcome their struggle? The hidden culture of aggression in girls can be a hurtful, lonely place. But it is in others' stories that we can hear and see ourselves. We know we are not alone. We know, too, that there is hope. We know it will not always feel the way it does right now.

In this new edition of *Odd Girl Out*, I am proud to share all that I have learned with you. The stories, including yours, must continue to be told.

When I was eight years old, I was bullied by another girl. I remember very little about that year. My memory is fractured by time and will. I was in the third grade, wore pigtails, and had a lisp. I was known to my teachers as a "rusher," the girl who tore through long-division worksheets and map quizzes, making careless mistakes I was told I could avoid. But I loved to finish first.

So did Abby. She was my popular friend, not a particularly close one. I still don't know why she did it. First she whispered about me to my best friend, who soon decided she'd be happier playing with other girls. When we went to dance class after school at the local community center, Abby rounded up my friends and convinced them to run away from me. Into the center's theater I would sprint after them, winded and frantic, eyes straining in the sudden darkness. Down over rows of slumbering chairs and up on the stage, I would follow the retreating patter of steps and fading peals of laughter.

Day after day I stood in half-lit empty hallways, a stairwell, the parking lot. In all of these places I remember standing alone. In the early evenings before dinner, I cried to my mother while she cooked.

The sorrow was overwhelming, and I was sure I was the only girl ever to know it. This is what I remember most.

Sixteen years later, I was attending graduate school in England. It was raining the day I rode my bike to the library in search of answers about what had happened with Abby. Exactly what pulled me there is hard to say. Something about the memory seemed terribly off-balance to me. On the one hand, I could remember few details. On the other, the anguish of being abandoned by all of my friends and of losing my closest at Abby's hand felt real and raw. It was something that never receded gently with the rest of my childhood memories. I wanted—I needed—to fill in the blanks.

That day, I carried with me the memory of a late night at college, when a casual midnight snack led to six of us confessing that an Abby haunted our past. It was exhilarating to discover we'd all been through the same ordeal. Like me, my friends had spent years believing they were the only ones.

Armed with that knowledge, I pedaled carefully along the slick streets, certain there would be volumes of books waiting to explain how and why girls bully each other. When my first few computer searches turned up next to nothing, I chalked it up to rusty research skills, or rushing. Then I called the librarian over for help. As it turned out, I'd been doing just fine on my own.

In a sea of articles on boys' aggression and bullying, there were only a small handful of articles about girls. There were no accessible books. No guides for parents. No cute survival manuals for kids. As I sat reading the articles, I could not see myself or Abby in what most of these researchers called bullying. I was first surprised, then frustrated.

I sent out an e-mail to everyone I knew in the States and asked them to forward it to as many women as they could. I asked a few simple questions: "Were you ever tormented or teased by another girl? Explain what it was like. How has it affected you today?" Within twenty-four hours my in box was flooded with responses from all over America. The messages piled up as women told their stories into cyberspace with an emotional intensity that was undeniable. Even on the computer screen, their pain felt as fresh and unresolved as my own. Women I never met wrote that I would be the first person ever to hear their story. It would be a long time before I knew it was because I was the first to ask.

Silence is deeply woven into the fabric of the female experience. It is only in the last thirty years that we have begun to speak the distinctive truths of women's lives, openly addressing rape, incest, domestic violence, and women's health. Although these issues always existed, over time we have given them a place in our culture by building public consciousness, policy, and awareness.

Now it is time to end another silence: There is a hidden culture of girls' aggression in which bullying is epidemic, distinctive, and destructive. It is not marked by the direct physical and verbal behavior that is primarily the province of boys. Our culture refuses girls access to open conflict, and it forces their aggression into nonphysical, indirect, and covert forms. Girls use backbiting, exclusion, rumors, name-calling, and manipulation to inflict psychological pain on victimized targets. Unlike boys, who tend to bully acquaintances or strangers, girls frequently attack within tightly knit networks of friends, making aggression harder to identify and intensifying the damage to the targets.

Within the hidden culture of aggression, girls fight with body language and relationships instead of fists and knives. In this world, friendship is a weapon, and the sting of a shout pales in comparison to a day of someone's silence. There is no gesture more devastating than the back turning away.

In the hidden culture of aggression, anger is rarely articulated, and every day of school can be a new social minefield that realigns itself without warning. During times of conflict, girls will turn on one another with a language and justice only they can understand. Behind a facade of female intimacy lies a terrain traveled in secret, marked with anguish, and nourished by silence.

This is the world I want the reader to enter. It is where, beneath a chorus of voices, one girl glares at another, then smiles silently at her friend. The next day a ringleader passes around a secret petition asking girls to outline the reasons they hate the targeted girl. The day after that, the outcast sits silently next to the boys in class, head lowered, shoulders slumped forward. The damage is neat and quiet, the aggressor and target invisible.

Public awareness of bullying has grown in recent years, propelled by the tragedies of youth gun violence. The national conversation on bullying, however, has trained its spotlight mostly on boys and their aggression. Defining bullying in the narrowest of terms, it has focused entirely on physical and direct acts of violence. The aggression of girls, often hidden, indirect, and nonphysical, has gone unexplored. It has not even been called aggression, but instead "what girls do."

Yet women of every age know about it. Nearly all of us have been bystanders, targets, or bullies. So many have suffered quietly and tried to forget. Indeed, this has long been one of girlhood's dark, dirty secrets. Nearly every woman and girl has a story. It is time to break the silence.

I set out to interview girls between the ages of ten and fourteen, the years when bullying peaks. On my first day, I worked with several groups of ninth graders at a coed private school on the East Coast. My plan was to encourage an informal discussion guided by a list of questions I'd written down. Standing before each class, I introduced myself, explained my own history with bullying, and told the girls what we'd be discussing. Without fail, the girls would do a double take. *Talking about* what? *During class?* They snickered and whispered.

I started each session with the same question: "Do you think there are differences between the ways guys are mean to each other and the ways girls are mean to each other?" The whispering stopped. Then the hands flew like streamers. Suddenly, they couldn't talk fast enough. Their banter was electric. The girls hooted, screeched, laughed, snorted, and veered off into personal stories, while notes flew around the room, accompanied by rolling eyes and searing and knowing glances.

It was exhausting. My carefully organized list of research questions grew stale in my hand.

Not a single one of my group discussions that day went according to plan. This, it turned out, was a good thing. I quickly understood that trying to box the girls' voices into my prearranged questions would make them think I was an authority figure, and this was the last thing I wanted to be. I wanted *them* to be the authorities. After all, they were living what I was trying to understand. It wasn't a tactic so much as an instinct.

The girls responded in kind. Over the months that followed, we traded e-mail and instant message handles, talked about music groups, new shoes, summer plans, and crushes. They showed and told me things their teachers and parents couldn't know about. We sometimes strayed from the topic at hand to talk about the pressures of school and family.

Over time, however, I realized there was another reason for the ease we felt with one another. Most people who talk to kids about bullying approach the issue with the same message: Don't do it. Be nice to each other.

I came from the opposite place. My assumption was not that the girls ought not to be mean, but that they were; not that they should be nice, but that they weren't. I was there not to stop them, but because I wanted them to help other girls find a way to deal with it. If they wanted to participate in the group discussion, fine; if they didn't, they had to sit quietly and they couldn't bother the ones who did. Either way, I told them, they'd get a free snack out of it.

More often than not during the sessions, a girl would tell her own story of victimization. She might begin by replying to one of her classmates' remarks, and then, as though taken by surprise, slide into a slow, tearful remembering of her pain. Although I knew I was in the classrooms only to conduct research, I was overwhelmed by feelings of protectiveness toward these girls.

For this reason, I adhered to an informal discussion format, going with the girls where they wanted to go. Like the women I met on the Internet, many of the girls had never been asked about this part of their lives. Like me, they seemed to feel that they were all alone, the only ones to have gone through this. I met their sadness at the level of my own. They had chosen me to hear their stories, and I wanted to honor their voices. I also wanted them to realize it happened to me and plenty of others. It felt inhumane to move over and through their pain and on to the next question on the list. Sometimes I got through all my questions, sometimes I didn't. If my work suffers in any way, the responsibility is mine, and it's one I am happy to take.

During this period, I was guided by the work of psychologists Lyn Mikel Brown and Carol Gilligan, to whose pioneering research with girls I owe a huge intellectual debt. With a group of colleagues, Brown and Gilligan developed a "Listening Guide" to use in their interviews.[3] The method emphasizes flexibility and harmony with the interview subject, and it discourages orthodox interview protocols. Instead, researchers are to "move where the girls [lead]" them. The method is especially important to girls who might otherwise stay quiet in the presence of an interviewer who appears to have an agenda. Staying with the girls' voices, rather than emphasizing one's own, "can help girls to develop, to hold on to, or to recover knowledge about themselves, their feelings, and their desires," according to Brown and Gilligan. "Taking girls seriously encourages them to take their own thoughts, feelings, and experience seriously, to maintain this knowledge, and even to uncover knowledge that has become lost to them." With such an emotional issue as girls' bullying, this seemed more than appropriate.

As I sought out more schools to work with, I got mixed responses from administrators. Most were relieved to have me talk with their students. Staff had been mystified by the intensity of the girls' anger toward one another. They were bewildered and overwhelmed by the episodes unfolding around them.

The smaller towns and some private schools were less welcoming. Their refusal to grant me access, though never explained, seemed to me a sign of anxiety that the truth would be discovered about their girls: that yes, indeed, they *were* capable of being mean. In a society raising girls to be loving and "nice," this was no small exposure.

Because of the sensitive nature of the discussions, I made another decision. To get a comprehensive account of the problem of girl bullying, I had originally planned to travel to as many different cities as I could. After a few intensive sessions with the girls, I knew this would be impossible. To earn their trust, and the faith of their teachers and parents, I would need to become a part of their communities. For this reason I chose to stay in three parts of the country for extended periods. I was rewarded with almost unconditional access and support by many of my host schools. Two schools even reversed their policy of not permitting researchers on campus to allow me to work with their girls.

In exchange for their generosity, I promised to change the names of the girls, staff members, and schools. Other than giving an economic and racial profile, I use very few details to describe each school. I worked with a total of ten over a period of one year. In a major middle-Atlantic city, I visited three schools: the Linden School, a private school with mostly middle-class students, 25 percent of whom are minority; Marymount, a private all-girls school with a predominantly middle-class population and about 20 percent students of color; and Sackler Day School, a suburban middle-class Jewish day school. In a second Northeastern city, I visited Clara Barton High School, an alternative high school, and Martin Luther King Elementary; both schools had predominantly black, Puerto Rican, and Dominican populations. I also worked at the Arden School, a laboratory school with a mostly middle-class population that is 20 percent minority, and Sojourner Truth, an all-girls school with a majority black and Latina student body. Finally, I spent several weeks visiting the elementary, middle, and high schools in Ridgewood, a small town in northeast Mississippi.

At each school, I conducted group and individual interviews with students and interested staff and parents. At some schools, interviews took as many as three or four hours. At other schools, where time for the interviews was more limited, the meetings were shorter. At two of the urban schools, I struggled to connect with some students and parents. The families were mostly poor, and some did not have telephones, although I am sure my presence as a white, middle-class woman deterred an unknown number of others. Some students and parents expressed interest, then did not return my call or meet me at the appointed time. At every school I was disappointed, though not surprised, to find no parent willing to discuss a daughter who bullied.

In addition to girls and their parents, I interviewed approximately fifty adult women by phone and in person. I include their stories because time and therapy have given them broader, more nuanced perspectives on their ordeals. Their voices present a marked contrast to the stories of young targets and bullies.

Although I sought guidance from the methods of Brown and Gilligan, this book is not the product of a formal research experiment. In it you will not find statistics or scientific conclusions about girls and aggression or information about boys. Few would argue that boys have access to a wide range of ways to express their anger. Many girls, on the other hand, are forced to cut themselves off from direct aggression altogether.

Odd Girl Out is the first book devoted exclusively to girls and nonphysical conflict, and it tells the stories of aggressors and targets of what I call "alternative," or unconventional, aggressions.

In no way do I want to imply that only girls behave in these ways. Boys most definitely engage in alternative aggressions, though reportedly at later stages of childhood than girls. Nor am I suggesting that *all* girls do it. Although I set out to map the hidden culture of girls' aggression, it was always clear to me that not all white, middle-class girls lock conflict out of their relationships. Overwhelmed by what I was discovering, I neglected to talk with more girls who do feel comfortable with anger and conflict. I regret that.

I will use the term "girl bullying" throughout the book to refer to acts of alternative aggression. Yet I am arguing not that girls *feel* angry in fundamentally different ways than boys, but that many girls appear to *show* anger differently. Girls' aggression may be covert and relational; it may indeed be fueled at times by a fear of loss or isolation. That does not mean, however, that girls do not want power or feel aggression as passionately as their male peers.

In their important book *Best Friends, Worst Enemies: Understanding the Social Lives of Children,* Michael Thompson and colleagues point out that every child wants three things out of life: connection, recognition, and power. The desire for connection propels children into friendship, while the need for recognition and power ignites competition and conflict. My point is that if all children desire these things, they will come to them, and into learning how to acquire them, on the culture's terms, that is, by the rules of how girls and boys are supposed to behave.

When I began this journey three years ago, I wanted to write so that other bullied girls would know they were not alone. As I spent more and more time with the girls, I realized I was also writing to know that *I* was not alone. I would soon discover that the bullying I endured in third grade was only the tip of the iceberg. I discovered that I harbored pain and confusion over many relationships in my childhood.

Around the circles of girls I met with, I could see I wasn't the only one who felt this way. The knowledge that we shared similar memories and feelings, that someone else understood what we had previously held inside, was amazing. The relief was palpable, and it opened unexpected doors that we were able to enter together. If we began the journey at the memory of bullying, we ended up asking, and answering, more questions about the culture we live in, about how girls treat each other, and even about ourselves than we had ever thought to imagine alone.

When *Odd Girl Out* was first published, the little research that existed on alternative aggressions was buried in academic journals. It went unnoticed in the media frenzy over school shootings. Public commentary continues to suggest that bullying is most dangerous between boys or when it culminates in physical violence. In chapter one, "The Hidden Culture of Aggression in Girls," I explore what may be unique about girls' aggression and analyze school attitudes toward girl bullying.

This chapter also examines the phenomenon of covert aggression between girls. A great deal of girls' anger flows quietly beneath the radar of teachers, guidance counselors, and parents. It is not, as one woman told me, "something you find in your child's drawer." Girls, ever respectful, tend to aggress quietly. They flash looks, pass notes, and spread rumors. Their actions, though sometimes physical, are typically more psychological and thus invisible to even an observant classroom eye. There is the note that is slipped into a desk; the eyes that catch, narrow, and withdraw; the lunch table that suddenly has no room. Girls talk to me in this chapter about how and why they act in secret.

The barbs of a girl bully go unnoticed when they are hidden beneath the facade of friendship. In chapter two, "Intimate Enemies," I explore dynamics of bullying and emotional abuse between close friends. The importance of relationship and connection in girls' lives, along with the fear of solitude, leads many of them to hold on to destructive friendships, even at the expense of their emotional safety. Aggressors, on the other hand, are hurting the close friends they appear to love.

Although I set out to understand severe episodes of bullying between girls, I quickly discovered that everyday episodes of conflict can be just as harrowing. In chapter three, "The Truth Hurts," girls answer the question, "When you are angry or upset with someone, do you tell them about it?" They unpack their fears of direct conflict with one another and explore the indirect acts they choose instead. Girls dissect the politics of how and why they gang up on each other. They explore how repressing anger and avoiding confrontation can lead to disastrous consequences.

Some of these disasters are now digital. Social media, such as e-mail, online chat, and texting, offer the perfect alternatives to the direct conflict so many girls disdain. Cyberbullying has become vicious and wide-ranging, while girls have become virtual addicts to their gadgets in the drive to stay connected to their friends. In chapter four, "BFF 2.0," I lead readers through the sprawling landscape of girls' digital relationships and report on the unique challenges of these new communication channels.

Of all the insults girls can hurl at each other, one of the worst is getting called a girl who thinks "she's all that." In the chapter of the same name, I ask girls why they can't stand it when someone appears conceited or full of herself. If this is indeed the age of girl power, why would someone else's success bother them? The girls open up about why they keep jealousy and competition secret from one another, and along the way introduce me to a code they use to communicate uncomfortable feelings.

I count myself among the many women and girls who have demonized the girl bullies in their lives. At some point, I began to wonder what it would be like to see Abby today, and I imagined the questions I might ask her. In chapter six, "The Bully in the Mirror," several former and current bullies talk about why they hurt and betrayed their friends. Listening to their stories, I consider my own past, wondering why so many of us are quick to separate ourselves from the "mean girls," and how this may affect our ability to address the problem of girl bullying.

The culture's socialization of girls as caretakers teaches them they will be valued for their relationships with others. In chapter seven, "Popular," I challenge some of the current research on what makes girls popular. In particular, I look at how the politics of girls' relationships can lead to mistreatment and aggression. I explore why some girls may be nice in private but mean in public and why other girls simply abandon their friends.

Not all girls avoid conflict. Aggression may be biological, but the face of anger is learned. Although I found alternative aggressions most severe among white, middle-class girls, I spent time in other communities where assertiveness and direct conflict are valued in girls. In "Resistance," I explore the history and practice of direct conflict and truth telling in African American, Latino, and working-class communities. Although girls from these specific communities are at the center of this chapter, the reader should not take this as a sign of their exclusion from others. *Odd Girl Out* focuses on life under rules of feminine restraint that all but refuse girls open acts of conflict. Those girls are primarily, but certainly not only, white and middle class.

The attention shown targets and aggressors of bullying often means the situation parents face is overlooked. Parents and guardians of targets harbor intense feelings of shame and helplessness, yet they are as isolated from one another as their daughters. Often they can only watch as their daughters come home crying day after day. Called at work because of a stomachache that doesn't exist or watching their girl's increasing isolation, they are embarrassed that their child is scorned. Some blame themselves, while others are angry at their daughter's passivity. Girls, if they confide the problem, often beg their parents not to intervene, fearing retribution.

In chapter nine, I explore how parents find themselves thrust into a world not unlike their daughters'. They want to help their children but fear making things worse. They are first torn, then muzzled, by their own confused feelings. Even as they struggle to help their child, they fear confrontation with another parent. Some choose to wait for the problem to pass or the phase to end.

When it's time for action, read chapter ten. "Helping Her Through Drama, Bullying, and Everything in Between" has my answers to the most pressing questions parents have asked me over the last decade. You will get my best thinking on what to say, how to say it, and the optimal course of action. You will also hear the voices of women and girls who told me what they wished their parents had done to make their lives easier during their ordeal—and why so many of them refused to tell their parents the truth.

When should your daughter get a Facebook account or cell phone? What kinds of limits should you set on use, and how do you talk to her about technology? For the answers, see chapter eleven, "Raising Girls in a Digital Age." Readers will learn what every parent of a girl should know about safe, ethical, and responsible use of social media.

Over the last decade, I have spent countless hours with educators and administrators—indeed, I have become a teacher myself. We work on the frontlines of the battle to end bullying. It is a complex and confusing war to wage. In chapter twelve, "The Road Ahead for Educators and Administrators," I share effective intervention and prevention strategies for classroom teachers and school leaders.

Are girls' problems with conflict confined to friendship and bullying? In the conclusion, I visit girls at a leadership workshop and discover unexpected parallels between their identities as girlfriends and girl leaders. Remembering the girls of chapter two, I explore links between girls' behavior in abusive friendships and the trauma of relationship violence. Finally, I consider the loss of self-esteem that besets girls around adolescence. Since alternative aggressions explode between girls around this time, I suggest potential connections between the two.

Because I wanted the girls to feel comfortable saying anything, teachers almost never joined my interview sessions. At one woman's insistence, I allowed her to sit in the back of a classroom I was visiting. Thirty minutes into a lively discussion about the ways girls are mean to each other, she was sitting stiffly, her face tightening in anger. Finally, she raised her hand.

"You know," she said, "not all girls are mean. Girls are wonderful! Women are the most important friends you'll ever have, and I don't think it's fair to talk only about the bad parts of girls." Although I could not agree with her more, the remark haunted me. It would be a grave mistake for the reader to interpret this book as a condemnation of girls and women. Nothing could be further from the truth.

Our culture has long been accustomed to celebrating the "niceness" of girls. The stories of *Odd Girl Out* may therefore unsettle some readers. But my attempt to name the aggression of girls should not be read as an attempt to disparage them. For the purposes of this book I interviewed only girls who identified as aggressors or targets. Not all girls bully, nor do they inflict injury in such severe ways.

I want to make clear that my deep affection for girls and women has guided this project every step of the way. Throughout my life, women and girls have nourished me with strength, wisdom, and care. I credit a great deal of my own success to older women mentors, many of whom were invaluable in helping this book come to life. And without the women closest to me, I would never have had the courage to arrive at many of the personal insights I share in this book.

Writing this book changed my life. I was astonished to find how many of my own fears and questions about relationships were echoed in the girls' remarks. Their stories forced me to look hard at my own fears of conflict, especially my need to be a "good girl." It is my hope that readers will be able to confront their own fears and pose their own questions. Such a journey of reconnection is certainly not easy, but it is well worth the trip.

CHAPTER *one*

the hidden culture of
aggression in girls

The Linden School campus is nestled behind a web of sports fields that seem to hold at bay the bustling city in which it resides. On Monday morning in the Upper School building, students congregated languidly, catching up on the weekend, while others sat knees-to-chest on the floor, flipping through three-ring binders, cramming for tests. The students were dressed in styles that ran the gamut from trendy to what can only be described, at this age, as defiant. Watching them, it is easy to forget this school is one of the best in the region, its students anything but superficial. This is what I came to love about Linden: it celebrates academic rigor and the diversity of its students in equal parts. Over the course of a day with eight groups of ninth graders, I began each meeting with the same question: "What are some of the differences between the ways guys and girls are mean?"

From periods one through eight, I heard the same responses. "Girls can turn on you for anything," said one. "Girls whisper," said another. "They glare at you." With growing certainty, they fired out answers:

"Girls are secretive."

"They destroy you from the inside."

"Girls are manipulative."

"There's an aspect of evil in girls that there isn't in boys."

"Girls target you where they know you're weakest."

"Girls do a lot behind each other's backs."

"Girls plan and premeditate."

"With guys you know where you stand."

"I feel a lot safer with guys."

In bold, matter-of-fact voices, girls described themselves to me as disloyal, untrustworthy, and sneaky. They claimed girls use intimacy to manipulate and overpower others. They said girls are fake, using each other to move up the social hierarchy. They described girls as unforgiving and crafty, lying in wait for a moment of revenge that will catch the unwitting target off guard and, with an almost savage eye-for-an-eye mentality, "make her feel the way I felt."

The girls' stories about their conflicts were casual and at times filled with self-hatred. In almost every group session I held, someone volunteered her wish to have been born a boy because boys can "fight and have it be over with."

Girls tell stories of their anger in a culture that does not define their behaviors as aggression. As a result, their narratives are filled with destructive myths about the inherent duplicity of females. As poet and essayist Adrienne Rich notes,[4] "We have been depicted as generally whimsical, deceitful, subtle, vacillating."

Since the dawn of time, women and girls have been portrayed as jealous and underhanded, prone to betrayal, disobedience, and secrecy. Lacking a public identity or language, girls' nonphysical aggression is called "catty," "crafty," "evil," and "cunning." Rarely the object of research or critical thought, this behavior is seen as a natural phase in girls' development. As a result, schools write off girls' conflicts as a rite of passage, as simply "what girls do."

What would it mean to name girls' aggression? Why have myths and stereotypes served us so well and so long?

Aggression is a powerful barometer of our social values. According to sociologist Anne Campbell, attitudes toward aggression crystallize sex roles, or the idea that we expect certain responsibilities to be assumed by males and females because of their sex.[5] Riot grrls and women's soccer notwithstanding, Western society still expects boys to become family providers and protectors, and girls to be nurturers and mothers. Aggression is the hallmark of masculinity; it enables men to control their environment and livelihoods. For better or for worse, boys enjoy total access to the rough and tumble. The link begins early: the popularity of boys is in large part determined by their willingness to play rough. They get peers' respect for athletic prowess, resisting authority, and acting tough, troublesome, dominating, cool, and confident.

On the other side of the aisle, females are expected to mature into caregivers, a role deeply at odds with aggression. Consider the ideal of the "good mother": She provides unconditional love and care for her family, whose health and daily supervision are her primary objectives. Her daughters are expected to be "sugar and spice and everything nice." They are to be sweet, caring, precious, and tender.

"Good girls" have friends, and lots of them. As nine-year-old Noura told psychologists Lyn Mikel Brown and Carol Gilligan, perfect girls have "perfect relationships."[6] These girls are caretakers in training. They "never have any fights...and they are always together....Like never arguing, like 'Oh yeah, I totally agree with you.'" In depressing relationships, Noura added, "someone is really jealous and starts being really mean....[It's] where two really good friends break up."

A "good girl," journalist Peggy Orenstein observes in *Schoolgirls,* is "nice before she is anything else—before she is vigorous, bright, even before she is honest." She described the "perfect girl" as

> the girl who has no bad thoughts or feelings, the kind of person everyone wants to be with....[She is] the girl who speaks quietly, calmly, who is always nice and kind, never mean or bossy....She reminds young women to silence themselves rather than speak their true feelings, which they come to consider "stupid," "selfish," "rude," or just plain irrelevant.[7]

"Good girls," then, are expected not to experience anger. Aggression endangers relationships, imperiling a girl's ability to be caring and "nice." Aggression undermines who girls have been raised to become.

Calling the anger of girls by its name would therefore challenge the most basic assumptions we make about "good girls." It would also reveal what the culture does not entitle them to by defining what *nice* really means: *Not* aggressive. *Not* angry. *Not* in conflict.

Research confirms that parents and teachers discourage the emergence of physical and direct aggression in girls early on while the skirmishing of boys is either encouraged or shrugged off.[8] In one example, a 1999 University of Michigan study found that girls were told to be quiet, speak softly, or use a "nicer" voice about three times more often than boys, even though the boys were louder. By the time they are of school age, peers solidify the fault lines on the playground, creating social groups that value niceness in girls and toughness in boys.

The culture derides aggression in girls as unfeminine, a trend explored in chapter four. "Bitch," "lesbian," "frigid," and "manly" are just a few of the names an assertive girl hears. Each epithet points out the violation of her prescribed role as a caregiver: the bitch likes and is liked by no one; the lesbian loves not a man or children but another woman; the frigid woman is cold, unable to respond sexually; and the manly woman is too hard to love or be loved.

Girls, meanwhile, are acutely aware of the culture's double standard. They are not fooled into believing this is the so-called postfeminist age, the girl power victory lap. The rules are different for boys, and girls know it. Flagrant displays of aggression are punished with social rejection.

At Sackler Day School, I was eating lunch with sixth graders during recess, talking about how teachers expected them to behave at school. Ashley, silver-rimmed glasses snug on her tiny nose, looked very serious as she raised her hand.

"They expect us to act like girls back in the 1800s!" she said indignantly. Everyone cracked up.

"What do you mean?" I asked.

"Well, sometimes they're like, you have to respect each other, and treat other people how you want to be treated. But that's not how life is. Everyone can be mean sometimes and they're not even realizing it. They expect that you're going to be *so* nice to everyone and you'll be *so* cool. Be nice to everyone!" she mimicked, her suddenly loud voice betraying something more than sarcasm.

"But it's not true," Nicole said. The room is quiet.

"Anyone else?" I asked.

"They expect you to be perfect. You're nice. When boys do bad stuff, they all know they're going to do bad stuff. When girls do it, they yell at them," Dina said.

"Teachers think that girls should be really nice and sharing and not get in any fights. They think it's worse than it really is," Shira added.

"They expect you to be perfect angels and then sometimes we don't want to be considered a perfect angel," Laura noted.

"The teacher says if you do something good, you'll get something good back, and then she makes you feel like you really should be," Ashley continued. "I try not to be mean to my sister or my mom and dad, and I wake up the next day and I just do it naturally. I'm not an angel! I try to be focused on it, but then I wake up the next day and I'm cranky."

In Ridgewood, I listened to sixth graders muse about what teachers expect from girls. Heather raised her hand.

"They just don't..." She stopped. No one picked up the slack.

"Finish the sentence," I urged.

"They expect you to be nice like them, like they supposedly are, but..."

"But what?"

"We're not."

"I don't go around being like goody-goody," said Tammy.

"What does goody-goody mean?" I asked.

"You're supposed to be sitting like this"—Tammy crossed her legs and folded her hands primly over her knees—"the whole time."

"And be nice—and don't talk during class," said Torie.

"Do you always feel nice?" I asked.

"*No!*" several of them exclaimed.

"So what happens?"

"It's like you just—the bad part controls over your body," Tammy said. "You want to be nice and you want to be bad at the same time, and the bad part gets to you. You think"—she contorted her face and gritted her teeth—"*I have to be nice.*"

"You just want to tell them to shut up! You just feel like pushing them out of the way and throwing them on the ground!" said Britt-ney. "I wanted to do it like five hundred times last year to this girl. If I didn't push her, I just walked off and tried to stay calm."

Try as they might, most girls can't erase the natural impulses toward anger that every human being knows. Yet the early research on ag-gression turned the myth of the "good," nonaggressive girl into fact: The first experiments on aggression were performed with almost no female subjects. Since males tend to exhibit aggression directly, re-searchers concluded aggression was expressed in only this way. Other forms of aggression, when they were observed, were labeled deviant or ignored.

Studies of bullying inherited these early research flaws. Most psy-chologists looked for direct aggressions like punching, threatening, or teasing. Scientists also measured aggression in environments where indirect acts would be almost impossible to observe. Seen through the eyes of scientists, the social lives of girls appeared still and placid as lakes. It was not until 1992 that someone would ques-tion what lay beneath the surface.

That year, a group of Norwegian researchers published an un-precedented study of girls. They discovered that girls were not at all averse to aggression, they just expressed anger in unconventional ways. The group predicted that "when aggression cannot, for one reason or another, be directed (physically or verbally) at its target, the aggressor has to find other channels." The findings bore out their theory: cultural rules against overt aggression led girls to engage in other, nonphysical forms of aggression. In a conclusion uncharacteristic for the strength of its tone, the researchers challenged the image of sweetness among female youth, calling their social lives "ruthless," "aggressive," and "cruel."[9]

Since then, a small group of psychologists at the University of Minnesota has built upon these findings, identifying three subcategories of aggressive behavior: relational, indirect, and social aggression. *Relational aggression* includes acts that "harm others through damage (or the threat of damage) to relationships or feelings of acceptance, friendship, or group inclusion."[10] Relationally aggressive behavior is ignoring someone to punish them or get one's own way, excluding someone socially for revenge, using negative body language or facial expressions, sabotaging someone else's relationships, or threatening to end a relationship unless the friend agrees to a request. In these acts, the aggressor uses her relationship with the target as a weapon.

Close relatives of relational aggression are indirect aggression and social aggression. *Indirect aggression* allows the aggressor to avoid confronting her target. It is covert behavior in which the aggressor makes it seem as though there has been no intent to hurt at all. One way this is possible is by using others as vehicles for inflicting pain on a targeted person, such as by spreading a rumor. *Social aggression* is intended to damage self-esteem or social status within a group. It includes some indirect aggression like rumor spreading or social exclusion. Throughout the book, I refer to these behaviors collectively as *alternative aggressions*. As the stories in the book make clear, alternative aggressions often appear in conjunction with more direct behaviors.

beneath the radar

In Margaret Atwood's novel *Cat's Eye,* the young protagonist Elaine is seated frozen in fear on a windowsill, where she has been forced to remain in silence by her best friends as she waits to find out what she had done wrong. Elaine's father enters the room and asks if the girls are enjoying the parade they have been watching:

> Cordelia gets down off her windowsill and slides up onto mine, sitting close beside me.
>
> "We're enjoying it extremely, thank you very much," she says in her voice for adults. My parents think she has beautiful manners. She puts an arm around me, gives me a little squeeze, a squeeze of complicity, of instruction. Everything will be all right as long as I sit still, say nothing, reveal nothing.... As soon as my father is out of the room Cordelia turns to face me.... "You know what this means don't you? I'm afraid you'll have to be punished."

Like many girl bullies, Cordelia maneuvers her anger quietly beneath the surface of her good-girl image. She must invest as much energy appearing nice to adults as she will spend slowly poisoning Elaine's self-esteem.

Some alternative aggressions are invisible to adult eyes. To elude social disapproval, girls retreat beneath a surface of sweetness to hurt each other in secret. They pass covert looks and notes, manipulate quietly over time, corner one another in hallways, turn their backs, whisper, and smile. These acts, which are intended to escape detection and punishment, are epidemic in middle-class environments where the rules of femininity are most rigid.

Cordelia's tactics are common in a social universe that refuses girls open conflict. In fact, whole campaigns often occur without a sound. Astrid recalled the silent, methodical persistence of her angry friends. "It was a war through notes," she remembered. "When I wouldn't read them, they wrote on the binding of encyclopedias near my desk, on the other desks; they left notes around, wrote my name on the list of people to send to the principal." This aggression was designed to slip beneath the sight line of prying eyes.

Most of the time, the strategy works. Paula Johnston, a prosecutor, was dumbfounded at the ignorance of her daughter's teacher when Paula demanded Susie be separated from a girl who was quietly bullying her. "[Susie's teacher] said, 'But they get along beautifully!'" Paula snorted. "I asked her to move Susie, and she moved one in front and one behind! She would say, 'Everything's wonderful; Susie's adorable,' and meanwhile, Susie's in the library hiding."

A Sackler sixth grader described her attempt to expose a mean girl to her teacher. "[The teacher] said, 'Oh my gosh! You in a fight? How can that be!'" At every school I visited, I heard stories of a teacher being told of a girl's meanness, only to respond, "Fight? She'd never do that!" or "I'm sure that's not true!" or "But they're best friends!"

Covert aggression isn't just about not getting caught; half of it is looking like you'd never mistreat someone in the first place. The sugar-and-spice image is powerful, and girls know it. They use it to fog the radar of otherwise vigilant teachers and parents. For girls, the secrecy, the "underground"[11]—the place where Brown and Gilligan report girls take their true feelings—are hardly unconscious realms. In the film *Cruel Intentions,* Kathryn cloaks her anger in syrupy sweetness. In a bind, she decides to frame another student because, she purrs, "Everybody loves me, and I intend to keep it that way." Later, surreptitiously snorting cocaine from a cross around her neck, Kathryn groans, "Do you think I relish the fact that I have to act like Mary Sunshine 24–7 so I can be considered a lady? I'm the Marcia-fucking-Brady of the Upper East Side, and sometimes I want to kill myself."

In group discussions, girls spoke openly to me about their intentionally covert aggression. When I visited the ninth graders in Ridgewood, they threw out their tactics with gusto, prompting the semicircle of bodies to lean forward, nearly out of their desks, as eager affirming cries of "Oh yeah!" and "Totally!" filled our fluorescent-white lab room.

Walk down the hallway and slam into a girl—the teacher thinks you're distracted! Knock a girl's book off a desk—the teacher thinks it fell! Write an anonymous note! Draw a mean picture! Roll your eyes! Send an instant message with a new username! Steal a boy-friend! Start a rumor! Tell the teacher she cheated!

"You step on their shoe. Oops!" Jessie squealed in a girly-girl singsong voice. "Sorry!"

"You walk past someone and you try to bump them. You say, '*Ex-cuse you!*'" The girls laughed in recognition.

"The teacher says she didn't mean it, she just bumped into her," Melanie explained, "but the girls, they *know* what it is because it happens so much."

"Girls are very sneaky," said Keisha. "Very."

"We—are—sneaky!" Lacey crowed, emphasizing every word.

The next day, the Ridgewood sixth graders met. The freight of the good-girl image still weighed heavily upon them, and they lacked some of the boisterous energy and sarcasm of the ninth graders. Their voices were hesitant and halting. Amy was brave.

"The teachers don't say anything. They don't expect it. They don't think we're doing anything, but..." She paused.

"But what?" I asked. I was getting used to sentences abandoned midway.

She was silent.

"The teachers think girls behave better," Elizabeth explained.

"Does that make a difference in how people get in trouble?" I asked.

"Some people call each other names and stuff and the teacher wouldn't believe it. They would say, 'So-and-so did this to me,' and the teacher would say, 'No, she didn't.' Some teachers have pets, and you say, 'She called me a bad name,' and the teacher says, 'No, she wouldn't do a thing like that.'"

Leigh said, "Some girls act real good around the teachers, and then when they do something bad, the teachers don't believe it because they never seen them do it."

"Boys don't care about getting into trouble. They think they're all bad and don't worry about it. They don't care if they got in trouble, but girls don't want anyone to know they got into trouble,"

Maura said. "Girls worry about how they're going to look. They have more of a nervous system than boys." The room tittered.

Tina raised her hand. "A girl in my class passes notes and never gets in trouble for it. Around the teacher she acts all sweet and stuff."

"Everybody writes notes," Sarah Beth added. "Teachers are so stupid. They don't get it. You can see it. It's easy."

Kim said, "Girls can be passing notes during class and the teacher will find out about it. She won't get them in trouble because they're like one of her best students. Most of the girls in her class are but the boys usually aren't."

Torie sat up on the back of her chair, elbows on her knees. "If girls are whispering, the teacher thinks it's going to be all right because they're not hitting people. If they punch, they get sent to the office. Teachers think they're not hurting you," she said, looking cautiously at her classmates, "but they are."

At once I was reminded of scary movies in which only children can see the ghost. The adults pass through the same rooms and live the same moments, yet they are unable to see a whole world of action around them. So, too, in classrooms of covertly aggressing girls, targets are desperately alone even though a teacher is just steps away.

Sixth period was about to end. Jenny's stomach clenched harder with each loud click of the wall clock. She never jumped when the bell rang. Although she prided herself on her good grades, Jenny stopped paying attention five minutes before class ended. Still, at 1:58 her heart started to race. By 1:59 she was short of breath.

Through the cracks between her straight brown hair she watched the other seventh graders get up. As usual, she pretended to be slow and preoccupied. She shuffled her pencils noisily in the cool metal air inside the desk, buying time. In a moment she would be free to leave.

Ever since Jenny arrived two months ago from San Diego, the popular clique at Mason Middle School had decided two things: first, that she was a major threat to their status, and second, that they were going to make her life miserable.

She had moved reluctantly with her family to the small ranching community in Wyoming four days after the end of sixth grade. In San Diego, Jenny had gone to a huge city school and had mostly Mexican friends. She spoke fluent Spanish and loved the warmth and friendship of Mexican culture. She never minded being one of the only white students in school.

That everything was different in Mason was an understatement. There were eight hundred white people in the whole town. Everybody knew each other's business, and outsiders were unwelcome. So it didn't matter to Brianna and Mackenzie that Jenny's entire family had grown up right in Mason. Even though Jenny spent her summers riding tractors through their families' fields with her grandfather, the town alderman, she may as well have been born on a spaceship.

Brianna and Mackenzie were the queen bees, and they presided over the seventh grade. Brianna was the prettiest, Mackenzie the best at sports. Their favorite hobby was having a boyfriend. Jenny wasn't really interested in a boyfriend, but she still liked hanging out with the guys. Mostly she liked to play soccer and basketball with them after school. She liked to wear jeans and T-shirts instead of makeup and miniskirts.

She had barely introduced herself when Brianna and Mackenzie gave her a code name and started calling her Harriet the Hairy Whore. They told everyone Jenny was hooking up with the boys in the woods behind the soccer field. Jenny knew that being called a slut was the worst thing in the world, no matter where you lived. No one was even kissing yet. It was the lowest of the low.

Brianna and Mackenzie started a club called Hate Harriet the Hore Incorporated. They got every girl to join except two who didn't care. All the members had to walk by Jenny in the hallway and say, "Hhiiiiiiiiii. . . ." They made a long sighing noise to make sure she knew they were sounding out the initials of the club: HHHI. Usually two or more girls would say it and then look at each other and laugh. Sometimes they couldn't even say the whole thing, they were laughing so hard.

Then Brianna got the idea to charge into Jenny as she walked the hallways. The other girls followed suit. Wherever Jenny was between classes, a girl would body slam her, knocking Jenny's books, and sometimes Jenny, to the ground. If someone was watching, they'd pretend it was an accident. Even though Jenny was small for her age, only four foot eleven, she decided to start smashing the others first, figuring they'd stop. They didn't. She ended up with a lot of bruises, missing papers, and an uncanny ability to predict when the bells would ring. There was no teacher in the hallway to see.

She tried to shrug it off the first few days, but by the end of the week, Jenny burned with embarrassment and fear. What had she done? It seemed like Mackenzie and Brianna had suddenly made it their goal in life to ruin her. Nothing like this had ever happened before. In San Diego, she had three best friends. She had always been good at everything but not because it was easy. She strove for success in everything she did. In her head she heard her father's voice: "If you try hard enough, you can do anything." This was her first failure.

It was her fault.

She knew she'd never touched a boy, but maybe there was something really wrong with her. There were two other new girls in seventh grade, and they were doing just fine. They worked hard to fit in, and they did. They bought the same clothes and listened to the same music as everyone else.

Jenny closed her eyes. They also let Mackenzie and Brianna and the others determine who they would be. Jenny didn't want that, at any price. She wanted to keep speaking her mind. She liked her California clothes and Mexican embroidered shirts. Maybe she didn't want to try hard in the ways you had to in seventh grade. Her father was right.

Jenny began to weep quietly in her room not long after she realized there would be no end to her torture. She managed to wait until her homework was done, and then she cried, silent always, her sobs muffled by her pillow. There was no *way* she'd tell her mother, and certainly not her father. She felt nauseous just thinking about telling her parents she was such a reject.

Every day was an endless battle. She was exhausted trying not to cry, stiffening her body against the hallway attacks, sitting through lunch after lunch alone. There was no one else to be friends with in the grade because everyone, the few that there were, was against her. Her cousin was a year ahead of her and felt sorry for Jenny. Sometimes she let Jenny hang out with her clique. It was small consolation that they were the popular group of the eighth grade. In fact, it seemed to make Brianna and Mackenzie even angrier.

One night Jenny's sadness left no room for her fear, and she picked up the phone. Jenny called Brianna, Mackenzie, and a few other girls. She asked each of them, "Why do you hate me?" They denied everything. "But why are you doing the Hate Harriet the Hore club?" she pleaded.

Their voices were light and sweet. "We don't have a Hate Harriet the Hore club!" each one assured her, as though they were telling her the earth was round. They were so nice to Jenny that for a second she didn't believe it was really them. Then she could almost feel her heart surging up through her chest. The next morning, she actually looked forward to getting out of bed. It would be different now.

Then she got to school.

"Hhhiiiiiiiii . . . !" *Slam.*

Jenny blinked back tears and locked her jaw. She hated herself for being surprised. She should have known. The strange thing about it was, even though she was used to it, this time her heart felt like it was breaking open. Brianna and Mackenzie had seemed so genuine on the phone. And Jenny, stupid, stupid Jenny, she muttered to herself, had imagined herself at their lunch table in the back of the cafeteria. "Stupid, stupid, stupid," she repeated through gritted teeth, raising her books as a shield as she made her way into homeroom.

One day, months later, searching through desks after seeing the girls pass it around in homeroom, Jenny found the petition. "I, Mackenzie T., promise to Hate Harriet the Hore forever," it said. Every single girl in the class had signed it, and it was appended with a long list of reasons why everyone should hate her. Jenny's eyes bore into the paper until the words blurred. She suddenly felt dizzy. The weight of her anguish was too heavy. She couldn't take it anymore. Jenny felt like her world was crumbling. She went to the principal.

Mr. Williams called Brianna, Mackenzie, and some of the others into his office. They glared at her for weeks but said nothing. HHHI was officially disbanded.

Jenny struggled through seventh grade alone. Because the meanness of her peers was almost invisible, not one teacher had noticed or intervened on her behalf. Because she was a new student, it was difficult to observe changes in her behavior and character. Her parents had known something was wrong, but had they asked her how she was, Jenny told me, "I would have told them, 'Fine.'"

HHHI never resurfaced and Jenny adjusted well over the next several years. She became captain of the softball team and pep club president, but her pain stayed fresh and hidden as she waited patiently for revenge.

Brianna, her chief HHHI tormentor, had begun dating the most popular boy at Cheyenne High School in fifth grade. That was the way things were, Jenny said. "You pretty much picked who you were going to date when you were ten or eleven and that's who you dated until you left Wyoming." Eric was captain of the basketball team and everything else that was important at Cheyenne. Brianna had lost her virginity to him and wanted to marry him.

Jenny's chance came in the fall of her junior year, when she was asked to manage the boys' basketball team. She quickly became friends with Eric. "I made it my goal to steal him from her, and I did," Jenny said. "I know for a fact it had nothing to do with him. It had everything to do with taking what was important to her." Jenny and Eric dated secretly for a month before Jenny made him call Brianna from her bedroom and break up with her. I asked Jenny how it made her feel.

"I just had this feeling of victory. I wanted to rub it in her face. I felt really good that I had hurt her back," she said. "It's vindictive and it's sad, I know, but to this day I hate this girl and I wanted to hurt her." Today Jenny is thirty-two, and she feels neither shame nor remorse, only the anger that still smolders some twenty years later.

relationship and loss

At first glance, the stories of girls not being allowed to eat at the lunch table, attend a party, put their sleeping bag in the middle, or squeeze inside a circle of giggling girls may seem childish. Yet as Carol Gilligan has shown, relationships play an unusually important role in girls' social development. In her work with girls and boys, she found that girls perceive danger in their lives as isolation, especially the fear that by standing out they will be abandoned. Boys, however, describe danger as a fear of entrapment or smothering. This contrast, Gilligan argues, shows that women's development "points toward a different history of human attachment, stressing continuity and change instead of replacement and separation. The primacy of rela- tionship and attachment in the female life also indicates a different experience of and response to loss."[12] The centrality of relationship in girls' lives all but guarantees a different landscape of aggression and bullying, with its own distinctive features worthy of separate study.

To understand girls' conflicts, one must also know girls' intimacy, because intimacy and anger are often inextricable. The intensity of girls' relationships belongs at the center of any analysis of girls' ag- gression. For long before they love boys, girls love each other, and with great passion.

Girls enjoy unrestricted access to intimacy. Unlike boys, who are encouraged to separate from their mothers and adopt masculine pos- tures of emotional restraint, daughters are urged to identify with the nurturing behavior of their mothers. Girls spend their childhood practicing caretaking and nurturing on each other. It is with best friends that they first discover the joys of intimacy and human connection.

Yet ours is a culture that has ignored the closeness of girlfriends. Many people believe girls should reserve their true emotions for boys, and that girls should channel their caretaking toward husbands and children. Anything up to that life stage is assumed to be practice, if not insignificant.[13]

In fact, it is the deep knowledge girls have of relationship, and the passion they lavish on their closest friends, that characterizes much of their aggression. The most painful attacks are usually fashioned from deep inside a close friendship and are fueled by secrets and once-shared weaknesses.

Moreover, the relationship itself is often the weapon with which girls' battles are fought. Socialized away from aggression, expected to be nice girls who have "perfect relationships," many girls are unprepared to negotiate conflict. As a result, a minor disagreement can call an entire relationship into question.

What do I mean by this? In a normal conflict, two people use language, voice, or fists to settle their dispute. The relationship between them is secondary to the issue being worked out. But when anger cannot be voiced, and when the skills to handle a conflict are absent, the specific matter cannot be addressed. If neither girl wants to be "not nice," the relationship itself may become the problem. And when there are no other tools to use in a conflict, relationship itself may become a weapon.

Since relationship is precisely what good, "perfect" girls are expected to be in, its loss, and the prospect of solitude, can be the most pointed weapon in the hidden culture of girls' aggression.

During her interviews with adults, sociologist Anne Campbell found that where men viewed aggression as a means to control their environment and integrity, women believed it would terminate their relationships.[14] I discovered identical attitudes in my conversations with girls. Expressing fear that even everyday acts of conflict, not to mention severe aggressive outbursts, would result in the loss of the people they most cared about, they refused to engage in even the most basic acts of conflict. Their equation was simple: conflict = loss.

Like clockwork, girl after girl told me twenty variations on the following remark: "I can't tell her how I feel or else she won't want to be my friend anymore." The corollary works like this: "I just don't want to hurt anyone directly, because I want to be friends with everyone."

Fear of solitude is overpowering. In fact, what targets of bullying recalled most to me was their loneliness. Despite the cruel things that happened—the torrents of vulgar e-mail and unsigned notes, the whispered rumors, the slanderous scribblings on desks and walls and lockers, the sneering and name-calling—what crushed girls was being alone. It was as though the absence of bodies nearby with whom to whisper and share triggered in girls a sorrow and fear so profound as to nearly extinguish them.

Girls may try to avoid being alone at all costs, including remaining in an abusive friendship. "You don't want to walk alone at recess," a sixth grader explained when I asked why she wouldn't stay away from a mean friend. "Who are you going to tell your secrets to? Who are you going to help and stuff like that?" An eighth grader, recalling a television documentary, remarked plaintively, "If a female lion is alone, she dies. She has to be part of the group."

As girls mature, the prospect of being seen alone by others becomes just as daunting. They know that "perfect girls" have "perfect relationships." "Walking through a hall and feeling like everyone's looking at you is the worst," a Linden ninth grader told me. "People who are alone are pitied and no one wants to be pitied. They're secluded. Something's wrong with them. Being seen as a loner is one of our biggest fears." Driven by the fear of exclusion, girls cling to their friends like lifeboats on the shifting seas of school life, certain that to be alone is the worst horror imaginable.

Every child, boy or girl, desires acceptance and connection. Most boys would not prefer or even tolerate being alone. Yet as girls grow up, friendship becomes as important as air, and they describe the punishment of loneliness in dramatic terms. "I was so depressed," Sarah explained. "I sat in class with no friends. Everything I cared about completely crumbled." A fifth grader said of her solitude, "It was like my heart was breaking."

it's just a phase

When thirteen-year-old Sherry's friends suddenly stopped speaking to her, her father, worried for his devastated daughter, approached a friend's mother to find out what happened. She was underwhelmed. "Girls will be girls," she said. It's typical girl behavior, nothing to be worried about, a phase girls go through. It will pass. "You are making a mountain out of a molehill," she told him. "What are you getting so upset about?"

Her remarks echo the prevailing wisdom about alternative aggression between girls: girl bullying is a rite of passage, a stage they will outgrow. As one school counselor put it to me, "It's always been this way. It will always be this way. There's nothing we can do about it." Girl bullying, many believe, is a nasty developmental storm we have no choice but to accept. Yet the rite-of-passage argument paralyzes our thinking about how the culture shapes girls' behavior. Most importantly, it stunts the development of anti-bullying strategies.

The rite-of-passage theory suggests several disturbing assumptions about girls. First, it implies that there is nothing we can do to prevent girls from behaving in these ways because it's in their developmental tea leaves to do it. In other words, because so many girls engage in alternative aggressions, they must be naturally predisposed to them. Bullying as a rite of passage also suggests that it is necessary and even positive that girls learn how to relate with each other in these ways. Rites of passage, after all, are rituals that mark the transformation of an individual from one status to another. So the rite of passage means that girls are becoming acquainted with what is in store for them later as adults. Because adult women behave in this way, it means it's acceptable and must be prepared for. (Many despairing mothers I spoke with, as well as those who shrugged off the bullying, confided a sense of consolation that their girls were learning what they'd come to know sooner or later.)

The third assumption emerges directly from the first two: it suggests that because it is universal and instructive, meanness among girls is a natural part of their social structure to be tolerated and expected. And there is one final assumption, the most insidious of all: the abuse girls subject each other to is, in fact, not abuse at all.

I have heard schools decline to intervene in girls' conflicts because they do not want to interfere in the "emotional lives" of students. This philosophy makes two value judgments about girls' relationships: it suggests that unlike aggressive episodes between the sexes, which are analyzed by lawyers and plastered on evening news programs, problems between girls are insignificant, episodes that will taper off as girls become more involved with boys.

Second, it trivializes the role of peers in children's development, turning into school policy the myth that childhood is "training for life," rather than life itself. A strategy of noninterference resists the truth of girls' friendships, remains aloof from the heart of their interpersonal problems, and devalues the emotional intensity that leaves permanent marks on their self-esteem.

Yet there is an even simpler reason why schools have ignored girls' aggression. They need order in the classroom. On any given day, the typical teacher is racing against the clock to meet a long list of obligations. She must complete her lesson plans, fulfill district and state standards requirements, administer tests, and occasionally find time for a birthday party. Like an emergency room doctor, the teacher must perform triage on her discipline problems. Disruptions are caught on the fly and met with swift punishment. Generally, boys are more disorderly. Girls, ever the intuiters of adult stress, know that passing a nasty note or shooting mean looks like rubber bands is unlikely to draw the attention of an exhausted teacher who is intent on completing her lesson plan.

When she sees a perpetrating girl, a teacher has little or no incentive to stop the class. Taking the time to address relational discord is not always as easy as yelling at a boy to remove his peer from the trash can. As a sixth grader explained to me, "Teachers separate the boys." Relational problems, however, demand attention to something that is more complex. Invariably, the teacher is far more concerned with the boys flinging balls of paper and distracting the other students.

Schools lack consistent public strategies for dealing with alternative aggressions. In the absence of a shared language to identify and discuss the behavior, student harassment policies are generally vague and favor acts of physical or direct violence. The structure of school days also complicates teacher intervention: in many schools, for instance, lunch aides supervise at recess, when bullying is rampant.

Since alternative aggressions have been largely ignored, their real-life manifestations are often seen through the lens of more "valid" social problems. For example, at many schools, the threat "do this or I won't be your friend anymore" is considered peer pressure, not relational aggression. In academic writings, researchers explain girls' manipulation of relationships as a form of precocity or a way to "establish central position and to dominate the definition of the group's boundaries." Some psychologists classify teasing and nasty jokes as developmentally healthy experiences. They call rumors and gossip spreading "boundary maintenance."[15]

Also common is the assessing of the targets of meanness among girls as having a social skills deficit. According to this school of thought, bullied children are obviously doing something wrong if they are attracting the social abuse of others. This usually puts the onus on the target, who must toughen up or learn to integrate socially. Perhaps she is responding to social situations inappropriately, failing to "read" the feelings and attitudes of others correctly. Perhaps she needs to pay more attention to clothing trends. Perhaps she is too needy, daring, as one book lamented, to say "Let's be friends" instead of the more subtle "Let's go to the mall this weekend."

Relational aggression in particular is easily mistaken for a social skills problem. When a girl is nice one day and cruel the next, or is possessive, or overreacts to another child, the behavior can be inter-preted as a sign of delayed development. This is an especially insidious problem because the targets may be encouraged to show patience and respect to their aggressors. In the course of things, the aggressive as-pect of the behavior is lost, and the aggressor is left alone.

Most disturbingly, what the target understands to be true about her own feeling of injury is denied by adults. Since aggressors are often friends, girls, ever compassionate, spring easily to the rescue with their endless understanding when shown human mistakes. Annie, who is profiled in chapter two, remembered Samantha, the girl who made her cry all night, with whom she was still friends. "Right now Samantha has a lot of friends and is more socially skilled," Annie explained. "But back then she wasn't really.... If she had a friend, and if they said some slight thing to her, she would think that it was the most offensive thing that anyone's ever said to her. I don't think I really ever said [this was wrong]. I think she was trying to keep the friendship just as she could have it." In order to be a good friend, Annie showed compassion for Samantha's social limitations while shelving her own painful feelings.

Misdiagnosing bullying as a social skills problem makes perfect sense in a culture that demands perfect relationships of its girls at any cost. Social skills proponents claim that the best interactions are sit-uation appropriate and reinforced by others, reflecting abilities in which girls are already well schooled. Indeed, the majority of female bullying incidents occur at the behest of a ringleader whose power lies in her ability to maintain a facade of girlish tranquillity in the course of sustained, covert peer abuse. She also directs social consen-sus among the group. As far as the social skills school is concerned, then, girl bullies appear from the outside to be doing A-plus work. At one school trying the social skills solution, for example, the mean girls were simply urged to be more "discreet."

The trouble with the social skills argument is that it does not question the existence of meanness, it explains and justifies it. As a result, it has helped alternative aggressions to persist unquestioned.

As they try fiercely to be nice and stay in perfect relationships, girls are forced into a game of tug-of-war with their own aggression. At times girls' anger may break the surface of their niceness, while at others it may only linger below it, sending confusing messages to their peers. As a result, friends are often forced to second-guess themselves and each other. Over time, many grow to mistrust what others say they are feeling.

The sequestering of anger not only alters the forms in which aggression is expressed, but also how it is perceived. Anger may flash on and off with lightning speed, making the target question what happened—or indeed whether anything happened at all. *Did she just look at her when I said that? Was she joking? Did she roll her eyes? Not save the seat on purpose? Lie about her plans? Tell me that she'd invited me when she hadn't?*

Girls will begin summoning the strength to confront alternative aggressions when we chart them out in their various shapes and forms, overt and covert. We need to freeze those fleeting moments and name them so that girls are no longer besieged by doubt about what's happening, so that they no longer believe it's their fault when it does.

CHAPTER two

intimate enemies

Ridgewood is a blink-and-you-miss-it working-class town of 2,000 in northern Mississippi. Big enough to have its own Wal-Mart but too small for more than a few traffic lights, Ridgewood is bordered by dusty state roads dotted with service stations and fast-food chains. It is the largest town in a dry county where the mostly Baptist churches outnumber the restaurants. The majority of the town is white, although growing numbers of African American families, mostly poor, are beginning to gather around its edges. Families have long made comfortable livings at local factories here, but threats of an imminent recession have given way to layoffs and a thickening layer of anxiety.

Ridgewood is a fiercely tight-knit community that prides itself in its family-centered values and spirit of care for neighbors. When a tornado cuts a fatal mile-wide swath through town, everyone heads over to rebuild homes and comfort the displaced. Ridgewood is the kind of place where grown children make homes next to their parents and where teenagers safely scatter onto Main Street without looking both ways, drifting in and out of the ice-cream parlor and game room after school. Year-round, going "rolling," toilet papering

an unsuspecting peer or teacher's home, is a favorite pastime, sometimes supervised by parents.

By ten o'clock one October morning in Ridgewood, it was already
eighty-two degrees. The Mississippi sun was blindingly bright, and
the earth was dry, cracked, and dusty. We were having a drought. I
was late getting to school, although the truth is in Ridgewood it
doesn't take longer than a song on the radio to drive anywhere.

I raced through the front door of the elementary school, sunglass
frames in my mouth, spiral notebook in hand. Cassie Smith was waiting. Tall and big-boned, prepubescently round, she had blond hair
that waved gently in strings toward her shoulders, kind green eyes,
glossed pink lips, braces, and a soft, egg-shaped freckled face. She
was missing sixth-grade band class to be with me. Cassie met my eyes
squarely as I nodded to her—I'd been laying low here, trying not to
expose the girls who volunteered to talk to me—and we headed
silently down the long, blue-gray corridor, down the ramp, underneath a still, rusty red fan, and toward the plain, cluttered room I
had been using for interviews. Children were mostly oblivious to us
as they slammed lockers and whirled toward class in single motions,
their teachers standing stiff as flagpoles in the doorways. We passed
class projects in a blur: elaborate trees decorated with sunset-colored
tissue paper to welcome the autumn, which had actually been more
of a summer than anything.

I motioned for Cassie to sit. We made a little small talk. She was
whispering so softly I could barely hear her.

"So," I said gently, leaning back in my chipped metal folding
chair. "Why did you want to come talk with me today?"

Cassie inhaled deeply. "This is happening *right now,* okay?" she
said, as though to admonish me that I was not just some archaeolo-
gist come here to sift through dirt and bones. "My best friend
Becca," she began, staring fiercely at her fingers, which were playing
an absentminded game of itsy-bitsy spider against the lead-smeared
tabletop, "I trusted her and everything. She called me and asked if I
liked Kelly, who is our good friend. Becca said that Kelly talks bad

about me and everything." Cassie sounded nervous. "I really didn't want to say anything back about Kelly because I didn't want to go down to her level." On the phone, Cassie tried to change the subject.

But when Becca called, Kelly had been over at her house. When Becca hung up, she told Kelly that Cassie had called her names. Kelly called back and told Cassie off.

Now, at school, Kelly was teasing Cassie relentlessly—about what she was wearing (she wore that outfit last week) or not (she needs tennis shoes); about how stupid and poor she was. Cassie didn't know what to do.

Cassie and Becca had been best friends since first grade. Last summer, Kelly moved to Ridgewood from Texas, and this fall she'd started hanging around Becca. At first they were all three quite close, with some tension between Cassie and Kelly. And then, Cassie said quietly, over the last few weeks, "Kelly kind of forgot me. They started to get really close and they just forgot me. And then they started ganging up on me and stuff like that."

"How?" I asked.

"They ignored me. They just didn't want to talk with me or any-thing..." Her voice caught and her eyes filled with tears. I squeezed past some desks to the teacher's table and leaned over to grab a box of tissues.

"Did you try and talk with them about it?" I pulled out a tissue and handed it to her.

"No," she said. "Like, after lunch we have a place where we meet and stuff. We have to line up and go to class. That's when everybody starts talking. We get in a circle and just talk. And they'd put their shoulders together and they wouldn't let me, you know, in the circle or whatever. They would never talk to me, and they would never lis-ten to what I had to say. Stuff like that." She was whispering again.

"I don't think I've ever done anything to them." Her voice shook. "I've always been nice to them."

Lately, it had only gotten worse. Kelly, by now no stranger in the school, had been warning other girls to stay away from Cassie. Becca was saying that Cassie was insulting Kelly behind her back, and Kelly was passing notes that said Cassie lived in a shack and was too poor to buy Sunday clothes.

"So how are you feeling?" I asked.

"Like I don't want to go to school," she whispered, sinking into her red fleece vest.

"Why not?"

"Because I don't know what they'll do every day."

"What have they done so far?" I asked.

"They'll be like, 'Cassie, get back, we're going to talk about you now.'"

"They'll say that?"

"No, they'll just"—she was getting frustrated with me—"*I can tell*. They don't have to say anything. They'll whisper and look at me, and I know they're talking about me."

"Have you talked to your mom?" I asked.

"I talk to my mom but it just . . . I don't really want to worry her a lot." She began to cry again.

"Does it worry her?"

"It kind of makes her mad because—she says I should ignore them. But I *can't*. They just keep on."

"Why is it hard to ignore them?"

"Because they're like, running over you, you know? And I can't concentrate. They're like—they look at me and stuff like that. They stare at me. I can hear them saying stuff and whispering and they look right at me."

Cassie struggled with the absence of a language to articulate her victimization. As the silent meanness of her friends attracted no teacher's attention, Cassie was filled with a helplessness that was slowly turning into self-blame. Without rules or a public conscious-ness of this behavior, Cassie's only sense that what was happening was real (or wrong) was her own perspective. For a ten-year-old, that would not be enough.

———

Relational aggression starts in preschool, and so do the first signs of sex differences.[16] The behavior is thought to begin as soon as children become capable of meaningful relationships. By age three, more girls than boys are relationally aggressive, a schism that only widens as children mature. In a series of studies, children cited relational aggression as the "most common angry, hurtful...behavior enacted in girls' peer groups," regardless of the target's sex. By middle childhood, the leading researchers in the field report that "physical aggressors are mostly boys, relational aggressors mostly girls."

Relational aggression harms others "through damage (or the threat of damage) to relationships or feelings of acceptance, friendships, or group inclusion."[17] It includes any act in which relationship is used as a weapon, including manipulation. First identified in 1992, it is the heart of the alternative aggressions, and for many girls an emotionally wrenching experience.

Relational aggression can include indirect aggression, in which the target is not directly confronted (such as the silent treatment), and some social aggression, which targets the target's self-esteem or social status (such as rumor spreading). Among the most common forms of relational aggression are "do this or I won't be your friend anymore," ganging up against a girl, the silent treatment, and nonverbal gesturing, or body language.[18]

The lifeblood of relational aggression is relationship. As a result, most relational aggression occurs within intimate social or friendship networks. The closer the target to the aggressor, the more cutting the loss. As one Linden freshman put it, "Your friends know you and how to hurt you. They know what your real weaknesses are. They know exactly what to do to destroy someone's self-worth. They try to destroy you from the inside." Such pointed meanness, an eighth grader explained to me, "can stay with you for your entire life. It can define who you are."

Where relationships are weapons, friendship itself can become a tool of anger. You can, one Ridgewood sixth grader explained, "have a friend, and then go over there and become friends with somebody else, just to make them jealous." Nor must the relationship be withdrawn or even directly threatened: the mere suggestion of loss may be enough. One girl may stand among a group, turn to two friends and sigh, "Wow, I can't *wait* for this weekend!" One girl may pull another away from a group "and tell them secrets, right in front of us," a Mississippi sixth grader said. "When she comes back, people ask her what she said, [and] she's always like, 'Oh, nothing. It's none of your business.'" No rule has been broken here, yet it takes little more than this for a girl to inflict pain on her peers.

A combination of nonphysical, often furtive aggression is extremely dangerous, in large part because it is impossible to detect. Relational aggression has remained invisible because the behavior resists the typical displays that we normally associate with bullying. Two girls playing quietly together in the corner might be two girls playing quietly in the corner—or they might be one girl slowly wearing down the other.

Teachers and parents may not be looking or listening for signs of a problem behind the facade of friendship and play. Who can blame them? Nothing *looks* wrong. It is tempting to interpret signs of trouble as the passing "issues" that afflict all normal childhood relationships, but in some cases, turning the other way can be a terrible mistake.

"Nonverbal gesturing," a fancy word for body language, is a hallmark of relational aggression. Denied the use of their voices by rules against female anger, girls like Becca and Kelly have instead learned to use their bodies. Nonverbal gesturing includes mean looks, certain forms of exclusion, and the silent treatment. It also drives girls to distraction. For one thing, body language is at once infuriatingly empty of detail and bluntly clear. It cuts deep precisely because a girl will know someone is angry at her, but she doesn't get to find out why and sometimes with whom it's happening. In girls' worlds, the worst aggression is the most opaque, creating a sort of emotional poison ivy that makes it hard to concentrate on anything else. Teachers become characters in "Peanuts" cartoons, their lecturing unintelligible. Words swim on the page. The target of this silent campaign looks around the room and everything—a look exchanged, someone writing a note—has crooked, wildly irrational new significance, like reflections in a funhouse mirror.

The day after I met Cassie, I spoke with some of her fifth- and sixth-grade classmates about ways girls can be mean without saying a word. Kayla, chubby with sparkling blue eyes, was nearly falling out of her seat hopping and waving and making pleading, wordless noises. I smiled inwardly: This was always my "problem" in class.

"Yes?" I asked.

"Girls can look at you, and you know they're mad!" she exclaimed. "They don't have to say anything. You look at them and they roll their eyes and they have little slits in them."

Miranda, sitting primly with an arrow-straight arm in the air, added that girls "whisper and you get jealous. They look at you while they're whispering. They might point and start laughing. You see their lips moving."

"So," I said, scanning their faces, "how do you feel when you think you're being whispered about?"

A tiny, tinny voice rose up from a chair in the corner of the room. "It's a funny feeling," Cerise said.

"What do you mean?"

"Like they don't care about you or what you do."

"See, girls don't tease," Tammy explained. "They talk behind [your] backs, they giggle and point at [you]. They start rumors and they totally ignore [you]. Even if they're not teasing, it's still obvious that they don't like you."

As I moved from class to class, from school to school, I learned that the worst kind of silent meanness is the only one with a name: the silent treatment. In this, the most pointed kind of relational aggression, one girl ceases speaking to another and, with little or no warning, revokes her friendship. The target, often unaware of why her friend is angry, is consumed by panic and the fear of permanently losing the friendship.

"When you ignore," an Arden eleven-year-old explained, "they"—meaning the target—"get scared over every little thing. They don't understand what's going on."

"Oh, yeah," a classmate chimed in. It's the worst thing you can do. You gain a lot of power and they come crawling back." A twelve-year-old remarked, "Giving someone a look makes [the targets] paranoid. [They] overanalyze it." A Ridgewood eighth grader explained, "You try to find out why they're mad at you and they just kind of laugh at you. They toss their hair and look away." "When someone glares at you," a Linden freshman told me, "it makes you feel lower and deteriorates your insides. Oh God, you think, what are they doing? You ask them why they're mad and they don't say anything. You have no control. It gives them power."

One of the more chilling messages conveyed through silence and staring is that, in eleven-year-old Mary's words, "you're telling them you're not worth my time or me talking to you. It's the worst thing. You're saying, 'I don't want to argue it out.'" Silence throws up an impenetrable wall, shutting down the chance for self-expression and more importantly, the opportunity to play a proactive role in one's conflicts.

Not getting to find out why someone's mad often has the unfortunate effect of making targeted girls believe that whatever's gone wrong is surely their fault—if only they could deduce the unwritten rule they broke. Already prone to self-dissection, girls are only too willing to take up the challenge. Filled with dread, seeking some measure of control, they search for the mistake they're sure they made. In this way, the simple act of silence or a nasty look can take on a life of its own, continuing well beyond the moment it is shared.

To the aggressor, the silent treatment can be a quick, easy path around a direct confrontation. Putting it simply, a girl at Marymount remarked, "If you don't tell someone why you're mad, you can't get a rebuttal. You win." Girls on the receiving end will usually persist, begging for an explanation. But "when they come around, you just walk away," reported one girl. That's hard, her classmate explained, because if you're on the receiving end "you can try to tell them, try to say you're sorry, and they won't listen or solve the problem."

When confronted, girls often deny that they are angry, even as they project the opposite. Most women remember uncomfortably approaching a friend with the question, "Are you mad at me?" only to get a brusque or even cheery "No!" followed by a quick exit. The supplicant has to take the girl at her word, but she knows the score. As one ninth grader explained, "Last week, I asked my friend why she was mad—I had no idea why—and she said, 'I'm not mad at you.' Right then I knew she was mad at me." To survive in the social jungle, friends learn to doubt what they see and hear and instead search for a second layer of real feeling beneath a false exterior, a quality that comes to dominate girls' interactions.

Mean looks and the silent treatment are the ultimate undercover aggression. The least visible of the alternative aggressions, nonverbal gesturing slips easily beneath teacher radar, allowing girls to remain "good girls." Debbi Canter, a sixth-grade teacher in Ridgewood, said, "I see those looks flying around the room. I call them on it. And they look at me with those big, innocent eyes. 'What are you talking about?'" Indeed, some teachers justify their hands-off attitude toward girls' aggression because they can't confirm it. Middle-school assistant principal Pam Bank explained, "If I see a boy tapping his pen, I'll say, 'Stop that tapping.' But if I see a girl giving another girl the evil eye, I might say, 'Eyes on me.' I knew the boy was thumping on his pen, but I might not know for sure what the girl was doing."

Girls understand the futility of exposing nonverbal gesturing. Maggie, a Ridgewood sixth grader, said, "Teachers, most of the time, they're like, 'Don't worry, it will be okay, just ignore them.' But it's hard to ignore them. If they do it on purpose and they're right in front of you and they do something to make you really mad, it's hard to ignore them. And it hurts your feelings." Her classmate Emily told me, "If they're whispering, the teacher thinks it's going to be all right because they're not hitting people. She might think they're not hurting her, but if they're punching she might get on them and send them to the office." Kenni added, "Most teachers think, 'Oh, well, she's not hurting you. Don't worry about it.' But really they are hurting you. They're hurting your feelings."

In a social world where anger is not spoken, reading body language becomes an important way for girls to know each others' feelings. Yet the practice can have grave consequences. Bodies at rest are always in motion: no matter how hard a girl tries, it's impossible to be in conscious charge of every move she makes. Misunderstandings happen all the time. A girl passes her friend in the hallway, and her friend doesn't say hello. The girl is certain her friend is angry. Actually, the friend was deep in thought and never even saw the girl. It doesn't matter: a fight begins.

"People look at you and don't mean to, and you think something bad, and it starts something," a Mississippi freshman said. "If girls were more like guys and came out and said what they thought, a lot of stuff wouldn't get started." A Sackler sixth grader remarked, "If you, like, ignore me and don't talk to me so I don't know what's wrong, then maybe I'll turn against you."

Confusing body language can indeed lead to confrontations, albeit bewildering ones. Sixth grader Reena told me, "Last year, in my English class, there was this girl, and I wasn't that good friends with her, but one night she called me up and said, 'You've been mean to me and I want an apology.' And I didn't know what she was talking about because I never really was friends with her so I just said I apologized to her but I never really knew what it was for."

Silence deepens conflict intensity, as each side wonders what the other is thinking. As is often the case when girls avoid confrontations, there may be a long list of possible reasons and past squabbles to plumb. "You each have different ideas about what's going on," a sixth grader at Arden explained. "When you finally do talk, it's worse than when it started."

intimate enemies

Eyes frozen wide in horror, Veronica is gaping at the corpse of her best friend, whom she has handed a now-empty Drano cocktail.

"I just killed my best friend!" gasps the heroine of the film *Heathers.*

"And your worst enemy," purrs her accomplice boyfriend.

"Same difference," she moans.

The word *bully* evokes the image of an enemy, not an intimate, and yet it is often the closest girlfriends who are caught in protracted episodes of emotional abuse. The meanness can unfold secretly under a cover of intimacy and play. Young and ignorant of the signs of relationship abuse, targets struggle to reconcile their circumstances with what they have learned about friendship. Aggressors tend to be equally unaware that their "possessiveness" or "bossiness" is crossing a line. To the contrary, they are often deeply attached to their targets. In the course of these relationships, both target and aggressor often assimilate their behaviors into their concept of friendship. These stories of girl bullying are seldom told. They are a singular alchemy of love and fear, and they defy many of our assumptions about female friendship.

VANESSA'S STORY

Even in the first grade, Vanessa recalled, Stacy was popular and funny. Vanessa was instantly awed by her, and when Stacy asked her to be best friends, she was overjoyed to become part of her clique. Throughout elementary school, Vanessa would relish her status, and especially her power over Nicki and Zoe, who let Vanessa be second-in-command to Stacy. Not long after they became friends, Stacy started asking Vanessa to do things for her. At first, Vanessa felt important when Stacy singled her out, saying she'd like Vanessa if she did whatever it was she wanted at the time. Stacy seemed to leave Nicki and Zoe alone.

"I was very attracted to that," Vanessa, now twenty-seven, told me. Under this arrangement, Vanessa could look tough and still allow herself to be controlled. "I was an insecure kid, but I was confident on the outside," she explained. "And I wanted to be accepted by her, to be her. I wanted to be her second, you know. I wanted to be her right-hand girl."

One night during their frequent sleepovers, when they were nine, Stacy asked Vanessa if they could play dress-up. "I'll be the man, and you'll be the woman," she told Vanessa. That night Stacy kissed Vanessa, and Vanessa enjoyed it. Their sleepovers always included some dress-up for a while after that, and they never told anyone about the game.

In fifth grade, dress-up stopped. The game was never mentioned again, though Vanessa didn't forget about it. The memory became hers instead of theirs; for Vanessa it was strange to have a secret that only she thought about.

That year, Stacy's popularity skyrocketed. Not only was she the first girl in the grade to get MTV, but her parents were cool and let her and her friends eat junk food whenever they wanted. Stacy had the best bike, too. Over at her house, Vanessa told me, "We'd make crank calls. She was always really good and really vicious, and she knew exactly what to do to get the person really upset."

Most of all, though, Stacy was fun, and she had a lot of it by controlling her friends. "She had this way with the other girls," Vanessa recalled. "In a minute, she could make them do anything she wanted. She was the one who always had crushes on boys, and she would tell her friends to go up and tell them something so she didn't have to do anything." She made Vanessa steal candy for her from a local store. "Of course I did it," Vanessa said. "All I wanted to do was make her happy. And of course there was the underlying fear of being rejected by her."

One day, on the bus to school in sixth grade, Vanessa mentioned their old dress-up game. Stacy stared darkly at Vanessa. "What are you talking about?" she snapped. Vanessa stiffened as she watched Stacy turn away.

"Was she afraid?" Vanessa wondered years later. "I think that's when she felt I was a threat. I had this information on her. And that was the beginning of the end."

Stacy began writing songs about Vanessa. "They went something like, 'Vanessa is fat, Vanessa wears a bra.'" Vanessa was the first in the grade to develop breasts, and she had also put on some weight. "There were these limericks. And they would snap my bra all the time," she said. "The boys wouldn't. The girls would."

Nicki and Zoe didn't hesitate to back Stacy up. "They were very creative in the way they would torture me. They would steal my notebooks and they would just write all over [them], 'Vanessa is fat,' 'Vanessa wears a bra,' 'Vanessa sucks,' and all this stuff. In the wintertime they would scratch it into the ice on the bus, and we'd ride around town like that."

The ironic thing, Vanessa recalled, is that Stacy was the only other person developing breasts at the time. "But it was all focused on me," she said. "At the time I thought it was because I was gross and ugly and they didn't want to have anything to do with me. Now I think Stacy saw a lot of things in me that reminded her of herself, and it scared her. I was a bit too close to her. The other girls didn't look at all like her, they didn't act like her, but most of all, they didn't know her secrets."

Vanessa's closeness with Stacy seemed only to inflame Stacy's cruelty. Nevertheless, Vanessa clung to her. "Every day I'm hearing these songs, and every day I'm hanging out with them," she explained. "I'm going to lunch with them. I'm going after school to their houses. It was like I was her best friend, and yet I was her total target."

The girls promised that it was just a joke. They told Vanessa they needed to write a song and that she was just so easy to write about. Vanessa wanted to believe them, so she did. "I didn't have any other friends," Vanessa said. "I was so wrapped up in these people. There were other people I knew who were really cool, and I just—I was so wrapped up. I was so wrapped up in wanting to be part of this group because it seemed to me to be the center of power." Since Nicki and Zoe were affectionate whenever Stacy wasn't around, it was easier for Vanessa to stay with the group.

It also allowed the bullying to be built around the friendship and vulnerability Stacy sensed in Vanessa. One morning at school, before class started, Stacy somberly announced that her mother had died. Vanessa was devastated for her. She got Stacy lunch, told teachers she wouldn't be able to attend class, and covered for Stacy all day. "I thought, 'She finally needs me,'" Vanessa recalled. "She needs me as emotional support, not just to mess with. I was so excited because I'd take care of her, do anything for her."

At the end of the day, Stacy surrounded Vanessa with a large group of girls and told her she'd lied. You're a sucker, she said. "She had convinced the whole school to be in on this," Vanessa said, anger like gravel in her voice. "She wanted to show everyone that she could manipulate me to such an extent, and everyone else wanted to be involved. They all stood up behind the lie. Everyone. And watched me the whole day feel so sorry for Stacy."

Stacy never lifted a finger against Vanessa. She abused Vanessa quietly, deftly using third parties throughout sixth grade. She sent so many notes and messages through other willing girls that Vanessa, feeling surrounded by hate, stopped wanting to go to school. "Wherever you were," she recalled, "there would be a note waiting for you."

One day, the phone rang at Vanessa's house. It was from a trainer at a local gym, asking if Vanessa was still interested in the weight-loss program that she had signed up for. Her father had answered the phone. Vanessa had never been to the gym. Although this might have been a good opportunity to tell her parents about her peers' abuse, Vanessa pretended the call was a mistake.

When I asked Vanessa why, she replied swiftly.

"I never wanted my parents to think that I was making bad decisions," she explained. "I think deep down inside I knew. I knew this wasn't good for me and that Stacy was mean. But you never want to admit your mistakes to your parents, especially when you're eleven, and you're just starting to feel like you can make your own decisions." It was a comment I would hear often from the adult women I interviewed.

Vanessa's mother, who had begun suspecting her daughter's victimization, didn't help. When Vanessa refused to listen to her mother's warnings about Stacy, her mother countered with sarcasm and anger. Adding to the problem was her increasing pressure on Vanessa to lose weight. Her mother stepped up the encouragement, offering to put coins in a can every time Vanessa lost a pound and buy a new dress with the money.

When Vanessa's mother joined the critical voices of her "friends," Vanessa was left feeling alone, without any allies. That they targeted the area that Vanessa was most sensitive about—her weight—seemed to validate the abuse. As she told me, "There was no way I was going to my mother because I was so sure she'd say, 'Well she's absolutely right, Vanessa.'"

By seventh grade, Vanessa was depressed. She began wearing a black trench coat. Inside the pocket she kept a bottle of pills stolen from her grandfather's medicine cabinet. Vanessa imagined they were sedatives as she walked the hallways in school, sometimes holding them absently in her hand. At night she would stare at them, imagining her funeral. Fortunately, she reported, "I was too much of a wimp to do myself in." In school, her grades nose-dived from A's and B's to straight D's. She started hanging out with kids who smoked pot, and she began smoking cigarettes. Her parents were called in to a conference with her teachers, and that night they confronted Vanessa to ask what was wrong. "I said, you know, all the typical things," Vanessa recalled. "School's boring. I'm not interested anymore. All my teachers suck." Her parents believed her, and Vanessa pulled her grades up to the point where she knew she would be left alone. "At one point, it had gotten so bad," she told me, "that people were ripping my clothes in the hallway. I had a horrible pit in my stomach where I couldn't move and I just wanted to throw up everywhere I went.

"That was when I stopped trusting my parents," she recalled, "because I knew they just didn't get it. And if I had actually broken down and told my parents what was going on at that point, that no one was talking to me, that I was already having suicidal thoughts because I just thought I was totally ugly and fat and disgusting, absolutely uninteresting and so weak, and no one wanted to be friends with me, I don't know what would have happened to me."

————

From the earliest moments of their friendship, Stacy meted out love and acceptance only when Vanessa obeyed her. The purposeful control over the terms of a relationship is a signal aspect of relational aggression. At age six Stacy threatened her friendship over Vanessa's failure to play a game; a few years later, she would use it to make her steal. The style of coercion also evolved. Stacy controlled Vanessa for herself, but she soon graduated to making Vanessa perform acts that affected others. Stacy grew to use Vanessa and others as tools to express her own aggression without suffering the responsibility for it.

Vanessa was a valuable pawn in the collection of followers. "I wasn't a wimp and I wasn't quiet and I wasn't meekish and I wasn't stupid. I was funny, really witty, and I always had these comebacks." Stacy's cruel practical joke, Vanessa concluded, was her way of affirming that "I was just a pawn. I was simply like a representation of her power."

Vanessa's compliance with her bully's demands reveals a distinctive element of girls' bullying. Like most bullied children, Vanessa feared reprisal if she fought Stacy's control. But because she continued to associate with these girls as friends, she chose a damaged relationship over no relationship at all.

More and more, Vanessa's conception of her situation was unrealistic, hankering back to the sunnier days of their friendship. After the faked death of Stacy's mother, Vanessa could hardly contain her excitement and sense of relief that "finally, she needs me. She needs me. . . . She needs me as emotional support. . . ." For Vanessa, fear of being alone was an invisible hand keeping a corroded relationship alive, in spite of her intense pain.

Then, one day, Vanessa was filled with a peculiar sense of certainty about what she had to do. "The bottom dropped out," she recalled. "Either I was going to, like, kill myself or I was going to have to claim my space back." The next day, she walked straight up to Stacy and ordered her to be outside at lunch. Word got out, and by noon there was a big crowd assembled. Stacy was waiting.

"I said to her, 'I don't fucking care anymore. I have nothing to lose and I hate you and I hate everything you've done to me, and I think you're a totally evil person and I don't want to have anything to do with you. You can make as much fun of me as you want, but you know what?, like, it doesn't matter anymore.'"

Stacy snarled. She wasn't having any of it. "She pulled out every single insult. She said, 'Vanessa, you're going to regret this for the rest of your life, and no one's ever going to forgive you.'"

When Vanessa didn't flinch, Stacy followed up with a reply that exemplifies the bizarre union of love and cruelty in bullying among friends. She shouted, "Do you know what you're throwing away? You know I could have been the best thing for you forever. We could have been so good together. And yet you just throw it all away."

Vanessa was shocked. She said, "What are you talking about? There's nothing left." And after that, "I just didn't even look back." The spell was broken.

Today, Vanessa believes her relationship with Stacy had a major impact on her social and intimate life. After Stacy, she turned away from girls and became friends with mostly guys. When I asked why, I heard a response that was echoed repeatedly by women who were targets of girl bullies. "I think in a way it's because I don't trust women," Vanessa said. "I don't trust them with my fears." Vanessa believes that women criticize each other more than men do, and more frequently than men criticize women. And for Vanessa, as with countless others, it's not solely a matter of how often women criticize. Vanessa put it succinctly: "When a girl says something, for some reason, it's like it gets deeper. You take it personally. You can't just write it off."

Even when she has resolved her problems with other women, Vanessa can't shake the feeling that "they're going to get you again. And you've got your defenses up at all times." She added, "I'm so scared of their underlying motive and the potential breakdown of [the relationship]. Because the potential breakdown is what, you know, my real fear is. It's like, are they going to hate me? Are they going to make my life miserable? Are they going to just consistently call and write letters and tell me how awful I am and how awful I have been to them? And that my life will never again be happy?"

And yet, Vanessa said, she'll tell a man her deep secrets, even men she doesn't know that well, because she feels safer. Because girls had made her feel so sexually unattractive, she made sure to let me know she has made a point of sleeping with men on the first date, to silence the haunting feeling, instilled by Stacy, that she would never be "girlfriend material."

ANNIE'S STORY

When meanness and friendship become inextricable, girls lose the ability to distinguish between them. They may come to understand meanness as a component of friendship, learning to explain it away and even justify it. When abuse permeates friendship, some girls lose their ability to defend themselves against it.

Annie Wexler's long legs were flexing off the couch she was sharing with her mother, Petra. At fourteen, she looked every bit the girl athlete in white high-tops, blue mesh shorts, and a long, worn Adidas T-shirt. Her long hair was pulled back in a ponytail, and though her eyes looked tired on this dewy Sunday morning, she smiled cheerfully when I apologized for the hour of my visit. The house was still and large, blending into an affluent suburban bouquet of other still and large homes, the only sound the yellow lab clicking his tail insistently against the dark wood floor.

Annie's story began in the third grade, a time when there were already strict social rules. You were in a group—the nerdy one, the cool kids, the "okay" crowd—but you weren't friends with everyone. Annie was, as she put it, "kind of in between this one group of girls and this other group." She had two best friends, one from each clique. Samantha was a small, scrappy girl on the margins of one group in Annie's math class. "Rapunzel" was Samantha's favorite fairy tale, and she had refused to cut her straight brown hair since she was four. Annie loved to brush and braid it. Samantha sat happily for whole recesses at a time as Annie tried different hairstyles and then went running with Samantha inside to look in the girls' bathroom mirror.

Alison was popular and pretty, the center of her clique's attention. Her friends called her "Glitter Girl." Alison had just gotten her ears pierced, but she had been collecting earrings since she was six. Every day, something different sparkled in her ears. Alison's friends played foursquare in the same corner of the playground every day, and it was a game Annie loved. At recess, Alison brought a maroon ball out of her locker, which she had decorated with glitter and glow-in-the-dark stickers.

Samantha usually asked Annie to play at recess just after they arrived at school, and Annie usually said yes. Once, when she replied, "Well, I was going to play with Alison today," Samantha suddenly shot back, "Then I don't want to be your friend anymore."

Samantha's threats triggered intense arguments between the girls. Annie didn't want to lose Samantha, so she would run over to Alison and tell her that she couldn't play after all. Sometimes Annie insisted on playing with Alison. Samantha would say, "Well, you obviously don't like me, so I guess you don't want to be my friend. You can just go play with her. I don't care." And then, Annie recalled, "she'd go off crying." Afraid, Annie would gingerly approach Alison. The very next day, Samantha would come up to play with Annie as though nothing had happened.

Alison responded competitively to Samantha's behavior. She began to want Annie exclusively, so that if Annie was playing with her, and someone else approached, the request to play was always denied. "It always had to be one on one," Annie said. "Samantha and me. Or Alison and me. And I'd feel flattered that people wanted me."

Alison, powerful and charismatic, disliked Samantha. She and her friends started excluding Annie when she played with Samantha. Eventually, Alison started making the same threats. "If you don't play with me at recess," she warned Annie, "I don't want to be your friend anymore."

On the couch, Annie tucked her legs under her and sat up on her knees. "I always felt in the middle," she said. "Who was I going to play with? I might lose them both." She made the first of a few self-deprecating excuses that would be sprinkled throughout our conversation. "It's kind of hard for you to imagine," she began. "I mean, Samantha is not a big person. It's not like she came up to me and was like 'Grrr! You have to play with me!' She's this big!" Annie thrust two fingers stuck together at her mother, who nodded in agreement. "I'm not kidding. I was bigger than her and a full year older than her."

But, Annie said, "you'd always feel intimidated by her because she was this loudmouthed girl. She wasn't afraid to talk. She was gonna say what she thinks. She was always going to have her way. The right way was her way."

Annie sank down into the couch. "Yet I felt so taken over. If I didn't do this I would lose that friendship, and if I did go I would lose this friendship. They wouldn't allow me to be myself. If I would have just mentioned the slightest thing about getting sick of it, they would drop me. I thought I was kind of like getting smaller and smaller to them, not as a friend but just as a person."

Practically every day, either Samantha or Alison would end her friendship with Annie. In her journal every night, Annie said, "I would always write, 'I broke up with Samantha today,' 'I broke up with Alison today.' I know I used the wrong term for it." She laughed.

Annie was quiet for a moment, eyes fixed on her dog. "It feels really bad when someone says, 'I don't want to be your friend,' because then I would wonder, did I do something wrong? Am I just not a person you want to like, and just stuff like that. It's just so powerful in my mind. So many things go through my mind. Did I do something wrong? Am I just not likable?"

"I know it's kind of weird," she insisted (and of course it wasn't, but I wondered for the first time if Annie was anxious about what I might think of her), "I mean, you want to say, 'Why were you friends with this girl?' But it was hard for me to say 'I won't be your friend if you treat me like this' because I really wanted to keep both friendships."

Petra was shifting on the couch, crossing and uncrossing her legs, and had been for the last twenty minutes. She was eager for her daughter to finish. Above all, Petra told me, she was upset about Samantha. For nearly three years, Samantha smothered Annie. In between her threats she showered Annie with gifts brought to school: bracelets, rings, hair clips, stickers, souvenirs from trips to foreign countries. Samantha would make crafts and draw pictures, even take things from her mother (with permission) for Annie.

"But," Petra said, "if Annie crossed her and said I can't play with you today, or I'm playing with somebody else, then she would give her hate notes. 'You're a bitch.' 'I hate you.' And she'd write long notes asking why Annie wasn't her friend anymore."

At school right before winter vacation, helping Annie clean out her locker, Petra was shocked less by the mess than the contents. "We would haul out—I mean, a bagful of gifts and a bagful of hate notes." Petra threw all the gifts away. "I didn't want them in this house," she said bitterly.

Her voice rose in anger. "Every spare moment of school Samantha was on her—play with me, sit with me, sit with me at lunch, play with me after school. Annie would walk in the house after school at 3:30, and the phone would be ringing. It would be Samantha.

"What I thought was sick," she continued, "was the extreme of the I love you–I hate you thing. And I have to be honest. I saw it as potentially the ingredients for a stalker. I kid you not. I use that word. That's what it felt like. It felt victimizing to me, on Annie's behalf, that this girl was a stalker. Had the situation not faded away, I would have been concerned for her safety. Annie would get in the car upset, Samantha this and Samantha that, and we would no sooner walk in the house and there'd be either a message on the machine or Samantha was calling."

There were times, Petra recalled, when Annie would refuse to answer the phone. Or, Petra said, "when I needed to protect her, and I'd say, you know what Annie, I am not letting you talk on the phone today." Annie would agree happily.

Every day as she pulled into the school car-pool lane to pick Annie up, Petra was filled with anxiety. "I could almost tell by her face. It's like, 'Oh God, what was it today?' She would get in the car and be so upset. And it was frustrating for me because I knew as an adult what was going on. As much as we would say to her, 'Oh just tell her to shut up!' that's not who Annie was. She would say to me, 'I can't, I can't be mean.' That part was so frustrating because I thought, 'Nobody's going to treat my kid like that!'"

Approaching Samantha's mother seemed daunting. She was not a friend of Petra's, and Petra dreaded her response to the so-called problem. Imagining the conversation, Petra grimaced: "Who the hell are you to say this! My daughter is giving your daughter gifts! How can you say that's not a nice thing!"

Annie stepped in. "I don't have a weak personality. I'm very strong and I have good leadership qualities. I'm not just going to be sitting there. But it's so hard for me to say, I don't want you to do this anymore, and I don't like the fact that you're doing this to someone who's my friend."

As she became more isolated, Annie was more vulnerable to Samantha's suffocating attention. Annie was folding into herself in other ways, too. She became fearful of crying or showing emotions in front of her peers.

Finally, at the end of fifth grade, Petra told the school counselor that they needed a break. "I said to [the counselor], she can't be the only one to carry Samantha. It's not fair to Annie." (Petra did not tell Annie about her intervention until our interview.) Petra discovered only then that Annie was not Samantha's only target. Between third and sixth grade, several mothers had asked the counselor to separate their daughters from Samantha.

In sixth grade, Annie had an autograph book that she asked her friends to sign at the end of the year. Most kids wrote in their favorite color or movie, and then they wrote what they liked about Annie. "What I like about Annie is that she's so tall," Petra remembered. "What I like about Annie is that she likes to talk on the phone." And Samantha? "What I like about Annie is that I don't really like her and she's really a bitch. What I like about Annie is that we get in fights all the time but she's still my best friend and I like the fact that she gets over the fights."

Annie was so afraid of isolation that tolerating abuse felt like her only option. She also loved her friends. Like Vanessa, Annie tried to please her friend at any cost, wanting only to save the relationship. Her unremitting focus on staying friends with Samantha allowed abuse to take over the friendship.

With meanness so intermixed with friendship, Annie lost the capacity to tell the difference. Consider Annie's incisive description of Samantha's behavior: "This was her way of saying, 'I am your friend and I like you.' I think she was trying to keep the friendship just as she could have it."

The plight of girls who are targets of relational aggression is usually the hardest to address. When family members know about it, it's often difficult to comprehend a girl's refusal to resist. Annie remembered one night "so clearly. I was crying my head off, going, 'I don't know what to do. I can't do this.'" Annie's brothers were kidding around, and perhaps a little exasperated. They asked, "Why don't you just go over there and beat her up? You're ten times her size."

"They were like, 'Go kick her ass!'" Annie said wistfully. "But I wouldn't do that. I wouldn't just go over and be like, 'Hey! You know what? I don't like the way you're treating me.' I just felt so insecure. I was crying so hard." Annie recalled sitting in the family room, not knowing what to do. "I was nine then—for a nine-year-old girl to be having to go through friendship struggles already, it's . . . it wasn't just like, 'I'll see you tomorrow.' It was, 'I don't want to be your friend.' To have that thrown in your face all of a sudden is just so difficult for someone so young, and someone who really thinks that friendship is important."

Our culture's limited understanding of female aggression and intimacy makes it hard for girls to deal with their peer relationships in healthy ways. Most damaging is girls' inability to identify what Carol Gilligan and Lyn Mikel Brown call "relational violations," or dynamics of meanness or abuse.[19] Without an understanding of their unique experience of bullying, girls often end up blaming themselves for their own victimization. Consider Annie, whose interview was dotted with embarrassed explanations of how it was possible that she was bullied by someone half her size and a year younger than she.

That girl bullies are often likely to be the most socially skilled in a group complicates matters further. Like the popular girls profiled by researchers, these girls are mature and worldly. Less often discussed, however, is their intensely charismatic, even seductive aura. Girls like these have almost gravitational pulls on their targets. The friendship is mesmerizing, and often the target is gripped by dueling desires to be consumed and released by her friend. The target may rationally understand the relationship's problems, nod in agreement at her parents' entreaties to pull away, and then find herself inexplicably drawn to a bully's side. About a close friend who demeaned her and forced everyone she knew to ignore her, Chastity said, "She's the kind of person that whenever you'd meet her, you'd love her to death. She's the sweetest person. She'd hide her attitude so everybody loved her."

NATALIE'S STORY

In Ridgewood, Dr. Laura Fields, the city superintendent of schools, led me through a multipurpose room teeming with children lining up to leave. She strode confidently between the long brown benches, stopping to chat with students here and there: "How are you! . . . Good to hear it! . . . Now, don't you think you should close your backpack before you get on the bus? That's a good boy....What a lovely dress!" Some of the kids waved shyly. Others just stared.

Outside at the football field, I marveled at the crowd already gathered. This was the spiritual center of town. Football was just about religion here, and it was common for town residents, even those without school-age children, to drive forty-five minutes on the interstate to fill the stands at away games. Laura led me up through the bleachers, and I could feel people watching me. After we found seats, Laura began chatting with someone while I sat by awkwardly, queasy as I felt the bleachers sway.

The bleachers creaked as a woman plunked down next to me. Short and stocky, with dyed red hair and acid-washed jeans, a cheerful, hearty voice rose up from her belly. "I'm Susan Patterson, how're *you*. I'm real excited for you to speak with my daughter, Natalie." So much for blending in. She turned intense eyes on me and gave me a friendly smack on the shoulder, guy-style. "I think she'd be good for you to talk to."

Natalie seemed less sure. In the days that followed, I said hi to her at school and got little more than a fleeting look before her pageboy hair swung back toward the floor, her locker, anyplace that was not me. I wondered if her mom was forcing her to meet with me.

The day of our interview, I slid into a desk next to her. Natalie was thirteen years old and in the eighth grade. She was wearing blue jeans with a matching jacket and a white T-shirt underneath.

Today Natalie would introduce me to a secret, repeat-offender girl bully in Ridgewood. She was the last one you'd pick in a lineup: picture your typical girl-next-door cheerleader captain. Reese had straight A's, a ponytail that swung like a metronome, and a face that would make Scrooge smile. I was introduced to her mother early on, a charming woman with a quick laugh and a reputation for being at the center of all things off the record in Ridgewood.

Natalie grew up with Reese. Their families had been friends, and the girls started playing in preschool. Natalie felt almost worshipful toward Reese, who always had a new game to pretend. She adored the time spent at Reese's house, which always felt more crowded than it really was.

In third grade, Reese started telling Natalie stories about having a brother who died or a pet that didn't exist. She'd come over to Natalie's house and criticize her outfits and the pictures on her bedroom wall. Natalie was hurt but figured if she changed her clothes and stripped her walls, Reese would stop. She didn't. At school, Reese started pretending Natalie wasn't there when they were around other girls, even though at home they were still best friends.

Reese was the girl version of the stealth bomber: she flew low and she was in and out before anyone knew who did it or what happened. Spectacularly sweet, she was one of the first to spring to mind when teachers ticked off a mental list of girls with good reputations. Which made her the last person most people even thought to look at. "She made good grades and didn't talk out in class," Natalie explained. "The teachers saw, oh, Reese and Natalie are friends, so they'd put us together in groups in class. We were quiet and we'd tell each other things."

But whenever they were grouped or paired together, Natalie clammed up. Reese berated and teased her. "I'd be the quietest girl in the grade because I didn't speak out," Natalie said. Although she had once loved to read aloud from her journal in class, Reese began exchanging looks with other girls, so Natalie stopped. Meanwhile, Reese projected an image to their peers of harmony and affection. "She was all the time trying to be my friend."

I asked Natalie if she'd ever spoken out against Reese. She looked at me quizzically. "I thought she was, you know, like the world. She was my *best friend*." She said this carefully, as if English was not my first language. "I didn't—I was just scared to say something to her because I was afraid she'd get mad at me or dislike me and start talking about me even more." The few moments when Natalie or one of their friends showed signs of resistance, "She tried to make everybody think she was just fine and that it was all me coming up with this stuff in my mind." Reese successfully convinced Natalie that she was not strong enough to fight, even if she'd wanted to. "She took advantage of me and I didn't take up for myself," she told me. "I would let myself believe that she was better than me."

That Natalie hid the problems with Reese from her mother was no surprise. Natalie's downcast eyes were a stark contrast with her mother's easygoing, how-ya-doing personality. Sometimes, when her mother asked if school had been good and Natalie said not really, Susan breezed on to the next subject. She was friends with Reese's mother—looked up to her, in fact—and Natalie never thought her mother would believe her. She was ashamed.

In sixth grade, Reese became close with Drew, who had just moved to town. Reese put Drew through an unusually public torture, and Natalie eventually reached out to her. After watching Drew cry every day at school, Natalie tried to show her that she'd felt the same pain. It wasn't easy. "She was afraid to trust me," Natalie said. "And I was afraid to trust somebody at first, too. I thought I'd never trust anybody again because I put my whole trust in Reese. And she just totally went behind my back and talked about me. She told people everything I had ever told her. So I thought I could never tell anybody anything again. I didn't even tell my mama and my daddy anything."

When I asked Natalie if her friendship with Reese affected her in any way, she was modest. "I think it has affected me just a little," she said. "I used to be loud and funny and everything, but now I barely talk. I used to be the funny person with my friends and everyone would laugh at me. I used to stand out wearing funny clothes but I don't do that anymore because I'm afraid that Reese or somebody would make fun of me or talk about me."

"How does that make you feel?" I asked her.

"When I think about it, it makes me feel like I want to just cry. But I don't because I know that if I cry I'm letting her get to me and I just don't do anything." Natalie had befriended new girls and felt a world of a difference in these new relationships. But fear of new confrontations with Reese lingered.

As she sat before me, Natalie's face was anguished, but the pain was hardly fresh. It seemed stamped there. She had been on the verge of tears the whole time we were talking, reporting the facts with clarity and steadiness.

When we were done, I turned off the tape recorder. I told her how strong and wonderful I thought she was, and how brave. Natalie stood quickly to leave, and I felt intuitively that she would go somewhere else to cry. It was all I could do not to jump out of my chair and hug her, but I knew that was not what she needed. It was what I needed. Listening to her was like looking down into a deep well of sorrow, and the memory of Natalie stayed with me long after I left the building.

CHAPTER *three*

the truth hurts

At 1:15 P.M., my first group of eighth-grade girls at Marymount were looking like they might pass out. It was the right-after-lunch-and-I-need-a-nap class period. On the floor, the girls were drooping against one wall, refusing to make a circle, leaning into one another like reeds. It was March, and outside there was a hint of spring. Though it was no more than sixty-five degrees, many were wearing shorts or tank tops.

I pulled out the Oreos, and as if on cue, they sat up and began to munch. Relieved by these signs of life, I began the discussion by asking them to describe the perfect girl. They looked at me quizzically.

"Like in magazines. Movies. *Dawson's Creek*. Stuff like that."

A few hands went up. Hoping to foster a casual atmosphere, I had asked them to speak without raising their hands. Old habits die hard.

"Skinny!" one says.

"Pretty!"

Okay, I thought. And then: "Nice!"

"What do you mean, nice?" I asked, looking up from my notebook.

"She always has friends."

"She never gets in fights."

"Everybody loves her."

So began my understanding of girls' everyday aggression.

"Okay," I said, stalling to think. "So if one of your friends has done something to bug you or make you mad, or sad, do you tell her about it?"

"No!" came a chorus.

"Why?" I asked.

Silence. I waited.

A girl in the corner took a breath. "Because then it's going to cause a big thing."

"What's 'a big thing'?"

"There's going to be a big fight about it," someone else explained.

"Everyone's going to get involved. It's not worth losing your friendship over something small."

"People make stuff up."

"What if," I asked, "you were just telling someone how you felt, because *you* felt bad? You know, to make yourself—your friendship—feel a little better?"

"Then you might hurt her feelings," one said. Nods. Locking eyes.

"Can you tell someone the truth and not be mean?" I asked.

"The truth hurts," a girl in the corner said quietly. "That's why I lie."

When I set out to write this book, I sought the stories of women and girls who had been targets or aggressors of severe episodes of bullying. Following the received wisdom of scholars and teachers, I conceived of alternative aggressions as behaviors found outside girls' "normal" social structure. When I met with my first groups of girls, I was broadsided with stories of everyday conflict that bore a striking resemblance to their descriptions of bullying.

Girls don't have to bully, at least as far as we have understood the word, to alienate and injure their peers. In fact, the word *bullying* couldn't be more wrong in describing what some girls do to hurt one another. The day-to-day aggression that persists among girls, a dark underside of their social universe, remains to be charted and explored. We have no real language for it.

Girls describe their social communities as worlds in which unresolved conflicts hang like leaking gas in the air, creating a treacherous emotional terrain in which discord is rarely voiced and yet may explode silently with the slightest spark. For many, if not most, girls, every day can be unpredictable. Alliances shift with whispers under cover of girlish intimacy and play. Many girls will not tell each other why they are sad or angry. Instead, they will employ small armies of mediators, usually willing friends who are uncomfortably caught in the middle or eager for the moments of intimacy that result from lending a hand to someone in trouble.

Alternative aggressions, and the nonassertive behavior they suggest, are as embedded in the daily lives of girls as makeup, boys, and media. A girl learns early on that to voice conflict directly with another girl may result in many others ganging up against her. She learns to channel feelings of hurt and anger to avoid their human instigator, internalizing feelings or sharing them with others. She learns to store away unresolved conflicts with the precision of a bookkeeper, building a stockpile that increasingly crowds her emotional landscape and social choices. She learns to connect with conflict through the discord of others, participating in group acts of aggression where individual ones have been forbidden.

In my conversations with girls, many expressed fear that even everyday acts of conflict would result in the loss of the people they most cared about. They believed speaking a troubled heart was punishable. Isolation, they cautioned, was irreversible, and so too great a price to be paid. As a sixth grader told me, "You don't want to say it to them and if you do, it's like, well, you might as well just walk off because they're not going to want to be your friend." Hannah, an

Arden seventh grader, explained, "If I tell my friends I'm angry at them, I'll have another enemy. It's a vicious cycle." In a world that socializes girls to prize relationships and care above all else, the fear of isolation and loss casts a long shadow over girls' decisions around conflicts, driving them away from direct confrontation. By taking uncomfortable feelings out of everyday relationships, girls come to understand them as dangerous to themselves and others, worthy of being carefully shielded or perhaps not disclosed at all.

Many girls are afraid of not being able to anticipate the response to their anger, so they resolve to maximize what they *can* control. One of the reasons girls like to write letters, an eighth grader told me, is that they "help us to organize our thoughts and get it out perfectly. If I say it to her face, I'm gonna break down, mess up my words, say things I don't mean." Some girls described writing letters that they burned or trashed in order to balance feeling angry and preserving friendship. Letters were preferable, eighth-grader Shelley said, "because if you have a conversation, they can see your face."

A one-on-one conversation is scary, an Arden seventh grader said, because "I don't know what she's going to say next. You don't want to lose the fight. You're scared the friendship's going to end. You don't know what they'll say. And if the discussion goes badly, she might get other people involved. That's why I don't talk." You can't just tell someone that they're being mean, her classmate told me. "You think, 'Oh my God,' [she'll] get mad at me, or [she] won't be my friend anymore. People are afraid she'll spread rumors. You don't know what that person's going to think."

The need to consider others' feelings at the expense of their own was a theme that ran through my interviews. No matter how upset they were, these girls said they would rather not hurt someone else's feelings. Their own needs seemed to them utterly expendable. They described shrinking problems and feelings into "little things," calling them "unimportant," "stupid," "not worth a fight," stowing them somewhere inside, an inner room that would one day be too small to contain them.

boom!

I went to Jennifer's house twice before she agreed to speak to me. The first time, I sat drinking tea with her mom, and the eleven-year-old girl's fuzzy slippers hung slightly over the cracked divide between the kitchen and the den. She was checking me out. The second time I visited, she nodded shyly. On the couch in the den, I was pleasantly surprised to find her animated as a dragonfly, hands streaking the air with energy. Rapid-fire, she said, "My friend and I always ask each other if we're mad at each other. Immediately after we go, 'No,' because you don't want to say, 'I'm mad at you.'"

"Why not?" I asked.

"Because then you make the other person feel bad because you know someone's mad at you."

"Is it important that you feel mad?"

"Yeah, but are you supposed to let it out at the person you're mad at?" she asked, as though she really did not know.

"Some people would say yes because your feelings count," I said.

"What about her feelings?" she asked.

"What about them?" I asked.

"I just...no. We don't talk about this. I don't know if best friends talk about this. This is private." I ceased and desisted.

With twelve-year-old Carmen Peralta, a wry Latina student at a private school in the Northeast, I was asking about what it's like to tell someone you're angry. She said she never did, and I asked why. "Because it sounds weird for one thing! 'Hey, by the way, I'm mad at you!'" she drawled sarcastically. Becoming more serious, she began to stall. "I won't say, 'I'm mad'—it just—I don't know—I don't like that way of dealing with things because it's weird—just to say, 'I'm

mad at you.'...It's kind of like *boom!*"—Carmen made a huge, satisfying noise—"to them. They're just like, 'What did I do?' And if
you say, 'Hey, I need you to know I'm mad at you,' it's just like
boom! I think they'll end up thinking less of you." For Carmen, conflict falls like a bomb inside friendship, apparently blowing it to
smithereens. Conflict for Carmen is outside words, outside relationship, indeed seems to have no comfortable place anywhere in her life.

Some girls face conflict by appealing to lifelong lessons in being
nice. In Mississippi, ten-year-old Melanie was explaining to her classmates why she couldn't tell Kaya she was mad.

"You can't do that!" she cried.

"Why not?"

"Because some people are really sensitive in our school, and if you
said something like that, they'd bust out crying."

"But you'd be saying how you felt, right?" I was pushing for a
reason.

"But then you'd be hurting some people's feelings."

"But what if you're *reeeeeeealllly* upset?" I asked, and some girls
giggled.

"Sometimes you tell your friends but [sometimes you don't] tell
anybody," she decided. Anyway, she said, you'll probably get a
chance later to be mad at them. "You'll go up to somebody and say,
'Oh you know, Kaya gets on my nerves. She told me that so and so,
and so and so.'"

"But why don't you go up to Kaya and just say, 'Hey, you made
me mad!'"

"Because," she said simply, looking at me with cautious eyes,
"you want to get back at them."

For most girls, anger and hurt become the elephant in the room.
As the feelings grow in size and intensity, so does the challenge of
restraint.

Her best efforts notwithstanding, Meredith at Arden thinks it's
useless to hold in her anger. "When you don't let one of your friends

know, it builds up inside you. There's bitterness inside you. It's hard for them and for you." Charlotte agreed. "You can't make the feelings go away. If it's hidden it gets stronger and it gets harder and harder to hold in."

One student told me when she felt angry she kicked her dog. Plenty more said they hit their siblings. Some students I interviewed described feeling depressed as they tried to sequester their anger. Others told stories of escalating fury. "You get angrier and angrier when you can't hold it in. Then you explode," said Emily at Marymount. "It gets bigger and you find even more stuff to dislike about that girl." Disturbingly, the more intense the problem, the more likely a girl may pretend that everything's cool. Said Nancy at Marymount, "I was so angry I couldn't tell her about it. It was easier not to say anything and for her not to know I was so angry."

Fear of speaking face to face usually ends up worsening girls' conflicts by forcing them to involve third parties. When Shelley couldn't get Sarah to talk directly about the problem between them, Shelley began asking others what was wrong with Sarah. But to the ignorant observer—say, Sarah—Shelley looked like she was going behind her back. Sarah was enraged. "But I'm getting advice!" Shelley exclaimed, echoing innumerable girls I spoke with. A Mississippi fifth grader saw it as damage control: "If you tell the person you're angry at yourself, they're going to be madder quicker than if you tell someone else. And then later you have time to think what you're going to say and what you're going to do." A sixth grader from the same school described it this way: "You're scared the person will take it the wrong way, so you try out different versions and opinions. Otherwise, you might get it wrong and make it worse." Unwittingly, they are doing just that.

Other girls believe anything is preferable to the loss of a relationship. In their minds, they are merely choosing a lesser evil. "Girls can break each other," Hannah said simply. "Instead, they cool off by gossiping behind their backs. Otherwise you could end the friendship." Some girls reported trying to circumvent the conflict process by expecting their friends simply to know, like mind readers or super-heroes with X-ray vision, that they were upset. Linden sophomore Lily Carter, whose quiet thoughtfulness gave the impression of her being far older than she really was, laughed shyly as she handed me a tiny pink journal that she promised would detail the social chaos of her middle-school years. She had already flagged the pages with yellow Post-it notes, and in the very first entry of seventh grade she wrote, "It's hard having my feelings bottled up inside. I'm a sensor. I sense things and give people hints to how I'm feeling." She later noted:

> It's strange kinda feeling that the people you've been friends with so long can't get the hints I give. You'd think they'd know. When I'm not with them, they NEVER ask if I'm mad at them or try to talk to me. They just ignore me, as if I don't exist or like "thank heavens she's gone." I'm MISIRABLE [sic]!

Like a boat adrift at sea, Lily was sending distress messages no one could hear. The more she used indecipherable speech and gesturing to communicate, the more alone and abandoned she felt.

When silent pleas are ignored, a girl's despair can turn swiftly to anger. Many girls reported feeling indignant because their friends didn't know how they felt. These girls felt it should be obvious from the clipped tone of their voices, the terseness of their notes, the nights they didn't call. Yet their friends never responded. And as the girls silently willed their friends to know their inner feelings, their rage doubled when their friends didn't.

not my fault

Why not just take the girl aside and tell her calmly, in a nice way, what's bothering you? It's a question countless parents, guidance counselors, and bullying experts have asked. So did I.

"I try that," a Linden ninth grader told me anxiously, "but she tells me something I did wrong and then it's my fault." It was a comment I would hear over and over again, from girls of all ages. "She'll turn it around," "she'll make it about me," or "she'll get everyone on her side." Because so many girls lack facility with everyday conflict, expressions of anger make listeners skittish and defensive. The sound of someone upset feels like the first sign of impending isolation, a kind of social thunder rumbling in the distance.

For these girls, absorbing anger is just as frightful as voicing it. The idea that they may be "at fault" or "wrong" makes them uneasy, and it can breed panic and impulsive decision making. In many cases, they grasp for whatever will move the harsh spotlight away from them and onto someone else; sometimes, using alliance building (explored later in the chapter), they grasp for the girl who will stand with them and assure them of continuous, unconditional friendship. Raised in a culture that prizes sweetness, what feels right to these girls is an anxious scramble to remain the "good" girl; to hold up a mirror to their friend and, instead of listening, point out a past infraction. Needless to say, such conflicts escalate swiftly, often leaving both girls filled with regret and fear.

i'm sorry

The surface of a girl fight can be silent and smooth as a marble. You know that if you've ever been the last person to find out someone's mad at you. Many girls use double doses of distance and silence to announce their anger, leaving defendants clueless about what they've done. Beneath the surface, of course, is another story.

Girls approach the rituals of fighting and peacemaking with an eerie rigidity. For many, the shared knowledge that they are "*in* a fight" is much easier than actually going to the trouble of having one. Freyda and Lissa's "fight" may entail passing each other in the hallway silently for days before anyone speaks. No matter that the source of their conflict is utterly trivial and that in the silence between them the conflict will swell, taking on a life of its own. As one girl waits for the other to give in and say she's sorry, both girls may lose track of why they are fighting at all. "When [girls are] angry, they won't listen, and if you don't talk, [girls will] build up with anger and then you won't remember why you're in a fight," explained a

Sackler sixth grader. "Sometimes it's over, but you have to keep going," an Arden sixth grader remarked. "You don't want to give up. You don't want to drop it. You don't want to be the loser."

When the fight is concluded, one girl has usually surrendered and apologized—via note, messenger, e-mail, instant message, or in person—while the other has "won." It is not uncommon for girls, especially preadolescents, to avoid processing what happened beyond the immediate apology and relief. Many sit on the sidelines of their own discord, skirting the substance of conflict and instead clinging to process—to the rituals of a fight's beginning, middle, and end. Lyn Mikel Brown and Carol Gilligan observed in girls an uncanny ability to say "I'm sorry" and give conflicts "almost fairy-tale-like happy endings, so that strong feelings of pain and indignation end abruptly with this final act of attrition."[20]

So the denouement is often as troubled as the fight itself. The prime directive for girls is to maintain the relationship at any cost; this, along with the accompanying fear of a lost relationship, is what drives almost every step of a fight. *Sorry* may be a universal code word for a truce, but it is often perfunctory and swift, casual and automatic, like saying "bless you" when someone sneezes. However it is delivered, via written, cyber, or human medium, sorry is a razor-sharp, clean slice through a fight, shutting it down as abruptly as pulling the plug on a blaring stereo. And because this perfunctory apology often comes when a fight has not yet played itself out, because it is driven more by the fear of a lost relationship than the need to clear the air, sorry is often a purely procedural event, calling for peace while the source of the conflict still festers, tucked away like a genie stuffed into a bottle, stewing unresolved until the next trigger comes.

One girl recalled her usual "make-up" line: "Let's just be friends. I can't understand why we got in such a stupid fight." Steering clear of the details, a sixth grader told me, avoids being brought too close to the precipice of her own anger. "Someone might say the wrong thing again," she explained. Others simply can no longer endure the isolation. "I didn't want her to stay mad at me," her classmate explained, "so I'd just say sorry." Anyway, another girl offered, if you wait it out, "your anger just melts away." A Ridgewood eighth grader said, "You forget about what you're mad about because you don't want to lose the friendship." Still another recalled an erstwhile friend who bullied her mercilessly, then approached her at school and inexplicably apologized. "It just happened," she said. "Sorry."

Carmen Peralta said being direct with friends doesn't work for her, since everyone she knows gives knee-jerk apologies instead of really talking about their feelings. "When a person tells you [she's angry], it makes you feel like you're going to say sorry automatically—automatically, not thinking. But if you don't say, 'I'm mad at you,'" she said, and instead speak without words, forcing the person to wonder why you are acting strangely around her, "the person will actually think about what [she's] doing wrong."

Sometimes Carmen does apologize, but she can't stand it that she's always the one to say it first. "Sometimes when I say, 'I'm sorry,' [it's because] I just feel more guilty [not because I] understand what the person's saying. I just figure, 'What the hell, I'll say I'm sorry and make it all better.' I don't think that does make it all better," she added, shrugging, "because I'll probably still act the way that's annoying the person."

Under these social conditions, a cycle gets put into motion. Old conflicts are printed indelibly into memories and, unresolved, are summoned for use in the next conflict. One of the most common grievances I heard from girls was: "We remember everything. We never forget." One girl explained why: "Boys duke it out. Girls, they don't finish [the fight]. It grows bigger. And there's another fight and the next one's huge. That's what leads to people not being friends anymore." A Sackler sixth grader said, "You go back to these teeny tiny things that you didn't talk about before. Then it gets bigger." Lisa, at Arden, said, "Girls always look back at what you did the last time."

just kidding

Girls who want to bypass conflict entirely may turn to other behavioral pathways. Humor is an especially popular way to injure a peer indirectly. Joking weaves a membrane of protection around the aggressor as she jabs at a target. A sixth grader described a classmate who easily got away with teasing. "She'd say something, the teacher would kind of look, and she's like, 'I was just kidding!'" At Linden, students talked about the moment in which teasing crosses over into insult. "Slut is the worst insult," said Erica. "Ho is said easily. Like, 'That's such a ho outfit.'" When the jostling goes into shaky territory, someone quickly exclaims, "We were just kidding!"

Rarely, if ever, does the targeted girl disagree. The fear of being called hypersensitive—*Can't you take a joke?*—is enormous. Nobody wants to hang out with someone like that, and everyone knows it. "What's the big deal?" can sting when you're trying to act cool. "When a girl is the butt of all jokes, she wants to tell her friends it hurts her," sixteen-year-old Ellie said. "She thinks, 'I know they're not doing it to hurt me.' And they deny it. But it beats at your self-esteem."

The feeling of being crazy plagues the target of these "jokes," as she must choose between the sting of her own feelings and what she wants to believe about her friends. Believing a friend while ignoring the hum of her own instinct is an important example of how a girl can "give up or give over [her] version of reality to those who have the power to name or reconfigure [her] experience," a major symptom of girls' loss of self-esteem observed by Brown and Gilligan.[21]

Fear of reprisal is not the only deterrent to speaking up. Tasha Keller had just gotten her learner's permit, and she was scarfing down a bagel at a deli as we talked about how she responds when girls use jokes to cover their true feelings.

"In the end you see how foolish it is to get upset," she said, her words muffled with chewing.

"Even though someone's being nasty?" I asked.

"If someone's joking around, you're not supposed to think it's such a big thing."

"Even if someone hurts your feelings?"

"If someone told you something that hurt your feelings, would you think that's worse than being beaten up? The bigger thing would have been if someone's beating you up at school. That's what you think of a bully as." She was practically lecturing me now. "You don't think of it as someone who's..." She paused, searching to describe the phenomenon that has for so long remained unnamed—"*nicely abusing* you also."

Some mainstream psychologists view the ritual of comic or casual peer insults as formative to child development. University of California at Berkeley professor Dacher Keltner argues that "teasers convey that they are joking through laughter, knowing looks and nudges, and tone of voice."[22] Here girls' social world is again seen through a male lens. With access to a much wider range of opportunities for direct aggression, boys' use of humorous one-upping can be clearly distinguished from "real" or serious moments of anger. For girls, whose aggressions are frequently conveyed in body language, and who mostly share in common the need to sequester anger, the use of humor serves a different purpose. "A lot of times," thirteen-year-old Jasmine told me, "what you say when you're joking is really what you mean but you're too afraid to say it." And, she added, "humor doesn't work unless both people know it's true."

ganging up

"It's weird how time erases things," muses the once-popular, now-outcast Julie in the film *Jawbreaker.*

"Time doesn't erase things," replies the once-outcast, now-popular Fern. "People erase things."

"People erase people." Julie sighs.

Nothing launches a girl faster, or takes her down harder, than alliance building, or "ganging up." The ultimate relational aggression, alliance building forces the target to face not only the potential loss of the relationship with her opponent, but with many of her friends. It goes like this: Spotting a conflict on the horizon, a girl will begin a scrupulous underground campaign to best her opponent. Like a skilled politician, she will methodically build a coalition of other girls willing to throw their support behind her. Friends who have "endorsed" her will ignore the target, lobby others for support, or confront the target directly until she is partly or completely isolated. "You kind of declare war in your own way," explained Daniella, a sixth grader.

Ganging up is the product of a secret relational ecosystem that flourishes in an atmosphere where direct conflict between individuals is forbidden. By engaging in conflict as a group, no one girl is ever directly responsible for her aggression. Anger is often conveyed wordlessly, and the facade of the group functions as an eave under which a girl can preserve her "nice girl" image. The loser usually ends up isolated from others, giving her exactly what she fears conflict begets: relational loss. The specter of isolation is often enough to make most people "forget" their angry feelings.

Girls use alliance building to short-circuit the link expected between anger and the loss of relationship. Victoria, interviewed by Brown and Gilligan, explains that when people get mad it helps to "pass [their feelings] on to someone else and it will keep on going around so everyone can pick corners." Kenya, a Ridgewood sixth grader, explained, "They are mad at their friend, and their friend's mad at them, and they need to go find another friend and get to know them better and tell them about their problem, and maybe that will help another friendship to start." In this way, alliance building becomes an event of friendship. It provides a way for girls to displace their aggression while remaining connected to others. No matter how intense the fight, a girl is assured of a friendship that will outlast it; the girls who rally to her side promise her that with their presence. In this way, the trials of conflict are transformed into a series of relationships to be negotiated, a skill at which girls excel.

Nikki, an eighth grader from Marymount, described how it works: "If I'm mad at someone, it's just a lot easier to tell everyone else and turn them against the person because then I'm the one who's right. If you just tell the person, one-on-one, then the two of you are out there to be judged by the whole grade, and you can't know if you are going to be the one who's considered right by the others."

During alliance building, discussions spread like wildfire through circles of friends, growing in intensity until they dominate the day. "First people tell each other; then they use the phone, then the Internet; it gets bigger and bigger; they cut and paste conversations [from instant messages]," recalled thirteen-year-old Rebecca at Marymount. One girl wins, her classmate Maria noted, when she "gets people not to like the other one."

Another girl described it this way: "I think it was mostly just like, nobody can get mad at me for something. I was the good friend. I wasn't the problem. I am like best friends with all of these people now that I didn't used to be friends with. I have everything that she thought she had. It was just like a sense of empowerment."

Alliance building also conforms to girls' tendency to stockpile old conflicts. The aggressor's strategy is to appeal to those who have a history with the target. Particularly where girls have known each other for many years, the aggressor can plumb a rich history of relational trouble.

Alliance building was in full swing among the Mississippi fifth graders. Danika explained, "Girls try to get information from you about your other friend, [who] is their enemy. Such as, do you like so and so?" I asked how it works.

"They take [the information] from you and say, 'Thank you.' Then you say you have to be right back, that you're going to see somebody, and you go tell [your friend]. It's just like collecting information from the enemy." The potential foot soldiers have usually been waiting for the right opportunity. Beccy explained, "One person can have a problem, talk to one person, and she's got something she remembers from last week."

This is classic indirection, since it allows girls to hold the conflict at arm's length as they watch others fight it. Girls have multiple incentives to become embroiled in each others' conflicts. First, alliance building offers a chance for girls to belong, even briefly, to an ad hoc clique. Jumping on another girl's bandwagon to show support in her time of conflict affords a rare moment of inclusion and comfort. Nikki remarked, "People don't know what we're fighting about, but they want to be in it. They want to be part of the gossip." Said her classmate Mallory, "It gives you something to belong to, and inclusion is such a big deal." Since the girl coordinating the alliance is usually vulnerable, stepping in with support is an opportunity to be a friend while racking up a future favor for when your turn inevitably rolls around. Needless to say, effective foot soldiers can take leaps up the social ladder. "If you take sides," Rachel explained, "you can become popular through them and be their friend."

Indeed, popularity itself is in large part defined by the ability of one girl to turn her friends against someone else. If isolation is trauma for girls, there is power to be found in relationships. Having girls on her side offers a girl a sense of personal strength. "It makes you feel more popular and like you have more power. You're in the right," explained Lauren at Marymount. Said eleven-year-old Mary at Arden, "It gives you a feeling of security. If you know people are gathering on your side, you think, 'Wow, I am powerful. I have a feeling of power.'"

Alliance building is a sign of peer affirmation, an unspoken contract that means, for the moment anyway, that a girl will not be abandoned. If she can turn everyone against a target, it is impossible for them to turn against her. "It's a way of getting people to say you're cool and strong," Dana noted.

So ingrained is alliance building in girls' lives that many I spoke with struggled to imagine life without it. "You don't do it on purpose," said Lauren, shrugging. "It's your natural instinct. I tell other people and try to make myself look good."

"When you can't tell anyone, you feel helpless," explained Dana. "You don't know who to go to. It builds up."

Of course, there are troubling social and individual costs to this activity. Lauren described how to attract more supporters when the marrow of a conflict thins: "You bring other stuff into it. 'Oh, do you see what she's wearing.'" And sometimes, invariably, "you exaggerate and don't tell the whole truth." She explained, "When more people get involved, there's a lot more pressure to win." In this way, alliance building encourages other alternative aggressions, including rumor spreading and secret telling. Alliance building can distort the conflicts, and it makes fights last longer than they would have if they had been played out directly.

For the target, the mass shutting down of one by many has consequences that reach far beyond the moment. "It's like your life is a pond," a seventh grader told me, "and a girl throws a stone inside it, and the ripples mess up your life." If fights are ultimately a contest of relationships, the facts of the conflict are easily dwarfed by the alliances forming around them. As a result, girls are often forced to question their own version of events, feeling crazy once again. "When I'm in fights with people, they turn it against me," said Cari at Marymount. "They say it's my fault. Everyone will say you have no right to be angry. They make you think you're crazy." By lobbing the conflict out to others to judge and decide, said her classmate Courtney, "You can never win. The entire grade takes sides."

When fights cannot be enacted and concluded directly, girls learn it may be easier to stay silent. Noura, interviewed by Brown and Gilligan, described a typical episode of gossip, explaining that if she disagreed with someone's perception, "that person would get mad . . . and so sometimes I just don't know what to say, and it's hard to say something." Gradually, like a circus leaving town, the lights go out of the voices, opinions, and feelings of these girls.

Most fascinating about the ritual of alliance building is how it validates the experience of aggression for girls. Girls understand that face-to-face, one-on-one aggression with another girl is unacceptable. "If you have no sympathizers, you're the bad one. You're randomly mean," says Courtney. Megan, who lost the support of her peers in a campaign against Melissa, concluded that she "felt foolish being mean to someone without my friends."

Together, however, it's another story. A plurality creates a safe space for girls to be mean in a culture that refuses to allow girls individual acts of aggression, making alliance building a rare intersection of peer approval with aggression. Alliances create underground net-works in which girls can be in charge of their own social norms, de-ciding together when the use of aggression is deserved.

A Sackler sixth grader explained alliance building as a way to cir-cumvent punishment. "You don't want to be blamed for it, and so you blame it on other people, saying 'Pass it on.'" Aggressive boys may be just as likely to seek refuge from punishment or guilt in a gang. The different rules of the aggression game, however, make it likely that angry girls will seek and need company. A study confirmed that the guilt girls experience during aggressive acts decreases signif-icantly when responsibility can be shared with other people.[23]

middlegirls

Even if a girl manages to avoid being on either end of a conflict, she may end up stuck in the middle of it, a position just as perilous. When it's clear girls have no choice but to be drawn into conflict, many adapt by resorting to a skill they know well, one they have long ob-served in the adult women around them. Over the treachery of tak-ing a side, they choose to be mediators, or what I call "middlegirls."

When a girl's friends are the two people fighting, being in the middle is often the riskiest place. With both girls lobbying for a friend's support, both friendships can become endangered, or de-stroyed. Julia from Arden explained, "If you have two best friends, you feel you have to pick sides. [But] if you pick one side, the other girl starts whispering. You feel defeated and you want to give up. You become the one at fault." What's more, suballiances can de-velop, increasing pressure on a girl in the middle to act. "Then there are so many people against you," Stacy said, "and you just get de-feated and stop."

Since girls often refuse to talk to one another when they're mad, middlegirls are critical players in the conflict process. By the time a middlegirl enters the lives of girls in conflict, the foes are usually run-ning scared. The middlegirl's prime directive is to broker a compromise between the rival parties. By acting as an affectionate diplomat of sorts, she effectively rescues both girls from their isolation.

But the consequences for the middlegirl can be mixed. For instance, in the course of her diplomacy, the middlegirl learns she will be valued when she maintains the health of others' relationships, a skill prized in the feminine character. "I feel really good about myself when I can get my friends to sit down and talk," an eleven-year-old told me.

The warring girls face equally uncertain outcomes. A middlegirl holds their social future in her hands, and she knows it. She can just as soon gut a friendship as she can stitch it back together. A middlegirl may have her own agenda with one of the girls. Perhaps, as one sixth grader told me, she will lie to avoid being caught in a crossfire that is getting dangerously close. In that case, she said, "[you] would be afraid that the person would start telling rumors about you and then telling lies and then they won't be your friend anymore."

In Mississippi, I was sitting with seventh graders talking about alliance building.

"Why do lots of girls get involved in a person's fight?" I asked.

"She gets to watch it," Beth said.

"They'll be able to go tell other people what happened. 'Oh I know what happened!'" Andra sneered.

"You might want to be somebody's best friend so you make the fight worse than it is," Angela added.

"Sometimes people change things and make someone even madder," Beth said.

"Why," I asked, "would someone want to do that?"

"Because they don't really like that person or anything."

"—because you want to make them fight."

"And the person in the middle can add to the rumors."

"What does she stand to gain?" I asked.

"The messenger might have added or changed the story because one of the girls had made her mad before," Beth continued. "She had done something to her but she was waiting for a chance to get her back."

Forced to prioritize others' relationships at the expense of their own, middlegirls can quickly become part of the conflict itself. A sixth grader at Arden described her often futile attempts to bring girls together. "No matter how much I try to help, they ended up getting mad at me anyway. The way they made peace is over being mad at me." A classmate of hers got burned by choosing not to take sides. "They both got mad when I was with the other one." A fifth grader at a private religious school wrote simply, "I got into a fight talking about a fight." The words of a classmate were telling in describing her social problems that year: "I had a fight *between* Adelia and Marina" (my italics).

Rebecca, a sixth grader at the religious school, explained it this way: "I think of it as a Ping-Pong game. A championship. And like, you're gonna win. And the middlegirl is the ball, and one friend's on one side and one friend's on the other. And you want to keep on bouncing back and forth because you don't want to stop on one side or the other but eventually you have to land somewhere."

The increasing importance of the middlegirl is a result of a social community in which open conflict is feared and forbidden. The middlegirl helps filter and tamp down the anger that would otherwise flow freely between girls. She is a human tool girls use to avoid the possibility that they will say something the wrong way, or speak words they don't mean. As an Arden seventh grader put it, "When two of my friends were in a huge fight, it had become necessary that I was there. It was about me, too. They needed me to control themselves." Girls in conflict use middlegirls to fence in their own anger, helping them to stay "nice" at the moments that most challenge their feminine identities.

The middlegirl role has built itself not only into the structure of girls' conflicts but into their friendships. One researcher found that the failure of a girl to mediate conflict among her friends was actually perceived by her peers as overtly aggressive behavior.[24] Like girls who take sides, middlegirls who step in to help someone out in their time of need are met with the sort of gratitude and affection that thrives in situations where one person has a disproportionate amount of power. "Sometimes," a Sackler sixth grader told me, "there could be a fight with a popular girl. And the only reason you're helping her is because she's using you and you think that's so cool. The middlegirl is really thinking it's good for her."

The phenomenon of alliance building evokes the image of a daily relational minefield for girls. Each and every day presents the possibility of a relationship's endangerment. Friendships must be consistently charted, tallied, and negotiated. In waging these underground campaigns, the features of friendship become corrupted.

In 2000, UCLA researchers identified sex differences in the human response to immediate danger. Where males opted for "fight or flight," females would "tend and befriend," often nurturing or seeking the support of others rather than attempting to aggress or escape. The study, which exposed the troubling bias of research toward male subjects and the "fight or flight" response, showed that in stressful situations, females often seek company.[25] The findings suggest that girls' tendency to seek group comfort when threatened is a historic phenomenon, the study of which may yield more information on female aggression.

cliques

In 2000, the television show *Survivor* gripped America with a contest of sixteen "real" people vying to be the last one standing on a precarious deserted island. At the end of each weekly episode, viewers watched the disturbing spectacle of once-chummy Survivors coldly voting one of their own off the island. Every week, fans waited eagerly to see who would be next.

With just three contestants remaining, Kelly, long predicted the winner, was voted off. But it wasn't her surprise loss that made headlines that week. It was a breathtakingly cruel farewell from her fellow player, Sue. Calmly, before a spellbound audience of 55 million, Sue warned, "If I was ever to pass you along in life again and you were laying there dying of thirst, I would not give you a drink of water. I would let the vultures take you and do whatever they want with you, with no ill regrets." Mouths fell open across the nation.

Survivor's rite of expulsion resembles a disturbing ritual in cliques of girls. With little or no warning a clique will rise up and cut down one of its own. For the targeted girl, the sheer force of this unexpected expulsion can be startling, unpredictable, and even devastating.

In clique expulsions, punishments range from pretending the girl never existed to embarking on campaigns of scorching cruelty. These expulsions may seem sudden, arbitrary, and just plain mean. Bystanders may well wonder how a group could turn against one of their own with such intensity. Yet if we listen to the voices of girls, it does not take long to understand the intensity. Their anger is explained not by a root evil churning deep in their hearts, a pathetically common explanation, but rather by the imperative to above all be nice. Because these girls lack the tools to deal with everyday feelings of anger, hurt, betrayal, and jealousy, their feelings stew and fester before boiling to the surface and unleashing torrents of rage.

ERIN AND MICHELLE:
TWO FACES IN THE MIRROR?

Dr. Diane Harrigan remembers the day she ran into a teacher at her daughter's school. As she escorted Erin to class late in the day—it was a victory when her daughter could muster the strength to come to school at all—the unfamiliar woman stopped and touched her hand lightly to Diane's shoulder. "I just want you to know," she said quietly, "I know what you're going through." The teacher's own daughter, now thirty, was so shaken by being suddenly abandoned by her best friends as a teen that when she unexpectedly spied the ringleader at a bookstore recently, she'd had to leave. "It's still hard," the woman said. Diane felt tears start. "I know," she replied.

"She was the only person that really got it in the whole school," Diane told me. A clinical psychologist, Diane was the first parent to call me after the letters about my research went out to her daughter's class. Her daughter Erin had been the target of a clique expulsion and was still suffering the consequences.

Michelle was angry. She'd been assigned to buddy the new girl, Erin Harrigan, the summer before fifth grade. After talking on the phone and instant messaging, Michelle thought that Erin seemed really nice. But the first week of class, Erin sailed around like she was the most popular girl in the grade, like she always had been. She marched right up to the cool clique at lunch, sparkling with self-assurance and grace. Michelle said hi to her in the hallway, and she was pretty sure Erin didn't say hi back. Now they were going to be in a fight.

As groups became more defined in fifth and sixth grade, Michelle wasn't sure where she fit in. Sometimes the social tide brought her closer to the cool girls, and other times she drifted into the faceless sea of regular kids. She watched Erin beat out Kelly as most popular girl in sixth grade, become best friends with Nicole and exclude Kelly, and attract the hottest guys. She felt the constant rub of anger. Erin was confident and boy crazy, and she knew it.

When Nicole moved away the summer after sixth grade, Erin sent Michelle an instant message. It was good timing. Michelle had been getting annoyed with her friends, and Erin was a welcome change. Michelle's bitterness was quickly swallowed as her new friendship swept her into the popular group. Erin's friendship was intoxicating, the transformation quick and clean. Suddenly, Michelle was cool.

Three years later, fifteen-year-old Michelle and I were talking over cups of tea at a café near her school. "Erin's the kind of person so that when you're first friends with her, it's like a drug almost," she said. "She just seems like such a good friend. She's so nice and fun, not to mention the fact that she's really popular, and you're like, why is she friends with me? She says everything that you want her to say and she acts like she's such a good friend and acts like you're the best thing ever to happen to her, and you're kind of excited because you're like insecure and you're her everything. That's what people generally want to be. They want to be important to somebody else." Reveling in her proximity to Erin, Michelle enjoyed the rush she felt at being at the center of everything exciting.

The girls' friendship soon seemed fated: they had all their seventh-grade classes together. Michelle spent less and less time with her other friends. Then, after the first science quiz came back, Michelle felt an unfamiliar pang of something—was it panic?—when Erin scored six points higher. She noticed Erin's frustration when the tables turned in class, and soon, secret over-the-shoulder glances exploded into full-blown competition. "She'd do well on a test, and I'd get really mad, or if I did better than she did, she'd get really mad," Michelle explained. Michelle worked so hard to beat Erin that she got straight A's, and "Every time she got a bad grade I was *so* happy," she said.

The girls remained best friends, even as Michelle felt unease watching her old friends drift out toward the periphery of their crowd. That spring, on the bus, Michelle told Erin she secretly liked Luke, a guy in their grade. The next day at lunch, Erin announced, "Well, you know, I like Luke, too." Michelle was surprised, then angry, but she found herself unable to say anything to her friend.

The next night, Erin asked Luke out.

"Once she found out [that I liked him], she decided that *she* did. And she could have him because he had always kind of liked her. She asked him out," Michelle said, still incredulous, "and he said yes. I was like, 'Whatever, I don't really care, I'm not going to get in the middle of this.' But," she added, "obviously it bothered me."

Still, Michelle held her tongue. The next day, simmering, Michelle made Erin give her back a bracelet she had borrowed, just as Erin was putting it on. Erin was silent. She glared. Michelle felt a cold shock of fear ricochet through her. "She was the scariest person to have mad at you," Michelle explained. "I really didn't want her to be mad at me." To smooth things over, she asked what was wrong, and

Erin snapped that she was sick of Michelle's bad attitude. Michelle told her softly, "I'm sorry. I don't want to be in a fight."

The girls' later conflicts would resemble this first one, and as Michelle pushed down with all her might on her own anger, the girls fought more and more. As before, Michelle explained, "If you were mad at her about something, she would turn it around so that it was your fault. It would always be my fault, my fault, my fault."

"I always thought of it as like a dictatorship," she continued. "Kind of like where she has total control. If you say anything different, then you're wrong and she's right. *She* doesn't do anything wrong—it's all you."

Michelle refused to tell Erin how she felt. "No!" she exclaimed. "Because I couldn't say it. I was afraid to say anything." She told Erin she thought they shouldn't be exclusive with each other, which allowed her some distance without as many fights. As Michelle grew closer with girls in another group, the one Erin didn't rule, Erin became fast friends with Jessica, another eighth grader. It made Michelle angry, despite her relief that she was finally away from Erin.

Hanging out with new girls in eighth grade, away from the hypnotic pull of Erin, Michelle quickly discovered many of them thought Erin was a bitch. Kelly was angry because her ex-boyfriend Denis broke up with her for Erin; she had also not forgotten losing the popularity contest three years earlier. Mira was stewing, too. She had been best friends with Jessica when Erin had cast her spell. Now, watching Jessica and Erin at lunch, she was alone.

As Michelle grew even closer with the other girls, she realized that she just didn't need Erin anymore. The girl was always thinking about herself. "She'll just be sitting here and everybody'll be getting ready and she'll be like, 'How do I look, you guys? Does this look okay?' Everything's about herself." If Michelle got a new purse, Erin would show off hers. "She has this egotistical thing," Michelle explained.

So one day, when Erin called to borrow history notes, Michelle found it almost easy to refuse and hang up abruptly. Erin called back "thirty times," but Michelle let the calls go. Although she didn't need Erin, she was still unwilling to fight her. The specter of their past conflicts still haunted Michelle. "She would have turned it on me. She would have made me upset!" she predicted. "She would have told me I was a bad friend. Everything would be my fault and I didn't want to give up because it wasn't my fault!"

In the meantime, Ashley had begun dating Luke, who still pined for Erin. One day, when Erin was over at his house, Luke kissed her. Erin says she stopped it, but a week later it happened again. Luke told Kelly. Erin told Jessica. As it turned out, Jessica had been nursing a long crush on Luke, and her adoration for Erin began to falter. But like Michelle, Jessica feared saying anything to upset her status as "Erin's everything."

The next weekend, after Erin scored the winning goal in the field hockey finals, Kelly watched Ashley hug her and noted their increasing closeness. That night, Kelly slept over at Ashley's house with Michelle, and everything changed forever.

"Ashley," Kelly said somberly. "I just have to tell you."

"What?" Ashley asked, leaning forward.

"Erin hooked up with Luke twice while you were going out."

Ashley's face twitched in shock and she began to cry. Then she started throwing things. "That bitch!" she yelled.

"This is *so* it," Kelly said quickly. "We're not talking to her anymore."

"This is *such* bullshit!" screamed Ashley.

"Forget it," Kelly said. "Let me handle this." She picked up the phone and called Erin. "Hi," she said. "You know what? Luke told me about you guys, and Ashley saw the e-mail. She knows everything. Okay? Sorry. I have to go. 'Kay . . . bye." She hung up and smiled. "She's *really* upset," she said. The phone rang, piercing the silence.

"Don't get it!" Ashley snapped.

"Don't worry," replied Kelly.

Finally, a reason to be angry. It was, Michelle added, "a reason Erin couldn't defend." And, she said, "Once one person got mad, it was kind of like everybody did." The next day, Erin called Michelle, who said she couldn't talk and hastily hung up the phone. Then Michelle called Jessica.

Jessica was just leaving. "And I said, 'Jessica, how do you feel that Erin did that to you?'" Jessica said she didn't know. "I said, 'Jessica, I'm not going to tell anybody anything you say, I just want you to tell me, do you ever feel like you're afraid to get mad at her and you're afraid to talk to her?'" Michelle described her own feelings of fear.

"That's *exactly* how I feel!" Jessica cried. She had, Michelle believed, "come to some sort of realization on the phone." Then Jessica stopped taking Erin's calls.

From then on, Michelle explained, "it was kind of like we had to go around convincing people, saying you don't have to be afraid of her, you know? You don't." When the girls arrived at school on Monday, everyone ignored Erin.

"We're all sitting together—*beaming!*—because we're so happy we don't have to have that kind of relationship [with Erin] anymore." Then Erin walked into class, wiping away tears as she sat next to a girl, Michelle recalled, "who she may have talked to once, who was kind of insecure, who was kind of overweight, and all of a sudden she became her friend, because she needed to have someone to sit with." The girls watched Erin spend lunch with people who had always wanted to be her friend, but whom Erin had talked about behind their backs. The sight of Erin eluding the isolation they had used to punish her enraged them. That, Michelle said, "is when it really started."

Kelly would just laugh at Erin when she walked by. "It was because of Denis," Michelle explained, "because of when Erin and Nicole had excluded [Kelly], and I mean—we were like sticking together." The group became especially tight in Erin's absence. "We got so close and would always be like standing together in the hall, sharing our Erin stories. 'She asked me for this, and I was just like *no!*' and it felt soooo good because we could finally—like—be—people."

The girls flooded Erin's e-mail account with angry messages. It seemed that everyone was in on it; even students who had no connection to the incident were volunteering reasons for shunning Erin.

Some called her a bitch. Ashley wrote that it made her sick to look at Erin.

At what point, I asked Michelle, were people planning on talking with Erin, even forgiving her and moving on?

"Oh, *no*!" Michelle said, surprised. "Nobody wanted to be friends with her anymore. They just wanted to see her suffer like she had done to everyone else."

But let's assume, I said, that Erin would do anything to be forgiven, that she'd promise to be a better friend.

"We *knew* her. We knew that she wasn't going to be. We were all sick of it and we just wanted to get away from it."

"What would you have rather happened?" I asked.

"Well, she was suffering, but she was getting friends. We wanted her to see what it was like. I mean, subconsciously, we wanted her to see what it was like to not have anybody there, because she needed to."

Every day the girls tallied their sightings of Erin's anguish. They shot her dirty looks when she passed by. "We were like, 'This is brilliant.' We'd just be so happy. Everyone was so happy that it was finally being taken care of."

"That was the end of it," Erin said, "and they were my world! They were my everything! I didn't care about my family; I didn't care about anyone else but that one group of people. Oh my God."

We were sitting on Erin's bed talking, and I had promised we would be done in time to watch *Dawson's Creek*.

"They *loved* to see me cry," she recalled. The girls would stand in a circle a few feet from Erin's locker. "Today is going to be *so* much fun!" they'd crow, casting sidelong glances at Erin. "They would just talk to each other right in front of my face and they wouldn't look at me. They'd be like, 'Come to the bathroom with me?' and I'd walk by in tears."

When Erin went home, her parents didn't understand. "I would come home and scream, *'Get away!'* I was like, my life is over. My life is over."

Erin had no idea what was going on. She knew she had screwed up, but she didn't understand why everyone was involved. The confusion spun her downward as her grades went from straight A's to straight C's. She'd never needed help with homework, and now her mother had to sit with her every night and pull the essays out of her. "I could not do anything," Erin said. "I lost all my confidence. They totally ripped me down to nothing. They told me how horrible a person I was. So I was just nothing anymore. I just remember telling myself, 'A month ago you were so happy.'"

Bewildered at the sheer intensity of her friends' anger, Erin became despondent. The light went out of her. "I wasn't anything anymore because they had made me who I was, so I didn't even know who I was. I was always depressed."

The hardest moments for Erin were when she saw all of them together, without her. It felt as though she had died and was now a ghost. "I wasn't there. There was no Erin anymore."

The girls broke into her e-mail account and changed her password to "Slut." Luke broke in and deleted his love letters so he wouldn't look responsible for their kiss. Not that anyone had blamed him to begin with.

Erin's mother was frantic. The more Erin stayed out of school, "the more she fell apart." Erin was lethargic and depressed. Like a top ceasing to spin, Erin simply stopped doing everything. "She seemed very childlike again. She sort of crumbled in our arms." Diane remembers pleading with her to come to school, coaxing her with anything that came to mind to get her to school before noon.

By the time they got there, even Diane was filled with dread. "Here were these kids who had spent the night at our house, who had eaten at our house—whatever—and they would act like I wasn't there. It was just so"—she inhaled sharply—"so aggressive! I couldn't understand how they could be so rude to another adult. They were so defiant, so hostile, the look in their eyes was just—I was really—" Her voice broke. "We were devastated for her."

Diane watched as her daughter wept uncontrollably every night. The days Diane couldn't arrive early to be in the car-pool lane when the last bell rang, she'd find Erin alone on the curb, her shadow almost touching her friends', who stood chatting close by. In the car, Erin would dissolve into tears. Embarrassed, she refused to tell her mother what happened with Luke. Diane found a psychotherapist she prayed Erin would confide in and began sending Erin every week.

"Erin tried to talk to us," Michelle said. "She's the kind of person that no matter how upset she is, she loves herself too much to hurt herself. Everybody knows that about her. She wrote Jessica these e-mails that were like little poems: 'I have no one. I have no life anymore. I lost you.'" Michelle sounded confused. "Like all these random, random things so you're like *what* is she doing? And we'd see them and we'd be like, that is *so* funny and we'd like forward them to each other."

When Erin told a male friend that she wanted to kill herself, he became alarmed and told the other girls. They laughed it off. "She was like, 'I don't want to live anymore!'" Michelle said. "She was doing it all for attention. We knew she wasn't going to."

One day, as Michelle and Ashley were shelving their trays in the cafeteria, Erin approached. She took a deep breath.

"I am really, really sorry about what happened with Luke. Please forgive me."

Michelle shrugged. "That's not what it was about. It was about the kind of friend you were to everybody." They walked off.

By then, there was no going back. "She was such a bad friend, but I didn't know it," Michelle told me, then paused. "She's like *evil!*"

Diane went to the guidance counselor almost every day. "They kept telling me, 'It's going to pass, it's going to pass, believe us, it's going to pass.' " It was only when a boy sent Erin an e-mail that began with "You disgusting whore" that the school called a meeting to set limits on student e-mail. Diane watched helplessly as her daughter took to bed, claiming headaches, crying at night that she wanted to die.

In May, at eighth-grade graduation, Erin stood alone with her family. Her friends linked arms and skipped away, mortarboards and gowns trailing like streamers, to parties that would last all night. "We left," Diane said. "I was crying. I had tears streaming down my face. It was so painful." In the parking lot, a mother approached Diane. The woman had commented to Ashley's mother about how hard this must be for Erin. "That girl got everything she deserved," Ashley's mother had replied.

Diane knew she was missing a huge piece of what had happened, but despite her tearful entreaties, Erin stayed quiet. That summer, Diane sent Erin to visit her family in California. On sleepaway camp buses, at friends' houses, even in kindergarten, Erin had been the intrepid girl who never looked back, not even to wave good-bye. In Santa Monica she disintegrated, calling her parents sobbing in the middle of the night, unable to sleep, hyperventilating with anxiety.

At some point over the summer, Michelle relented. "Part of me missed her, part of me felt bad, and part of me just like wanted to be a good person and talk to her." At Ashley's house one day, Michelle called Erin to ask for some money Erin had owed her for a long time. Michelle knew she was looking for a reason to call her, plus Ashley had wanted some shorts she had lent her, and Jessica wanted to say hi, too. The conversation was "nice." But there wasn't much to say.

Right before school started, Michelle was ready to start over, though she feared breaking the group's official silence. "I was like, 'Okay, it's a new year. I can let myself do this. I don't have to be worried about what my friends are going to say.' " Besides, she'd been having trouble with some of the other girls, and as it had been in seventh grade, Erin offered a willing ear.

Together, the two girls felt at once new and old, comfortable and tense. But by then Erin had made other friends, making Michelle's friendship with her too difficult to sustain. Michelle feared "getting sucked in" to the old dynamics that irked her before. Nowadays, Erin is "just another person we walk by in the hall." Reflecting about what happened at the end of eighth grade, Michelle said, "I was feeling kind of bad, like maybe we should have gone about it a different way. . . . It was just a big part of all of our lives. It was probably something that needed to happen." Anyway, Michelle told me, Erin hadn't really changed. Everyone agreed about that. Which made Michelle feel okay about where things were in the end.

In her mind, Erin felt she'd changed completely. "I'm such a scared person now," she told me. "I'm always worried about what people think about me. I'm always worried about what people are going to say about me behind my back. I never used to care! Because people talked about me all the time, and I just didn't care. I'm always worried about why people hate me," she said. "They made me like this now."

Trusting her new friends is daily work. "I'm better about it, but I still become a wreck just because I'm scared that it will happen again, or I'll be a bad friend."

Erin spent ninth grade narrowly avoiding being asked to leave her school. Her academic performance continued to falter, and she was tortured by anxiety, finding normally easy assignments overwhelming. She remained in intensive therapy and was diagnosed with anxiety and depression. Fearing a recurrence of her peers' anger, she refused to let them see her appear weak. "I was trying to prove to them I could be okay. I was like, no, I'm going to have just as much fun." So she hung out with seniors, got invited to parties, and managed to appear as cool as she had been. Unfortunately, school administrators found it hard to believe she was as depressed and anxious as her parents claimed.

Erin grew close with Kim again, and she began to feel confused as the friendship offered her a second glimpse inside her old clique. She missed them, and apparently, they'd missed her. "How come I still get upset and miss stuff from before?" she asked me. "It's bad because I should know. I'm like, 'Why am I still friends with you? After everything you've done,'" she said. "I'm a completely different person."

The most marked change in her, she told me, is the way she approaches her friends. Before, when she was popular, she'd felt the need to be perfect, to perform in a particular way for others. Now, she can see how the strategy backfired.

"I think that being perfect was [my] way. You have to go up [in status]. You don't even look. Your peripheral vision is—you don't even care about the people next to you because you have to be better than them.... In some ways you know people are looking at you. And you're kind of like a show for people to see. You know when you walk down the hall that people are like, 'Oh, she's cool.' But you don't realize that they're like, 'Oh, and she's a bitch, too.' You don't know you're a bitch. You deny things; you avoid things. You should know it, but you don't know it because it's a normal thing to do and if you don't do it you're out of there."

She is chagrined about the person she was, about the mistakes popularity led her to make, yet she struggles to understand the force of her friends' anger.

So does Diane. Watching Erin in the days after her friends retaliated, she could never have predicted the crushing impact their anger would have on her child. Today, she shares with me an abiding regret that she did not try harder to force the school into action. Even this year, as the school has questioned whether it is appropriate for Erin to continue at Linden, Diane has been awed at the school's willful ignorance of the incident that so clearly marred her daughter's confidence.

During her sophomore year, Erin finally righted herself academically, bringing home all B's and one A. It's an "amazing feat!" she crowed in a recent e-mail to me. And, she reported, she'd fallen in love.

Erin's story illustrates with terrible clarity the consequences of girls' repression of their true feelings. Over three long years, each of Erin's friends buried everyday bursts of jealousy, anger, competition, and betrayal deep inside her. The point at which their anger finally broke the surface of their silence is extremely significant. Of all the incidents that upset the girls, the only one that incited them into response had two important features: it was an event they could experience and act upon together, and it was a socially acceptable reason for female anger.

At home in a culture obsessed with romantic love, where talk shows feature women sparring in you-took-my-man catfights, the girls knew instantly that kissing Luke was a valid cause for anger. This was not like the awkward feelings of jealousy for not being popular or not having the guy you want like you; it was not the discomfort of secret competition over grades or the sadness of having been abandoned by a friend. This was clearly wrong, a misstep no one could deny.

The trouble was, once the girls got going, their anger got out of control. Every past grievance shot to the surface and crashed down on Erin. Because the girls had sequestered their feelings, hurt and jealousy were transformed into a dangerous well of rage. Michelle celebrated that no one would have to be afraid of Erin any longer. She might have added that no one would have to be afraid of conflict and anger, either.

Yet at the peak of their fury, what these girls wanted was nothing more than to isolate Erin. They didn't want to strike her, spread rumors about her, or confront her. They wanted her alone. When Erin tried to hang out with less popular girls, her friends were even angrier. "She was getting friends," Michelle said. "We wanted her to see what it was like to not have anybody there."

Michelle's willingness to speak with me about her feelings toward Erin was extraordinary. She is an example to all of us who struggle to express our own anger. Yet she's very much an ordinary girl: fun-loving, sensitive, kind, and smart. She is the very opposite of cruel. What she struggled with was how to negotiate her anger and still maximize her intimacy with the friend she loved most. The same can be said of Erin. She is hardly the "bitch" her friends made her out to be. She is instead a girl who got lost in the demands of her own pop-ularity and ended up making mistakes. Like Michelle, Erin is a lovely young woman, sparkling with laughter, wit, and a generous spirit that pulls everyone to her like a magnet.

The salience of relationship in girls' lives makes their practice of imposing isolation worthy of our attention. As we have seen, girls experience isolation as especially terrifying. Since girls earn social capital by their relationships with others, isolation cuts to the core of their identities. For most girls there is little more painful than to stand alone at recess or lunch.

Erin's fear of her new friends' anger is echoed in different degrees by many survivors of bullying. These girls described feeling unfamil-iar with the most basic rules of relationship, things taken for granted by any socially adjusted person. They no longer feel certain of what makes people angry or upset, not to mention how to tell when someone is feeling that way. Their emotional radar is incapacitated. This can turn a girl into a cautious ghost of her former self, stifled and silenced by fear.

The fear is felt by degrees among girls who struggle with everyday conflict. One of the chief symptoms of girls' loss of self-esteem is the sense of being crazy, of not being able to trust one's own interpreta-tion of people's actions or events. *Did she just look at her when I said that? Was she joking? Did she roll her eyes? Not save the seat on purpose? Lie about her plans? Tell me that she'd invited me when she hadn't?* The girls I interviewed confirmed a similar unrest, the disturbing belief that what they were sure they knew or saw wasn't that at all, but was in fact something quite different. In discord between girls, gestures of conflict often contradict speech, confounding their intended tar-gets. In such a universe, for a girl to trust her own truths, her own version of events, can be excruciatingly difficult. At the cusp of their most tumultuous years of development, girls cling tightly to one another to know, as one told me, "that we're not crazy." Yet it is their close peer relationships, and the rules against truth telling, that often trigger these feelings.

CHAPTER four

bff 2.0: cyberbullying and cyberdrama

Two twelve-year-old girls were sitting cross-legged on the floor of a bedroom, hunched over a stickered laptop. Leah and Ellie were Facebook chatting with Ellie's ex-boyfriend who, moments earlier, had asked if he and Ellie could get back together. His request prompted Ellie to screech.

"Calm down!" Leah said briskly. Ellie froze. Her face grew stony. She stood up and walked a few feet over to her own laptop. The room began clicking with stubborn, angry keyboard strokes.

"ur so obsessed with Lilly! y dont u guys get married? all u do is talk about Lilly, y r u even here?" Ellie typed.

Leah stared at Ellie. "You can't say that to my face? We're five feet apart!"

Ellie typed, "SHUT UP B——CH!!!!"

Leah kept talking. "You're kidding, right? You can't even call me a b——ch to my face?"

When we spoke, Leah recalled the scene and sighed over Ellie's behavior. "She can say anything to me over text and it won't matter. We're five feet apart and she calls me a b——ch on Facebook."

———

It is now impossible to parent, teach, or even talk about girls without considering the roles of technology and social media in their lives. The virtual world has become a place girls go to hang out, no different from a hallway, locker room, or cafeteria. What has changed is the efficiency of aggression: social media is a bathroom wall with a jet engine, giving kids the ability to launch their graffiti into a peer's bedroom or pocket.

Depending on who you ask, anywhere from one fifth to one third of youth aged eleven to eighteen have been targets of cyberbullying, or the "willful and repeated harm inflicted through the use of computers, cell phones and other electronic devices." Ask girls if they have been targets of passing online nastiness, and the number skyrockets.[26]

Technology makes cruelty chillingly simple. Angry at the friend who ignored you today? Click. Annoyed at the girl who is copying your look? Click. Jealous of the girl who is flirting with the guy you like? Click. There is no eye contact, no tone of voice, no immediate consequence. Social media offers a limitless arsenal of weapons: Start a Facebook group to punish the guy-stealing girl. Tag an embarrassing photo of her for everyone to see. Send a vicious text at midnight, then turn your phone off.

"The Internet erases inhibitions," writes *New York Times* reporter Jan Hoffman, eliciting "psychologically savage" behavior. All this in a world where adults and policy have been slow to catch on, and even slower to act. Parents are alternately intimidated and overwhelmed, while most schools decline to intervene in behavior that occurred "off school grounds."[27] Website and software developers are slow to respond to distressed families. Law enforcement mostly clings to the threat of bodily harm as its standard for intervention. Into this vacuum of regulation move the cyberbullies and targets, who operate with few deterrents.

If we can no longer talk about girls without talking about technology, the same is true in reverse: girls' distinctive fears and passions are digitized in BFF 2.0, girls' online social universe. Girls perpetrate and experience cyberbullying in ways that are uniquely *girl*. Social media lets you type instead of talk, offering girls an oasis from the direct conflict so many of them fear. Armies of girls who avoid face-to-face confrontation can now use their fingers to vent rage, betrayal, or anxiety. "Online," a high school senior told me, "you can say whatever you want to say."

But like a mirage that vanishes upon closer inspection, technology betrays girls. When they turn to social media to resolve their problems, they are more likely to interpret others' messages negatively and act aggressively. These girls, who might otherwise struggle in a direct conversation, become suddenly fierce, cruel "orators" online. Before social media, girls might exchange a phone call or two; now, there are blizzards of nasty texts. "Somebody can't come through the phone and beat you up," a seventh grader told me. "But somebody can beat you up over text all day long." Girls' false confidence and unbridled emotion ignite conflicts for which they are scantly prepared.

Social media plugs right into girls' obsession with relationships— and their fear of losing them: on the one hand, technology allows girls exhilarating, instant access to their peers. Yet social networking sites like Facebook also make friendships tangible and public,[28] allowing girls to compare and judge others' relationships: *She has 800 Facebook friends, but I only have 350. She got nine comments replying to her last wall post, but only two people bothered to respond to mine.* This is a new kind of "popularity math," a test of likeability where anything you post can be "liked" and rated by your peers.[29] Friendships in the online habitat have become yet another item to measure oneself against—like bodies, boyfriends, and grades—and so another painful source of jealousy, insecurity, and anxiety among girls.

Like bullying in real life, cyberbullying does not erupt from thin air. It is often the endgame of a drama that originated in the more mundane interactions that dominate girls' lives. In a recent study, Sameer Hinduja and Justin Patchin, founders of the Cyberbullying Research Center, found that 84 percent of cyberbullying targets reported being bullied by someone they knew, such as a friend, ex-friend, former romantic partner, or classmate. Less than 7 percent of youth in this same study reported being cyberbullied by a stranger. (The rest did not know who was bullying them.)[30] To really understand girls and cyberbullying, then, we have to examine their day-to-day online exchanges, where the fuse of cyberbullying gets lit. In this chapter, I journey through the sprawling virtual landscape of BFF 2.0, from its darkest corners to its most traveled byways.

Media and culture would have us believe that children are "digital natives," while their clueless parents and educators are "digital immigrants." This is a dangerous myth.[31] The idea that there is nothing at all strange or foreign to children navigating technology suggests adults are the ones who need educating. But social media involves at least two discrete sets of skills: the ability to manipulate the gadgets, and the capacity to interact safely and responsibly. The two are not related, and ease of use does not guarantee a grasp of its consequences.[32] Navigating the virtual world requires new skills that must be learned and practiced. Just as girls starting school need tools to resolve the challenges of their "real-life" relationships, girls online require the same.

Unplugging is never the answer, just as staying home from school will not resolve conventional bullying. The phone or computer is not merely a device. It's a window to a world that, for most girls, is as compelling and active as their "real" world.

cyberbullying

My mother picked me up after school on the days Abby made my friends run away from me. When the car door closed, I knew I was safe. Today, the end of school no longer offers relief. Cell phones and social networking sites tether girls to their bullies day and night, making cruelty impossible to escape. As Internet safety expert Parry Aftab has said, cyberbullying follows you everywhere: to grandma's house, to sports practice, to dinner.

The cruelty moves as swiftly as it does widely. Before social media, bullying was slowed by the pace of physical relationship: It took time for girls to catch up and share. There was also less time to talk. Today, texting is social background noise, an accompaniment to nearly every other activity girls do. Researchers report a significant increase in "multitasking," or using more than one form of media at the same time, among teens.[33] Information is abbreviated, omitting important subtleties of a situation or feeling. It is also churned out addictively; the average American teen sent three thousand texts every month in 2010, and the most slanderous texts went viral with whiplash speed.[34]

Girls live in their very own twenty-four-hour news cycle. Where the bell once rang at day's end, giving girls a chance to rest and recharge, texts and chats now fly at all hours, including the middle of the night, when we are all least reasonable. Some girls sleep with cell phones under their pillows or on their chests, so they can feel the vibration and awaken. It is not uncommon for a Facebook status update to read, simply, "text"; meaning, I can't be reached this way, so find me another way. Find me at all times.

Add to this a radical change in privacy in girls' lives. Much of girls' social interactions online are now played out in public. On Facebook, where the age of use continues to shrink, the live news feed format runs a vertical crawl of endless updates: how friends feel from moment to moment, who they interact with and who their newest friends are. At the center of each user's personal page is the Facebook Wall, a kind of bulletin board where friends can "tack" messages to say *heyyyyy, happy birthday, what's tonight's homework?* Moments better left private—a girl and her friends making plans that may exclude others, a friend who posts inside jokes or leaves cryptic messages that make others insecure—are now broadcast with a few simple clicks.

Imagine being a girl who feels socially insecure and seeing, on your friend's wall, a post that simply says, "OMG" [oh my God]. She may think, *What does* that *mean? Is something happening? Why don't I know about it? Is it about me?* Sitting alone in front of a computer, she becomes anxious and assumes the worst. She may begin contacting others for more information, starting a chain of gossip that could set off a conflict about an issue that does not even exist in the first place.

Few girls learn about the insecurity, hurt, or betrayal these public online interactions can inspire, or what might happen if they make assumptions based on what they are reading; instead, girls simply *do* it, because everyone else is doing it, and because it is an inevitable part of being a twenty-first-century girl. As communication becomes more impulsive, quick, and public, it also becomes coarser. This is not necessarily because girls are trying to be mean, but because turning private interactions public can alter their meaning and impact.

The change in privacy has given rise to new norms among girls, especially when they are angry. Before social media, the most ganging up girls could do after hours was via a three-way phone call. Today, social networking sites allow hundreds of people to watch and throw their two cents into the mix. What an adult grew up thinking belonged in a journal, or vented quietly to a friend, is today easily shared and commented on by multiple peers. Girls who might fear live confrontations in front of peers now unleash online status updates and away messages filled with anger, frustration, and threats: "I wish," wrote a middle-school girl on her public Tumblr, which is a kind of online journal, "everyone knew what a lying piece of s——t you are." Within twenty-four hours, hundreds of peers had either reposted the comment to their own page, or declared their loyalty by "liking" the comment. "[W]ow people should really grow up . . . no one likes people that are b——ches, and come up with different lies everyday to make themself [sic] look cool!" posted a high-school girl on Facebook. Into the fray jump peers whose comments (*"loveeee u girl" "OMFG" "haha"*) betray varying agendas: sympathy, loyalty, backup, revenge.

Like summer thunder, online fights can erupt with little warning. A single misinterpreted remark can start a war. After an eighth-grade girl commented, innocently enough, that a photograph of her group's alpha female resembled another girl, friends swarmed the page, attacking her. As the girls barraged her with insults ("how about you go behind doors and CUT yourself" and "wat makes u think we care about ur life"), another crowed, "shutdown," while the target tried to defend herself. Eventually the other girls began declaring their love for each other ("I love you...you guys are amazing friends ❤") while the target flailed. As one detective told the *New York Times,* "It's not the swear words. They all swear. It's how they gang up on one individual at a time. 'Go cut yourself.' Or 'you are sooo ugly'—but with 10 *u*'s, 10 *g*'s, 10 *l*'s, like they're all screaming at someone." The viciousness of the messages is deepened by the public intimacy between the tormentors.

In girls' social universe, information is power. But gossip needs an audience, and getting one isn't easy if you lack status. Online, the social rules change. Technology levels the playing field, allowing girls with less status in real time a chance to make waves online. Should you have trouble getting someone to notice you at school, you are just a few clicks away from the rapt attention of online eyes. Power and status distribute more equally in a world where anyone can write anything that others may believe and act on.

Several studies have found significant gender differences in cyberbullying. Sameer Hinduja and Justin Patchin of the Cyberbullying Research Center found that 26 percent of girls were targets of cyberbullying, compared to 16 percent of boys. Another study found that girls are nearly twice as likely as boys to have rumors spread about them online. Some 22 percent of girls surveyed by Hinduja and Patchin reported cyberbullying others, compared to 18 percent of boys.[35]

Both targets and aggressors show significantly lower self-esteem than peers who are not involved in cyberbullying. Those victimized by cyberbullying are more likely to experience anxiety, depression, school violence, academic trouble, suicidal ideation, and suicide attempts.[36]

The breathtaking cruelty unfolding online cannot be attributed to only its medium, or the lack of oversight surrounding it. The teen brain is still developing, honing its capacity to take healthy risks and consider the consequences of behavior. Coupled with the burning desire to fit in that beleaguers so many girls, we have a dangerous recipe indeed.

In the fall of eighth grade, Kelsey broke up amicably with her boyfriend, Aaron, in a largely white, middle-class, northeastern suburb of about thirty-five thousand people. A few weeks later, she regretted her decision. When her close friend and soccer teammate, Lauren, said she liked Aaron, Kelsey remained quiet.

"At first," Kelsey told me in our phone interview, "I got upset, but then I was, like, she's my friend and I want her to be happy." Kelsey kept mum and resolved to enjoy her friendship with Aaron, who had asked Lauren out.

Within days, Lauren was bristling at Kelsey's friendship with Aaron. She texted Kelsey. "She started to tell me to back off, he doesn't like you, he never did, you're not his type." Kelsey refused to end her friendship with Aaron. Lauren posted similar remarks on Facebook for her hundreds of friends to see and comment on.

As it turned out, Lauren and Aaron were short-lived. When Aaron confided in Kelsey about the breakup, Lauren was incensed. "She sent me," Kelsey said, "a seven-page text. It was, like, calling me these nasty names like dumb ho. Aaron wasn't my type, I needed to shut the f——k up, I was a dumb whore, I was ugly, I was fat, I wasn't worth anything [and] I should just go die." In the transcript of the texts, Lauren wrote, "oh and sweetheart be prepared for a rude awakening seeing your gunna have no friends and everyone will hate you sooo much after this one stupid hoe."

Lauren concluded by revealing that when she dated Aaron, "he always told me and my friends how ugly you were and how much he hated you lmao ☺ [laughing my a—s off]." Shaken, Kelsey refused to give in. She also cared about Aaron, who had suggested they begin dating again.

The drama intensified. Lauren enlisted the support of her friends, who sent a blizzard of vicious texts. Dana, one of Lauren's best friends, wrote that "I was a bad friend and that I wasn't worth anything, that she hoped me and Aaron were happy because I would have no friends and everyone would hate me."

Technology eclipses the stages of feeling and reflection that used to precede many conflicts between girls. In a typical conflict, there is shock and anger; there is sadness, confusion, and betrayal. All of these feelings, which girls used to have time to process and react to, are now bundled into quick, digital gusts of emotion. Girls do not take as much time, if any, to sit, reflect, feel, or think.

The sheer range of attacks that can be communicated so quickly is itself remarkable. Lauren's texts fell like an onslaught of arrows bearing multiple social poisons: relational aggression; an attack on her physical appearance; an attempt to undermine beliefs about her romantic relationship; the threat to destroy Kelsey's relationships and isolate her; and the encouragement to *kill herself*. All in a few hundred, swiftly typed characters.

At school, the conflict continued. The seamless integration between kids' virtual and real lives blew the spores of the online conflict into live conversation. Several students confronted Kelsey in the hall at school. They told her that she was a "useless whore" who did not deserve Lauren as a friend. Lauren herself approached Kelsey and her friends at a football game and yelled that she hoped Kelsey ended up dead on the side of the road.

As virtual conflicts migrate into the physical world, so do their ferocity: harsh words typed online become familiar and so more easily spoken. In this way, online communication norms desensitize the way kids communicate in person, upping the ante for aggression and bullying in both spheres.

When Kelsey and Aaron broke up, agreeing their relationship wasn't worth its price, Kelsey decided that she wanted to tell her soccer coach about the cyberbullying. Coach Rebecca had told the team she had a zero-tolerance policy for bullying. But she was also Dana's mother. When one of Kelsey's friends warned Lauren the texts were going to be reported, Dana's older sister texted Kelsey, threatening, "you know what, you better not show those texts to my mom it won't do anything so don't if you know what's good for you."

Kelsey backed off and tried to wait it out. A week later, there was another flare-up, and Lauren resumed her relentless texts. "I've done this once, I can do it again, try me b——ch," she wrote. "I will come after you, it won't be pretty, so do it again and things are going down." After each text, Kelsey denied the accusations, responded "okay," or wrote nothing at all.

But Kelsey was fatigued. Powerless to respond or make the daily texts stop, she became despondent. "I didn't feel like I could do anything," she told me. "I felt like if I told [the coach] about the texts, I would be, like, completely alone in school. So it kind of, like, scared me... I was just so done," she recalled. There was no refuge for Kelsey: at home, each vibration of her phone made her feel nauseated. School was unsafe, and she did not want to go. She became suicidal. "I had nothing left to live for," she told me.

When something is in writing, no matter its content, it becomes strangely believable, especially to the recipient. The written word carries the suggestion of gravity and truth. Kelsey explained,

> [Lauren] has spent some time putting this down. She's read it, and she knows what she's saying. She's not just angry and she's blurting out things. She's actually taking the time to think about them, and write them down, and send them to me. She actually, like, meant what she was saying... I felt, like, worthless and like nothing was ever really going to get better. I actually thought about how much easier it would be for people if I wasn't, like, alive anymore.

We seem more willing to believe what is in writing, perhaps because so much of what we do read—in textbooks, newspapers, and novels —comes from experts or other authorities. The irony is that what girls text out of anger is often anything but thought out or well considered. It is usually quite thoughtless—but try explaining that to a distraught girl. Cyberbullying has given written cruelty a platform, frequency, and impact it never had before. And unlike speech or gesture, or even printed text, online writing leaves a trail with infinite followers.

Though easier to report, written threats are not necessarily shared. The age-old fear of "snitching," and the retaliation that could follow, is timeless. Kelsey was afraid, and she refused to tell anyone besides her mother, even as the texts piled up.

For her part, Connie Jacobs was angry and protective, but measured. She knew she faced an uphill battle. If parents feel helpless in the face of conventional bullying, their resources shrink even further when bullying goes digital. In the absence of rules or protocol at school, and limited awareness of the behavior among parents, families are largely left to fend for themselves.

In our interview, Connie repeatedly mentioned that she had waited until she was calm enough to communicate with the other girls' parents. And she refused to see Kelsey as only a target. Connie knew Kelsey had contributed to the conflict by refusing to level with Lauren about her feelings for Aaron.

When Connie e-mailed Lauren's parents, she asked gingerly if they would have time to talk about what their daughters were "going through." There was no response.

It was one of Kelsey's best friends and teammates who finally showed Coach Rebecca the texts. Rebecca called in Lauren and admonished that she was "stupid to put [her feelings] in writing." When Kelsey's mother called to complain about the slap on the wrist, Rebecca said if she penalized Lauren, she would have to penalize Kelsey. To defend her position, Rebecca relayed evidence that Kelsey had behaved aggressively—stories that had come directly from her daughter Dana. They were, Connie told me, "thirteen-year-old reasons about why Lauren was justified in yelling at Kelsey. [Kelsey] told Lauren she was not going to go out with Aaron and then did. That's what Rebecca is repeating to me," Connie said, still amazed.

"She brought up every single lie that Dana told her that would make her story sound right," Kelsey said. Connie tried to balance agreeing with the coach that Kelsey bore some responsibility for contributing to the situation with the argument that no behavior warranted the persecution her daughter had now endured.

At this point, Rebecca pursued a new line of questions. Did you know, she asked Connie, that Kelsey wanted to kill herself? That she told the other girls a bruise on her face came from her mother? Connie paused. This was new. The bruise was sustained in a private dance class. Connie tried to remain calm and asked Rebecca how she knew Kelsey had said this. Did she hear it from Kelsey? "Well, no," Connie recalled Rebecca saying. "I heard from more than one source." Connie laughed wryly. "Right. These 'sources' now have a target, and that's Kelsey."

By law, Rebecca told Connie, I'm supposed to report the bruise to child protection authorities. "I didn't," she said, "because I don't believe [Kelsey], and I've known you for a while. I knew if I had reported it that it would have been hard on your career and really embarrassing." Connie, an aide in the public school system, was horrified. "She was threatening me. She was trying to tell me that she wasn't reporting the cyberbullying because she didn't really feel like it was a valid threat to Kelsey. She made that same judgment call in my favor a couple of weeks prior."

Rebecca sensed Connie's shock. "[Rebecca] told me, she said, you don't know your daughter. I was, like, 'I'm sorry, *you* don't know my daughter. I do know my daughter. I know she's not perfect, I know she's done some things, and I don't think you do.'" The call ended a few minutes later. Connie sat holding the phone, shell-shocked. "It's every mother's worst nightmare, to have someone question if you hit your children," she said quietly.

Connie backed off. Besides avoiding the humiliation of an investigation, a major tournament was just three weeks away. She did not want to see her daughter and Lauren expelled from the team. Throughout her conversation with her daughter's coach, Connie never once mentioned the texts that had come from Rebecca's own daughter. She laughed again, humorlessly. "You know, if you attack somebody's own daughter, it's not going to go well."

After her call with Rebecca, Connie sat down with Kelsey and told her how serious the situation could become. "I gave Kelsey complete amnesty to tell me if she had said [I hit her]," Connie remembered. She leveled with her daughter about the bruise. "Anything that someone can say to me about you, I need to know. We need to be a team. I need to know everything that somebody can say about you because it's going to come up."

Kelsey stared at her mother. "Absolutely not, Ma. You know how it happened. Why would I say that?" Connie hugged her daughter, relieved.

The next day, Kelsey stayed home from school. What made it so awful was that she saw her mother cry. "It was really upsetting to see my mom, who's kind of always been that strong person for me, like, I felt like it was my fault," she remembered.

It sounds as though you handled the situation pretty sanely, I told Connie, admiringly. "I did," she said, "but not in my heart." After her conversation with the coach, she attended the next three soccer practices to watch her daughter. "I no longer felt like Rebecca was protecting my daughter or had her best interests at heart," she said. Connie also decided not to tell school officials, waiting to see if the bullying would stop. It did. One of the girls involved apologized to Kelsey. Throughout, Connie gathered documentation. Eventually, she decided they would all "ignore the elephant in the room."

While the tone and language of cyberbullying has exploded, the mechanisms for response are inconsistent and flawed. Had Kelsey's school written a coherent policy on cyberbullying, Coach Rebecca might have been obligated to take steps to report the incident. Lacking this, Rebecca's loyalty to her daughter and her daughter's friends won out. The message sent to the untold number of children and parents who witnessed the drama? The school could not be trusted to protect its students.

Many schools continue to decline to intervene in cyberbullying incidents because they occur off school grounds. Yet as any school employee knows, what happens off campus comes right back into the school and disrupts the community. In 2010 multiple suicides were linked to cyberbullying, and state legislation began mandating that school districts include electronic aggression in anti-bullying policy. One such policy, in Westport, Massachusetts, bans cyberbullying that occurs near the school or at any school event, and on or off the property "if the bullying creates a hostile environment at school for the target, infringes on their rights at school or materially and substantially disrupts the education process or the orderly operation of a school." Still, most public schools are either unable or unwilling to make cyberbullying in a private home uniformly actionable. When neither families nor schools police cyberbullying, it becomes all too easy for a cyberbully to lash out.

The cliques at Lindsey Garrett's middle school were fearless enough to have their own names: the Kelly, the 9, the Catty Shack, to name a few. Lindsey floated among different groups, and her artsy look made her a novelty among the girls who obsessed over brands. Still, Lindsey was always nervous. She woke up at five A.M. to straighten her hair, put on makeup, and join the "beauty contest" at school.

She had opened her first Instant Messenger and AOL accounts in elementary school. In the beginning, she remembered, "It was really cool to me that I could even say hi to someone through the Internet." Not long after starting sixth grade, relationships began to shift, an inevitable rite of passage for middle-school girls. Lindsey's oldest and closest friend, Kate, began drifting toward Nicole, a girl in the emerging popular group. Lindsey panicked. "I was jealous," she told me. "Kate was my only friend at the time. If I was coming to middle school, I wanted Kate to be my friend."

Lindsey began instant messaging with Nicole, pretending she was angry at Kate. As Nicole responded supportively, Lindsey saved the messages, then showed them to Kate. "I was, like, making Nicole say all this stuff so Kate could see she was really mean," she recalled. Lindsey also cut and pasted some of Nicole's comments and edited them to make her seem meaner. "I basically wanted to destroy the relationship between Nicole and Kate." She was successful. Five years later, Nicole and Kate still do not speak.

Like gossip, which brings girls closer even as it destroys other relationships, cyberbullying and aggression carry their own rewards. By stockpiling written conversations, Lindsey accrued a reserve of virtual evidence that she used as currency in real life. She could compensate for her disadvantaged social position by leveraging social media. "I don't know, it was, like, when you see the writing, people believe it because it's, like, writing," Lindsey told me.

In middle and high school, the stakes of friendship drama increase; losing friends is not just an emotional downturn, but a change in your overall social security. Lindsey found that she could use technology to make others experience the feelings of insecurity and fear that were roiling her throughout middle school. "People were drawn to me. I would say, 'This person said this.' That's why I would copy and paste conversations and say, 'See, I have proof.'"

More ominously, social media eroded Lindsey's integrity, allowing her to maintain her sweet exterior while experimenting with power and aggression. "I was a huge, two-faced b——ch," she said, in a tone fraught with guilt and not a little awe. "[The Internet] was definitely, like, a face I could hide behind. By kind of saying what I would say online, it was something more than I would say to this person's face." If conventional bullying allows girls to fly beneath the radar of parents and teachers, cyberbullying gives perpetrators a chance to cloak themselves further, remaining unseen by their targets. As a moral vacuum, it lets girls take leave even of themselves. They no longer have to rationalize or face their own behavior.

In high school, Lindsey drifted away from the gossipy girls who formed her inner circle. She began dating a senior boy and, she says, became less petty and more mature. "I came into myself," she explained. "I mean, I'm still who I always was...I'm not saying I don't gossip but I just know how to do that." Lindsey understood that her strongest feelings should be shared with caution. Today, she vents only to her mother and best friend. She never shares her feelings online.

Now student body president of her high school, she is embarrassed by her prior aggressive behavior. "I was so manipulative. People didn't know I was so mean," Lindsey said. "I could go behind people's backs and, like, convince them of certain things and, like, people always believed me." At the same time, Lindsey is honest about the power and success she discovered as a cyberbully. It "felt good," she told me, to destroy Kate and Nicole's friendship, and there were still other relationships Lindsey admitted she sabotaged.

There is a reason why the middle-school years are the most notorious for bullying. Developmentally, girls (and boys) are moody and self-absorbed, emotionally explosive, easily embarrassed, concerned about status, and quickly swayed by the opinions of peers. They like to test the limits of authority. When this adolescent froth goes online, it's not pretty. As Lindsey says, "It was just like all my insecurities thrown onto a computer and thrown at people, and they didn't deserve that." A girl's developmental process is rarely considered in the face of a child's wish to "be like everyone else" who has a phone, a computer with access to Facebook, or an iPod Touch. In chapter ten, I advise parents about how to navigate this dilemma.

Teens, writes social media scholar danah boyd, not only use technology to bond, but also "to seek attention and generate drama," often to relieve insecurity about status and friendship. In this self-reinforcing cycle, technology makes you insecure, so you use technology to feel better, but often in the process generate more stress, which makes you more insecure. As if girls' lives weren't hard enough already...

Lindsey is now applying to college and was eager to tell me about one of the more creative questions on an application. "They asked me, 'If you could get rid of one invention in the world, what would it be?' My first instinct," she said, "was Facebook."

cyberdrama

In the beginning, technology was an adjunct to relationship. It helped girls connect, filling the gaps of contact that opened up between home and school. Today, technology is part of relationship itself. With gadgets more portable and accessible, the average person aged eight to eighteen spends nearly eight hours a day using an electronic device.[37] Like Leah and Ellie, at the beginning of the chapter, girls move fluidly between virtual and spoken conversation.

Real life is frequently experienced as a new opportunity to post or share online. As one high-school student I interviewed told me, the phrase "take a picture of me" now simply means "put it on Facebook." A college sophomore said, "People go to parties in college with the intention of just having [Facebook] pictures for the night. If someone makes a joke at a party, a person will be like, oh my God, that's the perfect title for my album." In 2009 a girl told *Teen Vogue,* "You're not dating until you change your relationship status on Facebook." A year later, "FBO," or Facebook Official, became the new measure of dating legitimacy.

Stand on the edge of any playground and you will see a scene play out day after day: most boys play games, and most girls linger on the edges to talk. The same is true online: social media is *social,* and girls use technology to connect and share. Girls typically send and receive fifty more texts a day than boys. Girls aged fourteen to seventeen are the most active, churning through a hundred texts a day on average. Girls are more likely than boys to carry their phones on them at all times.[38]

It is often said that technology simply magnifies the feelings and dynamics that were there all along. So, too, with girls. In real time, a girl's status is defined by her relationships: who she sits next to, which parties she is invited to, who she counts as her "best friend." Today, a socially aspirational girl must be the architect of her reputation online, on a new, uncharted plane of connection and coolness. A typical middle-class American girl sits at her laptop, chatting as the phone by her side vibrates with new messages (often while she's doing her homework). This balancing act requires a new kind of social expertise. It takes time, and it takes access.

This is why girls claim they "don't exist" if they lack a Facebook account. This is why parents sleep with confiscated laptops under their pillows; they know their daughters will do anything to get them back. And this is why girls show levels of rage and anxiety hence unseen when they lose phone or online privileges. It is precisely the value that girls place on their access to technology that illuminates its position at the heart of girls' relationships. It also underscores the need for us to pay attention to the everyday transactions of girls online.

The biggest mistake we can make is to assume that a girl "gets" technology in a way that an adult does not. Looks are deceiving. The world of BFF 2.0 has presented girls with new, unwritten rules of digital friendship, and it has posed a fresh set of social challenges. What does a one-word text mean when someone usually types a lot? What if you and your friend are texting the same girl, but she replies to only your friend? Does she like you less? How should you handle it? Online social interactions generate situations that demand sophisticated skills. Without them, girls become vulnerable to online aggression and worse.

A girl's adolescence is rife with moments of insecurity about identity and relationships. Online, girls discover a trove of tools that appear to ease those anxieties. If real life has dealt you a hand you mostly cannot change, a few clicks help a girl control her online appearance. Worried about weight gain or acne? Post a flattering photo as your profile picture. Want people to know you listen to cool music? List hip indie music festival pages under your favorite interests. Wish your peers saw you as "different in a cool way"? Upload an artsy still-life photo you took. Don't have a boyfriend, but want to show everyone that guys still like you? Change your profile photo to one of you and your best guy friend from camp.

A 2010 study by the Girl Scouts found that girls downplayed their confidence, kindness, and talents online in favor of highlighting how fun, funny, and cool they were.[39] The study suggested a girl's social media profile was a persona she constructed, a photoshopped billboard on the information superhighway. Unlike the messiness of real life, where you might come to school wearing the "wrong" outfit or say something awkward in class, a Facebook profile is a cool, controlled social avatar intended to stand in for *you*. Online spaces like Facebook and Tumblr are new social proving grounds for girls, rivaling the hallways where girls show off new clothes or friends. Unlike real life, the true self is more easily hidden online.

Lindsey explained how it works: "The statuses I put up, I want people to know I like those bands. I want people to know I think those bands are cool. You create your Facebook to make it seem how you want to come off as a person." She added, "People paint the picture of themselves on Facebook." This "painting" is more like an airbrushed version of yourself and your life.

Social media also offers a salve for the anxiety so many girls feel about relationship. It can provide the answers to burning social questions: *What do other people think of me? Do people like me? Am I normal? Am I popular? Am I cool?* A constant drumbeat of texts, especially from (and in front of) the "right" sort of senders, makes it clear that you are wanted, needed, and liked. Photos of you and your friends laughing, posing, and partying are a kind of social press conference, an announcement that *these are my friends, this is my tribe, I am part of something important.* Lindsey explained, "People take these pictures to show this is how I want you to perceive me. I go to these parties, I go to these events, you're not as cool." The constant ping of texts, chats, video conference calls, and new messages are quick surges of connection that emotionally nourish a girl throughout the day.

All this, however, has its cost.

The same tools girls use to alleviate insecurity are just as likely to inflame it. As relationship becomes more public, we learn things we would rather not know. Meghan, seventeen, called a friend to go to a movie. The friend said she didn't feel like it; later, Meghan read online that she had gone with someone else. Banned from the mall by her parents, fifteen-year-old Judith was seething when she spotted identical AIM (AOL Instant Messenger) messages from two best friends out shopping. "I'd prefer not to see that they were together," she told me. "I'd rather hear it the next day. Because I'm at home and I'm not doing anything, but they're together having fun." Social media forces girls to bear witness to painful realities of relationship that were previously hidden from view.

It is a new kind of TMI, or "too much information": publicly posted photographs of an outing or party you did not attend can send a girl into paroxysms of anxiety and grief. Reading a personal Web page (like Formspring, examined later in the chapter) with ruthless anonymous commenters is a masochistic but not-to-be-missed ritual. Where information is power, there can be no filter. Girls click to consume even the most searing social news because it is just a click away. And because they *can*.

As a result, girls learn to comb the electronic terrain both to connect and stand sentinel over their social security. Thirteen-year-old Jessica described her phone as a periscope that offered her intelligence on a conflict she was having with a friend.

If I didn't have a phone, I would have probably been more scared to go into school, like, that Monday because I wouldn't know what was going on. I wouldn't know who was mad at me and who wasn't, because I wouldn't have been able to talk and ask people. Like, I wouldn't have known if Saskia was on my side, if she was forgiving Jill again. I would know nothing. I would just know that Jill . . . was going to be so mean to me when I got back on Monday.

This world is not so very different from the video games many boys play. These games re-create dark, unpredictable worlds that reveal lurking enemies and rewards. So does social media. For the self-conscious or insecure girl, technology can become a crippling addiction, an insatiable hunger not just for connection but the elusive promise of being liked by everyone.

Away at college and separated from her best friend from high school, Samantha, nineteen, watched Susie drift away. Every day, Samantha logged on to Facebook in her cramped dorm room to track the growing closeness of Susie and a new girl.

"I remember the first time she changed the profile picture of me and her to the picture of them," Samantha says. "I see their statuses are about each other. There are videos. It just makes you feel like you're being replaced." Even when she needs a break from the drama, Facebook's live-feed format is relentless, telling all. "You don't even have to stalk," Samantha told me. "Facebook does the stalking for you."

Using social media like a seismograph to detect every up or down in a friendship, the smallest infractions are recorded and felt. Of course, girls are not only witness to their own exclusion or embarrassment. They react to it. Where there is more information, there is more opportunity for paranoia and conflict: drama rises from digital soil constantly fertilized and refreshed with new dirt.

Should Meghan say something to her deceitful friend? How can Judith handle her feelings of envy and anger? Does Samantha have the right to confront her best friend? Although these twenty-first-century episodes may be inspired by timeless emotions, most girls (and the adults who advise them) feel confused about how to respond.

In part, this is because social media has established new expectations and norms within friendship itself. Many girls now believe that, along with keeping secrets and providing support, being a good friend brings digital responsibilities. While some can be easily learned, others create confusion and unrest.

Consider birthdays. "You measure how much a person actually cares by which form of communication they use," Samantha told me. "Acquaintances will write on my [Facebook] wall. A friend will text me. A best friend will call." When Samantha's best friend texted her late in the day on her birthday, she was hurt. "It kind of makes you feel like an afterthought." With girls constantly connected, they may judge and dissect even the timing of a message.

On Facebook there is an unspoken expectation that if you write on someone's wall, giving them a social "boost" with your presence, they will return the favor. A girl may write on a cute boy's wall or "like" the senior girl's new profile photo, hoping to elicit a public reply for all to see. But the outcome will depend on your social status: The new measure of popularity is how much or how often you need to reply to these public notes. If you are flooded with online notes and posts, you need respond to only the "coolest" friends.

With much of relationship now taking place in the harried shorthand of texts, statuses, and chats, misinterpretation is constant. "You can't see the person, you can't read their body language or their facial expression," Erin, sixteen, explained. "Like, you don't know what their motives are. It could take someone fifteen minutes to reply to your message. You don't know if they're ignoring you, just not there, you don't know if they don't want to talk to you."

Erin described the discomfort of waiting to hear back from a laconic boy she was flirting with: "Why isn't he texting me back? Did I say something wrong? Did I insult him? Am I too sarcastic? Does he not like me? Why isn't he replying? What did I do wrong? Is he trying to make me feel this way for some reason, like for a chase or whatever?" It is exhausting just to listen to the heavy lifting Erin's mind endures for the privilege of online footsie. Real-time flirting can be equally rife with angst, of course, but technology infinitely multiplies the occasion for it.

What if a friend stops signing her texts "xoxo"? Does it mean she's angry? When it happened to Meghan, she grew anxious. "Once you start losing that at the end of conversations, you start wondering, is everything okay? Are we losing touch?" Meghan considered confronting her friend to ask if anything was wrong. Perhaps she was reading something into a minor alteration that had nothing to do with her. But maybe not. She wondered if she might be seen as needy, weak, or demanding. She was not entirely wrong to be worried: girl culture has yet to settle on an answer. There is no clear path. This particular brand of "girl problem"—a change in the tone of a text—is only a few years old.

So are the newly public platforms that allow girls to vent their feelings about problems with friends. Imagine logging on to Facebook or AIM and seeing this on the profile of someone you are feeling uneasy about: "some people really piss me off but i'd rather not be direct about it." This post, from a high-school girl, was instantly available to over seven hundred "friends." It inspired a flurry of curious comments from various peers, not to mention a surge of embarrassment, anger, and anxiety from the target.

The ubiquity of texting has inflected the dynamics of real-time friendship. Many girls think it is rude when a text is not instantly answered. It is now considered normal (if not outrageously rude) to text other people while you are spending time with a friend. The arrangement satisfies the texter's hunger to connect and offers her the impression of being in two—or seven—places at once. But the quality of such companionship is poor. As Amy, thirteen, told me, "My friends are always texting or calling their boyfriends or other friends whenever they're at my house. I feel like I'm losing my friend and her attention. It makes me feel so left out." Still, Amy remained silent. She did not feel entitled to speak up.

Each moment of insecurity, jealousy, anxiety, or anger online can ignite into something much bigger. All it takes is a quick, sarcastic text from Judith to start drama with her two friends at the mall. If Meghan decides to post a snarky message about her lying friend, it's a shot fired across the bow. Just a few years ago, these unique challenges and questions did not exist. But when a girl is sitting in front of a computer or phone, without the reassuring eye contact or comfort a present friend can provide, her feelings of paranoia, fear, anxiety, and insecurity may skyrocket.

Yet to ascribe the challenges girls face in BFF 2.0 to the medium alone would be a mistake. Social media may magnify emotions and facilitate cruelty, but it does not "make" girls act a particular way. For it is not just technology that is altering girls' friendships; girls influence the ways technology is used. They import and impose their distinctly girl values and habits online.

In ingenious ways, girls manipulate technology to reproduce the girl dynamics of real life. In person, one girl might make another one jealous by walking down the hall arm-in-arm with a new friend or love interest. Online, girls re-create this effect by posting vengeful, intimate photos. When Facebook ended the practice of allowing users to rank their "top" or best friends, girls compensated by using another Facebook mechanism to designate their closest friends as family members and even spouses. Just as boys whose parents ban war toys are known to cut a piece of toast into the shape of a gun, girls have made Facebook bow to their need for social hierarchy.

The unique communication rituals and habits of girls have also found homes online. In the hallway, an irritated girl mutters a clipped "hey" to signal something is wrong. On her phone, Lindsey texts her sullen "hi" with only the lowercase letter "h." "That would mean I'm angry," she explains. When all is well, "I'm [typing] 'hi what's up?'" And consider Erin, who takes the silent treatment into the twenty-first century by refusing to respond to a text when she is upset with someone. "When you have the option of not sending a message back, you have a sense of power. That is your way of saying, 'I'm in control of this relationship.'"

If the phrase "just kidding" wasn't bad enough in real life, it becomes even more cutting and confusing in BFF 2.0. Consider these messages: "HEY GET A NEW PROFILE PIC WOMAN LOL LUV YA," "shut up Amber ☺," "rosa, you're such a b——ch. Just kidding, you're not a b——ch. You're great." Are these senders really kidding? If you were a girl who received them, what would you think? Where real-time jokes can be sussed out for tone or gesture, these comments stand alone on a screen. They may be read by an insecure girl, a girl who bears a grudge against the joker, a confident girl, a distracted girl. Everyone has a different trigger point, and the opportunity for misinterpretation, and retaliation, is rampant.

Leah Martin, twelve, attends a public middle school in a middle-class suburb of a major East Coast city. During our telephone interview, she speaks so fast I can hardly follow her. My in box pings and pings; seated in front of her computer, she forwards links, chat conversations, and e-mails she thinks I'll want for my research, all without breaking stride in any sentence. She spins dizzyingly from one story to the next, and I scramble to keep up as she guides me through her social universe.

Most striking about Leah's life is a social hierarchy mediated by technology. Leah has a friend, Carrie, who she has met and now interacts with entirely via text message. Despite their frequent contact, when they pass each other in the hallways at school, they do not say hello.

They don't speak? At all? "It would have been awkward if I said hi to her," she explained, while I listened, agog. Leah had other friends who she only texted but still greeted, though "in person if we hung out it would be so awkward it's beyond belief. In person it's so awkward, I don't even want to talk to them." Then there was Andrew, a friend who told her he loved her in text messages but could not say it in person.

Leah volunteered to explain what she called her "food chain" of friendships:

My friends at the bottom of the food chain, like, I text them all the time but I don't socialize with them in person. Another level of friends is, you can be friends with somebody on Facebook but never have met them. I have over eight hundred friends on Facebook. I haven't met some of them. I don't know them. I don't talk to them. Then, my friends that I text and who are acquaintances. We say, like, "hi." Then I have good friends-ish: we text all the time and we hang out in person. And then we have, like, our best friends. You don't text them. You call them all the time. You talk in person and you can be completely honest with them. You text them but you talk on the phone and hang out every weekend. They are, like, your life.

If the girl mandate is to be constantly connected and have lots of friends, social media allows Leah to "overachieve." She can show off her success to her peers and reassure herself that she is far from alone.

Leah can also experiment with new, if slightly cringeworthy versions of relationship. On the one hand, her text-only friendships seem to substitute technology for authentic connection. On the other hand, who are we to judge? As long as she is safe and satisfied, why shouldn't Leah enjoy the thrilling reach of social media? Most tellingly, despite these new permutations of relationship, some things don't change: best friends are best when they are live and in person. The 2010 study by the Girl Scouts confirmed that 92 percent of girls would give up all of their social media friends if it meant keeping their best friend.[40] Your closest friends, as Leah says, "are, like, your life."

The fluidity between girls' online and virtual worlds allows them to recruit the tools of social media to execute offline agendas. Consider this Instant Messenger conversation[41] between Trisha and Leah. Trisha begins by instant messaging Leah, ostensibly to tell Leah that she has a new invitation to trick-or-treat on Halloween. It quickly becomes clear that Trisha has another agenda: she is in conflict with Julie, their mutual friend.

Trisha: leah i need to talk to you my phone is dead and i feel like
   charging it so please reply

Leah: hahaha okay whats up

Trisha: nvm [not very much] nora invited us to go trick or
   treating

Leah: do you want to go? did she only invite you or me too?

Trisha: both of us or you can go with julie idc [I don't care]

Leah: i wasnt invited to julies... but my other friends were
   suppose to come with me though if you want you can go
   with nora i wont be affended at all, but whats happening with
   julie? are you mad at her?

Trisha: nothing is happening with julie if she is going to like
   ignore me and s——t then i really don't care

Leah: yeah go trisha!!!!!! i love you and you and julie have been
   best friends forever everyting will work out

Trisha: truth is if things don't work out then its fine

Leah: youll still be best friends with me :D

Trisha: does julie say stuff about me

Leah: she just said you guys got into a fight today at lunch and
   now you wont talk to her

Leah understands that it is her obligation as a friend to invite Trisha
to vent and affirm that she is on Trisha's side. With Leah's loyalty
confirmed, Trisha ups the ante, asking Leah to betray Julie by dis-
closing anything Julie has said about Trisha. When Leah agrees,
Trisha reveals more:

Trisha: we didn't even get into a fight and she isn't talking to
   me and she is just like in my homeroom with deanna jen and
   elizabeth and they went to her show this weekend and they
   were like laughing and whispering and its just like oh hi julie
   whatsup like whos suppose to be your best friend them or me
   and i feel like she is just saying she is my best friend and not
   really meaning it and like she doesn't tell me anything so like
   i don't know if she really is

Leah: it doesn't really seem like you guys are that good of

friends which upsets me cause i love you both but i dont
really know if she actually likes us.

Notice how Leah has now begun to backpedal. She tries to play both
sides, affirming her friendship with Trisha but still saying she likes
Julie, too.

Watch how Trisha responds: detecting that she needs to work
harder to get Leah fully on her side, she takes aim at Leah's relationship with Julie by implying Julie has also betrayed Leah. Then
Trisha goes further, suggesting that Leah could never really know if
Julie was a trustworthy friend because she is fake and lies:

> Trisha: shes not my really good friend and i know she is not a
> true friend like she talks s——t about her friends and if you
> get to close to her she will tell people stuff about you and
> denies stuff when you confront her about it like she will say
> something about you and if like i tell you and you ask her
> about it she'll just deny it and usually people will just believe
> her because she isn't like me, like i will say whatever i want
> and i'll be mean to people and won't care and don't hang out
> with people i dont like but julie hangs out with them and just
> talks about them and she is nicer and trys to act innocent
> Leah: thats even worse what she does. thats os rude and mean.
> i dont even wanna know what kind of s——t she says about
> me because she probally says the same about you
> Trisha: like i know she says stuff about me and she has said
> something about you but like i'm not on best terms with her
> right now so i don't want you to think i am just saying that,
> like i don't want to be caught in the middle of anything
> because i go to school with her and will have to deal with her
> for at least two years so i might as well just if not be friends
> with put up with

Trisha has successfully triangulated, making Leah as much a target
of Julie as herself. Leah has moved from the role of supportive girl-

friend to the position of angry, jilted friend. She immediately spills the beans on just how much Julie talks about Trisha behind her back.

> Leah: thats so rude she trashing on both of us then denys everything this isnt okay trisha i always stick up when shes says s——t about you and like now she goes and say stuff about me? wow shes so insecure.
>
> Trisha: i just don't even know about her anymore and i just want to tell you before she trys to turn this on me
>
> Leah: i know i dont even care what she says. what do you reply when she says s——t? i wont get mad if you dont defend me not a lot of people do defend people
>
> Trisha: i always defend you because your my best friend and like its not cool if i just let people talk about you
>
> Leah: aww so do i i dont let her say s——t ❤
>
> Trisha: ☺ i gotta go i'll charge my phone and text yu later

In the conversation's finale, Leah not only affirms her loyalty to Trisha, but she timidly asks Trisha if she is willing to defend her. Trisha responds with the ultimate declaration of friend love—"your my best friend." Leah reciprocates. Within just a few lines of text, Leah goes from being the secure friend sought out for support to the supplicant seeking that same support, now fearful of a disloyal friend. Trisha has managed to recruit Leah to be a target with her and, in the process, affirmed their closeness as best friends.

There are few interactions that better illustrate how intertwined social reward and aggression are for girls. As Leah and Trisha degrade Julie behind her back, gossiping, which undoubtedly leads to in-person tension and conflict, they are deepening their own bond.

Some version of this same conversation might have occurred in a hallway or on a phone call. Yet isn't it easier to turn a girl against someone when you don't have to speak the damning words, or look a friend in the eye before you damage her relationship with your enemy? For instance, when I asked thirteen-year-old Jessica if it was easier to text when she was upset, she said, "Yeah. Because it's not, like, personal. It doesn't feel personal because you're just, they're just words...When I'm texting her, I wouldn't say it to her face because I know she would flip out more and there would be more to regret."

There is also this: Leah could share the conversation with me because she had stored it. Why? Would Julie someday see it? Social media has surely not invented these conversations. But it has altered their impact, speed, and ease.

The parasites of the social media world are websites and applications that let users post anonymous messages about others. In 2010 Formspring.me led the pack. Untold thousands of teenagers have accounts on the site, which allows your audience—almost always your classmates—to write anything on your personal page without being identified.

Formspring's power lies in its offer of an answer to the question, "What do people think of me?" Most girls open accounts hoping to read positive comments about their looks, personality, or talents. What they get is usually much worse:

> Okay so I just thought id help you out a little bit, okay, so ium going to try and say things in the nicest possible way...your not hot s——t. Alright so stop acting like it. Okay no one f——king likes you, its fake. No guys would ever like you, your a b——ch to a lot of girls, and say some pretty shady s——t, so if I were you I would f——king stop. Your f——king annoying. And if you haven't notest you have the hugest nose ever...i mean it what ever but yeah. & you made your self a formspring so don't except people to be nice on it. <3 bye b——ch.

Imagine walking the halls or sitting in class, never knowing if the person sitting next to you in math is the one pummeling you on Formspring. The site takes cybercruelty to a new low by making it appear consensual: When you register for your account, you literally invite others to bash you with their "honest" opinions. Because it appears consensual, it no longer seems like cybercruelty at all.

Girls are especially vulnerable to Formspring for several reasons. For girls obsessed with what peers are saying about them, the site seems too good to be true. Here, finally—girls believe—I will discover my true social worth. For girls who define success as being liked by everyone, Formspring lets hope spring eternal: You can open an account and maybe, just maybe, you won't get a mean comment. Or perhaps others will rally to your defense. You'll be that girl who everyone really loves!

Needless to say, it is a toxic, self-reinforcing cycle: If you are that desperate to know what your peers think, you probably lack the self-esteem to define your own value. The more you look outside of yourself for self-worth, by visiting the website, the more personal authority and confidence you give up.

Girls live in a social universe where truth is shielded and conflict is avoided. They flock to Formspring because it appears to bring those feelings to the surface. The site offers the illusion that users can do an end run around the girl underground. But Formspring invites people to be cruel without owning up, and users exaggerate, attack, and lie just because they can. They experiment with others' feelings as a game, just to see how they react. When there is no cost and no consequence to speech, people take leave of their ethics and good sense.

Yet too many girls buy into the fantasy that Formspring tells the truth. They do not pause to consider whether "truth" should be reconsidered if it is offered without responsibility or source. They are unable to tear themselves away. Shannon, thirteen, has been grounded several times for her refusal to get off Formspring. Each time her mother tracks down her page, she is punished. Desperate to know what her peers think, she fights every threat of grounding because she believes Formspring has something to offer that real life cannot: the truth about what others think about her and, so she thinks, a chance to repair her image and right wrongs.

Despite the breathtaking, casual cruelty that swarms the pages of Formspring, the girls who use it respond to their attackers with surprising indifference.

"I'd f*** you," posted one commenter.

"thanks I mean very blunt but still flattering," responded the account holder.

"YOU KNOW HOW YOUR ALLERGIC TO EVERYTHING.!! YOU SHOULD EAT A BUNCH OF PEANUTS AND HAVE AN ALLERGY ATTACK AND DIE..." said one poster. The account holder replied, "HAHA, you should eat some penis and choke on it and die! Take a HIKE KYKE."

"ur fat and hot and ur boobs r large," read one post.

"K," the page owner replied breezily.

How can girls be so blasé? It is not entirely clear. It is possible that aggression simply breeds more aggression: interpersonal norms online are radically different, with the bar for nastiness constantly being set, raised, and reset. For many girls, having a Formspring page seems to be a point of pride, a sign that you can handle the haters. You are tough enough to face the truth of what others think. But the reality is that most girls are hoping for something else. With every flip response, account holders authorize others to continue berating them.

Formspring has had predecessors like Juicy Campus and the Honesty Box feature on Facebook. It will likely have descendents and already has many cousins. Facebook is flooded with applications that tempt girls to find out what their friends have said about them. On my own Facebook page, I get a note every few days that a former student has answered questions about me. To further entice, the application reveals a long list of anonymously answered questions for me to preview. "Do you think that Rachel Simmons is a wannabe?" reads one. "Yes," someone has apparently written. "Do you think Rachel Simmons is cute?" (yes) "Do you think Rachel Simmons smells?" (no). And on and on. To find out who is taking the time to size me up, I have to "earn coins" by downloading other applications. Today, in my thirties, I roll my eyes. As a middle schooler? I would have fought bears to get those coins.

Perhaps that is the point. These website developers seem to know they are sinking their teeth into a juicy developmental moment: the insatiable hunger for acceptance. It is a longing some girls will do anything to satisfy, no matter the cost. I am reminded here of the children's book *Tuck Everlasting,* in which a young girl meets a family that has tasted the fountain of youth and now struggles with the challenge of eternal life. On Formspring, girls believe they have discovered a similar cure-all—for insecurity—but what they get is the curse of knowing too much. "You don't have to live forever," the narrator says in the film version of the book. "You just have to live." Similarly, girls don't need to be liked by everyone. Rather, they should just strive to be liked.

sexting

Sexting, or the sending of sexual images or text through electronic channels, broke the surface of American consciousness in 2009. Alarming surveys announced that as many as 19 percent of teens had sent a sexually suggestive photo or text, while 31 percent had received one from someone else.[42] Although this practice is not directly related to the hidden culture of aggression, girls use sexual images to humiliate each other. Sexting is also an important part of girls' relationship with social media, so I have chosen to explore it in this chapter.

The national conversation on sexting has cast girls as casualties of preying boys and an oversexualized culture. This is true, but only part of the story. In fact, sexting is a natural and predictable outgrowth of the relationship girls have created with social media. To suggest otherwise—that sexting is an exceptional phenomenon, or the sad story of a girl with low self-esteem—is to condescend to girls and ignore their context.

As I have shown throughout this chapter, girls are hardly passive vessels being manipulated by technology; to the contrary, girls lever-age social media to serve their drive to feel good about themselves, be liked, and achieve status. As girls approach adolescence, they engage with an entertainment culture that values women for their celebrity, bodies, and sexuality. At the same time, girls learn that attention from a high-status boy will vault them into the highest echelons of popularity. Enter sexting.

Erin Lambert is sixteen. With a pixie cut and sarcastic, quick tongue, she is a real-life Juno, the wisecracking, headstrong teenager from the eponymous film. She is both fierce and fragile, rolling her eyes brashly at her own regrettable sexts, but confiding that she longs to be told she is beautiful.

Erin tells me about two chat sites, Omeggle and Chatroulette, that connect her instantly with random strangers via webcam or text chat. No one knows who she is unless she tells them, and she can click to the next stranger should she grow uncomfortable or bored. Both of these sites crawl with men who touch themselves on camera and send explicit sexual messages. Erin doesn't care. She knows what she is looking for.

Girls have learned to use social media to feel closer to their friends. Now, they have figured out how to use it to feel beautiful and sexy. "I could go on Omeggle right now," she says, "and click to a couple of windows and be told, 'You're so gorgeous.'" Like many girls, Erin struggles to accept her face and body. She wonders if her body is attractive, even normal. She has had a few boyfriends, nothing serious. She agonizes in the mirror over her breasts, skin, and legs.

When Erin was fourteen, she showed her breasts over video chat to a friend of a friend. Recently dumped by a boyfriend, Erin met Steve at a party. The two Skyped for the next few nights. Steve pleaded with her for three hours. When I ask her if flashing him was fun, she says, "Kind of? To know that he really wanted to see me in a sexual way and knowing that he was trying really hard to do so. That was a little bit satisfying, I guess, to know I could make someone want that."

Yet she later felt "kind of, like, ashamed." It was, she said, "the first time a guy has seen you without your shirt on and I just wasted it." Still, she got something in return. Steve told her he liked her breasts, and it meant a lot to Erin. "At least I can be confident about them now because I know they're not Quasimodo boobs, like deformed and ugly and should be kept in a bell tower," she said wryly.

So you felt affirmed? I asked her. "Yeah," she replied. "It was nice to just kind of hear, like, you're okay. You're not horrid and disgusting. I think I just wanted someone to confirm that I wasn't worthless. And that I, like, could be attractive." The comfort of Steve's words lingered for two weeks, after which, she lolled mockingly, she was back to "all that low self-esteem stuff."

Was Erin's quick surge of affirmation from Steve so different from the charge a girl seeks when she sends out a text to a friend and waits anxiously for a reply? Both girls are using social media to summon reassurance: For Erin, it is about her body and sexuality; for another girl, it is about her likability or social worth. "I just wanted to know so badly that who I was physically was normal. And that it was like, something that could be loved and enjoyed and wanted." It is worth noting that before social media, Erin would have had to take real physical risks to earn this kind of feedback. On some level, sexting may be "safer" than the real-life alternative.

Yet the stakes for sexters are dangerous in a different way. Erin travels on thin ice in this world. When she met a boy from another country on Chatroulette, they talked every night for two weeks. Then he convinced her to take off her shirt. It was easier, she says, the second time, even though she still felt guilty. He asked if she wanted to see his penis; she didn't. "They're, like, weird-looking, man," she cracked. "It kind of looked like a hot dog." That Erin was not only uninterested but slightly repulsed suggests she was using the interaction for a purpose beyond sexual titillation or desire. When she explained why she did it, she says, "He was cute and funny and we flirted, so he would, like, tell me I was pretty and stuff."

Eventually, Erin completely disrobed on camera for Matt. "What if he's recording this?" she wondered. It turned out that he was. Through a mutual online friend, Erin discovered there was a digital file of her in the shower. Mortified, she sent a photograph of Matt's penis—which she had taken, she mentioned casually, "just in case"— to the mutual friend as revenge. (Not surprisingly, the effect was entirely different: "He was pretty well endowed so his friends just respected him more, it turns out.") She made him swear to delete it, though she will never know for sure if he did. Today, they are still friends.

Just as girls become desensitized to graphic language online, a similar indifference can develop around sexual exchanges. "After I did it the second time, it wasn't as awkward," Erin remembered. "I was, like, well, someone has seen [my breasts] before. I know they're not horrible. It was just a matter of, like, what if my parents walk in? What if he's a jerk about it?" She compared revealing her breasts to showing off a new haircut. "It's not like this huge big thing or, like, okay, I got a haircut. I show one person, and you're the first person to see my haircut. Then everyone else sees it. It's not a big deal anymore."

Even as she flirts with the danger of exposure, Erin is keenly aware of her power to "delete" the relationship. Unlike someone at school, who she might have to see every day, "you can delete [these guys] from your buddy list and then they're gone forever. You don't have to think about them if you don't want to." When she tells me this, Erin may be forgetting that an explicit video of her may be out there somewhere, immune to any delete button. Yet I am reminded of Leah's food chain of relationships: If she wanted to, she could easily "delete" her more trivial relationships with the peers she texts but never speaks to. Is this Erin's "food chain"?

Too often, the discussion of girls and sexting is occluded by moral judgment, alarm, and fear. I am not unconcerned about what girls like Erin do online, but to frame her behavior as pathetic, hypersexual, or warped prevents us from seeing that sexting is part of what came, unbidden though it was, from the world technology opened to girls.

Nor am I saying that girls sext only in response to external pressure. Girls are sexual beings and agents. They are curious, desiring, and passionate. Though we may be uncomfortable saying it, girls have long explored their sexual identities.[43] They have done it on their own, in relationships and flings, and through creative pursuits. For some girls, including Erin, the expression of desire online in the form of a sext is simply that. It comes not from a need to keep up, or be seen as attractive, but from desire and curiosity.

Insecurity, however, is an undeniably powerful factor in the decision a girl makes to sext. As an advice columnist for *Teen Vogue,* I find the most commonly submitted plea for help goes something like this: "Why don't guys like me? Why do all my friends have boyfriends? Am I weird?"[44] Just as girls agonize over whether they are thin or pretty enough, many worry they are not sexy or liked by boys. While girls have long lived in a culture inundated with heterosexual imagery, these messages have grown louder and more destructive.

In 2010 outrage over girls' sexualization was at an all-time high. An online video of seven-year-old girls gyrating in a dance routine set the Internet ablaze. American Apparel clothing ads of college-aged women were deemed pornographic, and seminude photographs of teen starlets Miley Cyrus and Demi Lovato were released. In a landmark 2007 report, the American Psychological Association linked sexualization, or objectifying and defining a person in terms of her sexual value,[45] to low self-esteem, depression, and eating disorders in girls. The study's authors attributed sexualization not only to media, but to adults and peers.[46]

Every day, girls consume messages that prescribe their power and value in sexual terms. Into this pressure cooker steps a girl with her cell phone. Just as technology democratizes gossip, giving anyone with dirt a chance for a fair hearing, sexting gives an overlooked girl a second, virtual chance to validate her sexual worth. This is a risk many girls are more than willing to take. By adolescence, dating or being liked by a high-status guy is a key component of social standing. Girls must maintain their sexual progress to prove themselves not only to boys, but to other girls, too.

I remember this well. In middle school, I was desperate to be asked to dance by the most popular boys. I never was. I was not much interested in hooking up with anyone, but I began doing it because the other girls in my group did. I worried that they would think I wasn't cool. I feared being left out. Would I have responded to the request of a popular boy for a photo? Would that have felt like a version of being asked to dance? If I lived in a world where what happened online was enmeshed with my real life, if the boy's request signaled that I was "liked," and if sending a photo meant I could reciprocate, I sure might have.

Sexting in particular illuminates how deeply technology has become embedded in peer relationships. For many girls, sexting is synonymous with flirting. When the right kind of boy asks for a photograph, girls translate the request as "I like you. I have a crush on you. I am interested." The boy's request is usually not experienced as lewd; when it is, most girls refuse to comply. (When an acquaintance of Erin's asked for a naked photo, she sent him a nude photo of an elderly woman she found on the Internet.)

If sexting plugs into girls' need to feel sexy, it satisfies boys' drive to feel manly. Imagine a "typical" adolescent boy's bedroom: Can you see the posters on the wall? Some of them are of cars and sports celebrities. Some are of scantily clad women. In 2010, Megan Fox was the pinup of choice. These posters do not just satisfy a boy's aesthetic; they affirm and communicate his heterosexuality, and therefore his masculinity. Just as girls face pressure to be hot for boys, boys face equally suffocating messages from media, adults, and peers about being a "player" who can "get" a hot girl to like and hook up with him.

Sexting takes the pinup off the wall and puts it into his phone. With a photograph of the "right" girl, he has new evidence of his successful masculinity. Unlike girls, who are often punished for their sexuality with epithets like "slut," boys get attention and social promotions for their sexual conquests. A sext gives a boy the chance to move up the boy ranks. When a boy asks for a photo from a girl, he may in fact like her. But he may also—or only—want something to show his friends. Once he forwards the message, or (as often happens) a friend grabs the phone and sends the image to himself, a girl's reputation is forever changed.

This is why talking with girls about sexting must focus on gender roles and how they influence behavior. Telling girls sexting, and they, are "bad" is thin gruel when it comes to behavioral change. Moreover, forwarding or sharing a sext must be understood as an aggressive act. In 2010 several state laws included sexting as a form of child pornography. Although this may help in prosecution and prevention, it deflects attention from the impact a sext has on a target's relationships and reputation, and the hostile environment that can result.

To suggest that it is only boys who forward sexual content is, yet again, to patronize girls and position them as targets. Online, girls police each other's sexuality by forwarding sexual images of girls they receive. In the twenty-first century, you call a girl a "slut" by sharing a humiliating image or text. Consider this posting on the Tumblr page of a high-school sophomore girl:

> Emmmm, why did somebody forward me a nude pic of some girl I know? SMFH [Shaking my f——king head] SHE'S SO STU-PID. SHOULD'VE LISTENED TO THE MTV COMMER-CIALS. BUT NOPE, SHE CHOSE TO DEGRADE HERSELF USING TECHNOLOGY. THAT WAS A BAD DECISION ON HER PART. OH WELL. I REALLY DON'T CARE CUS I HATE HER SO . . . I'M ABOUT TO FORWARD THIS S——T TO EEEEEVERYBODY.

Clearly, it eludes the writer of this post that she will now degrade the girl who she self-righteously accuses of degrading herself.

Erin remains conflicted about whether her online sexual activity is worth it. The intimacy she achieves online is gossamer, and she knows it. Nor can she find a way to hold on to the confidence she feels in the moment of virtual sexual connection. She struggles with the duality of her life. "I am sort of starting to feel that the only people who will appreciate [my sexuality] are the people I find on-line." She continues, "It's like, God, there must be something really wrong with me in person. I must smell really bad or something."

Erin's sexting in and of itself will be a problem only if she loses control over the images she sends, or relies solely on the Internet to develop her sexual identity and confidence. These "relationships" cannot ultimately fulfill her, and technology cannot be a substitute for relationship. Of her hundreds of friends on Facebook, Erin says, "I can look at a picture. It's like, yes, you're friends with all these people but you're not really friends with them, so I guess that makes you realize you're, like, very alone." Erin is discovering in sexting what she has already figured out about her online friendships: the further down the food chain you go, the less satisfying the connection becomes.

the paradox of online authenticity

When I think about girls' lives online, I am occasionally reminded of *The Wizard of Oz,* and the shriveled, fearful man who sat behind the controls of the great and powerful wizard. There are the girls using Facebook to project an image of careless cool; there are Formspring account holders who act indifferent in the face of cruelty; there is Erin, pursuing online trysts she is unable to find in real life; and there are the girls who spew uncharacteristic venom from behind digital screens. If there is now a seamless integration of girls' online and vir-tual lives, there remains a split between what girls do online and who they are in real life.

The question becomes whether or not we should view girls' on-line behavior as a courageous or creative extension of their personal-ities, or an unattainable fantasy of who they wish they could be. If a girl can express certain convictions or feelings only online, is she still being "real"? At what cost does this duality come to her integrity?

If girls squirrel away parts of their identities online, what will this mean for the selves they learn to present in real time? When I was in middle school, writing a note was my only alternative to direct conflict with a peer. Most of the time, I was forced to stand with butterflies in my stomach and blurt my feelings, as best I could, to the friends who had let me down. On some of those days, I lost my temper, uttering stupid things I didn't mean; on others, my courage dissolved into sobs. But sometimes, I hit those conversations out of the park. It wasn't easy. I had to try, fail, and try again. I had to wrestle with the messiness of relationship. I had to *learn*.

Today, girls can click and send around all that. It is a trade girls make with clear short-term reward but unknown long-term cost. Girls who type instead of talk are missing out on the in-person conversations they need to develop their social skills and communicate successfully. As they lean on texting to navigate their most difficult conversations, they are not getting smarter or more effective in real-life conflict. If anything, like muscles that atrophy without use, girls' social skills are being stunted. Technology may speed up relationship, but it will delay authentic connection. Ironically, like water that changes to steam, the drive to avoid conflict in real life may simply create much more of it online.

Social media is a temptation that offers the promise of something glorious but also exacts a painful price. At its best, social media allows girls to connect and explore their evolving identities. At its worst, it preys on girls' most painful insecurities. It becomes a weapon capable of pulverizing a child's reputation and self-esteem. Cyberbullying continues to confound adults and girls alike. Most schools talk to students about it, but few can do anything when an incident transpires in a private home. In the meantime, almost no one talks with students about what some call "digital citizenship." The day-to-day online interactions where children and teens play out their friendships—and begin the conflicts that mutate into cyberbullying—remain mostly unexplored. Girls are navigating this new terrain as best they can.

Still bigger questions remain: Is all this information valuable? Do girls need it? Aren't some things better left unknown, unseen, and unsaid in relationship? Although this book is an argument for girls to assert themselves more, it does not follow that everything must be said and known. A surprising number of girls agree. When I ask group after group of teens if their friendships would be better without technology, a majority of girls raise their hands. They say yes.

she's all that

From the outside looking in, Erin seems an unlikely candidate for bullying. Beautiful and popular, she is the kind of girl I might have worshiped in junior high. Yet Erin was punished in part because girls resented her social success. As I asked around after girls like Erin, I learned she was probably always a vulnerable target. Erin was a girl who "thinks she's all that."

At 8:00 A.M. in Mississippi, nineteen seventh-grade girls were slumped in their chairs, limbs dangling listlessly over metal and plastic and wood, cheeks pressing into the cool desktops. I felt like Atlas holding up the conversation, until I asked, "So, what is the big deal about a girl who thinks she's all that?"

The bodies rustled and looks slung around the room like arrows.

For once Amber didn't bother raising her hand. "They think they're better than all of us."

Christina added, "They put everyone else down."

"Sometimes they just push the girl out of the way and go after the boys. And they don't act like that to the boys."

"Mostly what they do is they try to flirt with all of their friends' boyfriends, and they think they can get anybody."

"They act like they're stuck up," Lacey said.

The next day, with the fifth graders, I asked, "Why don't we like the girl who thinks she's all that?"

"She thinks she's pretty!" one said indignantly.

"What's wrong with that?"

"She brags about it," Dee Dee said. "Most girls walk around like they're everything, prancing around, walking down halls saying 'I'm better than you are.'"

"What does she do when she brags?" I asked.

"My hair's so pretty," she sneered, imitating.

"Is that how she says it?"

"I'm prettier than you are. I'm just way better than you!" she replied in a sultry voice, then choked into giggles.

"Okay," I said. "Act it out. Let me see."

"They fix their hair during class. They prance around!"

"So let's see it," I urged. Raneesha jumped out of her chair and sauntered down the middle of the circle, swinging her behind dramatically.

"She's shaking her booty, right?" I asked. The girls roared. "So why don't we like that?"

The laughter settled gently like a sheet laid on grass. Silence.

"We may go somewhere, and she may be getting [the boys'] attention. And they may start liking her and not me," Dee Dee said.

"What's the right way to act, then?" I pushed.

"You just don't say it all the time," Lizzie said.

"Keep it to yourself."

"Act regular!"

"Act normal!"

"What's normal?" I asked.

"Just walk around not shaking your booty!" Lana said, frustrated.

"Act like everybody else."

"Act quiet," Raneesha said firmly.

"You can be friendly and happy and just...do things that everyone else does and don't hurt other people!" Lizzie exclaimed.

Two periods later, I asked the ninth graders to define a girl who thinks she's all that. Katie explained. "Say like you don't have as much money as them. They always get all the nice clothes and everything. They hang around the big groups and stuff. They think they're all that. They're like, well, you *wish* you could be in our group."

Lauren took up the slack. "Somebody's popular and they think they can get any boy in the school that they want, a lot of money and fancy clothes and stuff like that. She thinks she's so perfect."

"Yeah," Tanya said, "she's stuck up and she don't want to talk to nobody, but she might not be—you never gave her the chance to find out how she is."

"So why not?" I asked. "Why do we make those judgments?"

Heather again: "I was going to say she got it in her head that she thinks she's all that. She's snobby and stuff. She's got on Tommy Hilfiger and the other girls got on Jordache, and she goes up and says, look at my watch, I got it at such and such and it was $180."

"It's all about their attitude," Tanya said.

"You should be noticed," Kelly said, "but not calling attention to yourself. Have good posture and be confident and stand out but without saying anything."

"What's the biggest thing girls fight over?" I asked my first group of Ridgewood ninth graders. Toya raised her hand.

"If you go into a new school or something, and you come in decked out and got your hair down and stuff, other girls are going to be hating on you. They'll be like, she thinks she's all that. She too cute."

Tiffany added, "If you're at a new school they'll come up to you and be like, um, what's your name, why you tryin' to talk to my man, and all this stuff?"

"Why would girls do that?" I asked.

"They want to take you out!" Keisha crowed, and all the girls jumped in, their voices clotting indecipherably.

Today's girls come of age in a world that has replaced the glass ceiling with a space station. The twenty-first-century girl is a pro ballplayer, a CEO-in-training, a fighter pilot. She is anything she wants to be. Today, girl power is a cultural juggernaut.

And yet. The message that modesty and restraint are the essence of femininity persists. Contemporary feminist research shows that our culture continues to pressure girls to be chaste, quiet, thin, and giving, denying the desire for sexual pleasure, voice, food, and self-interest.[47]

In schools, the American Association of University Women found "the lessons of the hidden curriculum teach girls to value silence and compliance, to view those qualities as a virtue." Journalist Peggy Orenstein found that girls value in each other social characteristics of "sweet" and "cute," a term she found interchangeable with "deferential," "polite," or "passive." The good girl, Orenstein concluded, "is nice before she is anything else—before she is vigorous, bright, even before she is honest."[48]

Small wonder that singer Ani DiFranco is telling her legions of young female fans that everyone secretly hates the prettiest girl in the room. Or, she might have added, the most popular, the smartest, the thinnest, the sexiest, or the best dressed. Because, girl power or not, most girls know deep down that standing out can get you in big trouble. In *USA Today*,[49] a Virginia high-school teacher warned of a dangerous trip wire for girls at his school. Although a new student is usually ignored, he wrote, "as soon as she becomes a threat, especially if guys like her, she'll get ripped apart."

When I first started interviewing girls, I'd planned to organize their stories according to the qualities I assumed girls got punished for: the differently abled, the overweight, the poor, the haplessly uncool. I had not expected to find that girls became angry with each other for quite the opposite reason.

As most any girl knows, one of the worst insults is to be called a girl who "thinks she's all that." This girl, loosely defined as conceited, is considered a show-off, obnoxious, or full of herself. By fifth grade, girls are intimately familiar with "all that," an epithet that grows with them into adulthood, gradually evolving into the more genteel belief that "she thinks she's better than me."

How can you tell a girl who thinks she's all that? Well, it all depends.

The first people Stephanie met after switching schools were Marissa and Lori. Best friends since preschool, the girls made an odd couple: Marissa was the bubbly, magazine-cutout-cute cheerleader. Lori was stick thin and scrappy. Alphabetized seats in freshman homeroom fated Marissa and Stephanie to friendship.

Stephanie was pretty. She was no cover girl, but she had majestic height and a head of perfectly blow-dried, blond-streaked hair that made her, she said wryly, the "preppiest girl in school." She was also smart and a talented actor. Coming from the tiny, bland Catholic school where she'd been cooling her heels for the last eight years, Stephanie still felt queasy about starting at a much bigger place. Finding Marissa and Lori was a huge relief. When Stephanie got a crush on Josh after he headed a soccer ball into her locker, she sensed that things might just end up right.

On a Saturday night in late fall, Stephanie was invited for her first sleepover at Lori's. The three girls holed up in a makeshift mountain of pillows, sleeping bags, and junk food. While they were watching a movie and doing their nails, Lori's brother Steve came into the den with his friend Jeremy. Steve sat next to Stephanie on the floor. Everyone talked and joked for a while, the boys threw handfuls of popcorn at the girls, Lori got angry at Steve, and the boys left. The girls finished their movie and fell asleep on the TV-room floor.

On Monday, after study hall, Stephanie stood very still before her locker sensing something might have changed in a way she didn't understand. She felt dread. She opened her locker door. No notes from Marissa and Lori. She went to the bathroom. No one waiting for her there as usual. Stephanie drifted through the afternoon classes obsessing silently over what could be wrong, and why.

She decided to sleep on it. The next day, Marissa and Lori ignored her during homeroom, and her eyes nearly burned out of her head trying to hold their gaze. Later that morning, two girls informed Stephanie that people had been talking. Something was going on behind her back. Still, no one had spoken to her. Marissa and Lori were nowhere to be found. Yet everyone seemed in the know. Stephanie was out, gone from the group. No one would acknowledge her. She was invisible.

By fifth period, Stephanie was reeling. She didn't understand what had happened or why, only that she had no control over it. No friends. She slouched, sobbing and gasping, on the linty rug by her locker, hiding her face in her coat sleeves. What was going on? Was it because a geeky senior had asked her to the prom and she was only a freshman? (*She'd said no!*) Was it that she tried out for the play? Had Marissa not been joking when she'd called her a copycat for buying the same Gap pants? Maybe she'd been trying too hard. Maybe she needed to back away from people so they didn't get mad at her so quickly.

Soon Stephanie learned the truth. The whispers found her in the cafeteria as she sat alone behind a crowded table: At Lori's house she had flirted with Steve. Marissa had a crush on him and was furious. Stephanie was too stunned to move.

She had not flirted with Steve. She'd never *meant* to, anyway. It was Josh she thought constantly about. They knew it! What did it mean that she had flirted? What had she done, and when? And if she didn't know the answer, how would she ever know if she was doing it again?

No one would tell her. For the rest of the year, Marissa and Lori pummeled Stephanie with cruel, invisible abuse. On Valentine's Day, they sent her flowers from Josh. When Stephanie called to thank him, he was clueless and she died of embarrassment. The girls threatened to tell Stephanie's parents she smoked if she ever spoke to Steve again. When Stephanie did well on a test, they told people she cheated. They quietly advised the teacher to keep an eye on her. Lori wrote a letter to an enemy of Stephanie's, telling her Stephanie had called her ugly names, and the girl threw Stephanie against the wall, stuck her face up close, and threatened to kill her. Lori wrote a sexually explicit letter to Josh and signed Stephanie's name.

Now twenty-nine, Stephanie was sitting on a couch in her Washington, D.C., apartment, her mitt-sized mutt, Buddy, next to her. Sensing as only dogs can that I was there to ask tough questions, Buddy had indicated we were not going to be friends. Perched on a barstool, my feet tucked as high as I could get them, I asked Stephanie how her parents had handled it. She sighed.

"Do people get upset when they talk to you about this?" she asked.

"Sometimes."

"Okay. Because I'm getting upset." I offered her a tissue, which I had learned to carry with me. The dog growled. I curled my feet tighter around the stool as I told Stephanie that my closest friends waited years to confide their most painful stories. She continued.

Stephanie told me that she waited until after college to tell anyone about her experience. I was only the second person to know, but if it would help another girl, she'd do it. "I wouldn't take any amount of money to be fifteen again. Ever," she said, settling cross-legged on her couch. "I'm ready. I'm totally ready." She continued her story.

Over the next weeks and months, Stephanie refused to tell her parents. She didn't want them to worry or to see the punishment she was being forced through. Plus, she had friends from a nearby public school, so she never seemed as alone as she felt. Instead, she started dieting and exercising obsessively. "I thought if I lost twenty pounds it would all get better, you know?" It also seemed to Stephanie that if she could hide what was going on, it would all be less real. "If you handle this enough and if you just keep it inside, if you don't actually say out loud that everybody hates me, it's not true. You know what I mean? You build the armor around yourself."

But slowly, Stephanie turned inward as her confidence and self-esteem withered. Since she didn't understand what she'd done, since there had been no fight, no moment of confrontation, she decided it could be only her fault, that her habit of saying anything on her mind was a mistake. She talked too much; she was a flirt. The answer, she decided, was to disappear.

"I blamed myself for speaking. For confiding so much in them. For letting them know so much about me," she said. Stephanie no longer trusted people. "I saw the negative in everything people said to me." She stopped sleeping. She quit the swim team after she had an anxiety attack during a relay race. She left the house wearing her new team jacket and then tried to lose it at school. She didn't look anyone in the eye, a habit that would take years to unlearn. Fearing she'd be dissected by the other girls for wearing loafers, or a cheaper brand of sweater, or unmatched colors, it was all she could do to get dressed in the morning. When her mother bought sweaters for her uniform and Stephanie feared they were too loud, she wore them out the door and removed them in the school bathroom, shivering through the day.

"I did anything and everything to just try to be [unobtrusive]," she told me. "I didn't want to have anything. I didn't want anything to draw attention to myself at all."

If she found herself having feelings for a guy, Stephanie was terrified that someone would find out. "I didn't look twice at them," she told me. All she could think about was what people would say if they saw her. "I just closed down from people."

During this period, Stephanie began remembering the month before her life changed. She had never thought twice when Marissa and Lori were being rude to her. One time, the two girls had given each other the names of girls in a popular band, but Stephanie didn't get one. The week before the sleepover, they'd chalked all over the homeroom blackboard that she loved Josh, humiliating her. "We're just playing with you," they'd said. "It was always, 'We're just playing with you,'" Stephanie told me. "'Don't be so uptight.' 'Don't be such a tight ass.'"

She recalled how some weeks before, at a school dance, a hot guy from the boys' school had come up to her and asked if she wanted to dance. "All right," Stephanie had said. "Well, I don't," he sneered, laughing as he walked away. Earlier that week at a softball game, Stephanie had told Marissa and Lori she thought the guy was cute. She'd been so sure that letting it all slide would be easier than confronting them. She had forgiven them immediately. "I just never saw the signals," she explained.

Marissa and Lori played down the prank at the dance, making light of it. "They were like, 'Oh, Stephanie, we just thought you'd laugh.'" Fifteen years later, Stephanie told me, "I remember what I was wearing. I remember what it smelled like. I remember what song was playing. I remember everything about that moment. I remember every single time I saw him after that I could not speak."

Stephanie coped by creating what she calls an "alter personality." Monday through Friday she was tortured and afraid. Friday nights she went out with friends from another school and appeared to be having a blast. But the stress at school literally consumed her from within. At fifteen, she was diagnosed with an ulcer. Her parents were astonished. "So my mother's saying, 'What, doctor, why does she have an ulcer? She's fifteen years old,'" Stephanie recalled. "'Why is she puking and why is she throwing up food, and why [are] burps... coming out of her body that smell like ninety-year-old eggs that have been cracked open?'"

Someone suggested Stephanie see a psychologist. For twelve weeks, at the end of each forty-five-minute session, her mother thrust a wad of bills at the doctor as Stephanie watched. "She said she didn't want to write a check to a therapist, because she told me she didn't want it to come back and haunt me that I had seen someone." The weekly ritual did little to encourage Stephanie to talk about what was haunting her. Nor did it assure her that it was not her fault to begin with.

It all ended as quickly as it began. One day, the girls simply lost interest. But in the eerie silence that lingered in their absence, Stephanie only intensified picking apart everything she'd ever done in an effort to understand what triggered the nightmare.

Alone, Stephanie wandered through the halls at the beginning of sophomore year. The lockers and the rug were the same, but she knew she'd changed. "I didn't trust people at all . . . if they were nice to me, I didn't trust them at all. If one of the popular girls said 'Stephanie, I like your hair,' I thought they were being, like taking pity on me, like 'Oh, she's the big loser,' and rather than just being, 'Yeah, you have cool pants on and they're nice and everybody likes them.' . . . I didn't trust anybody with any of my secrets. No one. No one knew anything that I thought, [it] like had to be kept close. . . . I remember kissing someone at a dance at the end of that year, like the last dance of the school year, and being literally petrified to the point where it wasn't even healthy, because like what are people going to say if they saw me kissing, and I don't even remember who it was. I closed down from people. . . . Even when you think it's over. . . ."

By the end of sophomore year, Stephanie convinced her parents that the school didn't challenge her academically. She asked to transfer to the other public school, and they agreed.

At the new school, Stephanie became popular so swiftly that when she told me about it, she averted her eyes as though she thought I wouldn't believe her. By the end of October, she had half the junior class partying at her house on her birthday. The change was as instant as it was unbelievable. "I didn't understand it; I didn't try. I didn't know where it came from, and I was really, you know, becoming friends with people." Still guarded, she deflected her new friends' questions about transferring from her old school with the same answer: the classes had been a disappointment.

When Stephanie was invited to a ten-year reunion at the school she'd left, she mulled it over. "There was a part of me that hoped . . .

I could show up and be like, yeah, I'm a consultant and I live on my own and I have a great life and I feel fantastic, and I love every part of my body, I love every part of my skin, I love everything I do. And you know not because I'm faking it, not because I'm pretending, but because I'm genuinely, I'm like okay, everything's not perfect, but it ain't that bad. And that's how I feel right now. And I would love to, kind of like, show it to them, and that I can't believe it's still there. That the wounds were so deep fifteen years ago . . . I still wanted to kind of like say, you know, fuck you, look how cool I am now. You were totally wrong. And you have no idea how deep the wounds were. I didn't."

Despite what happened, Stephanie told me she is most grateful for the women in her life. "Women," she said, "are the strongest people in the world. Everything we do is harder and I really believe that. I think women are incredible creatures." Stephanie credits the women in her childhood for teaching her to hold fast to her own self-worth, no matter the obstacles. Thinking often of what she "owe[s] to the girls coming after me," she volunteers frequently with children. "I feel," she said, "like I have to always work with some connection to children for the rest of my life, simply because I think it's so important to tell them our stories and to witness what they're talking about and really make them feel comfortable talking about whatever they think is important." And it's women, she reminded me, who gave her back the strength to trust again. About her best friends, she said, "I know that I could give them my wallet and car keys and my dog and my boyfriend and I would get everything back."

As I discovered with the girls I interviewed, every clique can draw its own invisible lines. Not surprisingly, it is often the new girl in class who unwittingly crosses them, triggering resentment in her peers. Listen to Megan and Taylor, two ninth-grade classmates talking about their best friend Jenny when she first switched schools.

"Remember," Megan said, "when Jenny first came from [the school] where she was, like, the shit? And she came and before she made any other friends she had already gotten this cocky attitude. People didn't even know her. We were just talking about this—remember what a bitch she was?"

"Yeah." Taylor nodded. "She had so much confidence, too. And you come to a new situation, it's just like, why is she doing that? She has *no* place—"

"No right!" Megan interjected.

"—to be doing that. I remember before Jenny came she was telling me that she knew *so* many people. She acted like she knew everything. I don't know. That made me feel like, gosh, I don't know anybody. I don't have any friends. It's like, excuse me, what do you think you're doing?"

Or listen to a group of ninth graders in Mississippi, where I asked, "How do we feel about a girl who walks into the room who we don't know and who's pretty?"

"We automatically feel a hate towards her," Keisha said immediately.

"We feel offended," Toya offered.

"She's the most attractive person—," said Melissa.

"And she's new and she's going to be getting all the attention," Torie finished.

"We want her to be less confident so she won't talk to our boys," Keisha said. "Somebody new come in, they threatened by what they are. Look at her, this and that. She's going to take my friends, she's going to take my man."

I asked, "Do girls want other girls to be confident in general?"

"*No,*" came a chorus.

"No." It was Keisha.

Why not?

"Girls don't because they're threatened by what they are."

Every class, every school, pieces together its own definition of the girl who thinks she's all that. "All that" changes meaning depending on the events of the week. The school culture plays a role: in poorer schools, "all that" is often about luxury items like acrylic nails, hair extensions, and new sneakers. In wealthier schools, it may be more about flirtatiousness or conceit. The label cuts a wide swath across lines of class and race; no matter where I went, whether or not I brought it up, it always found its way into our discussions, and to great gusts of enthusiasm.

In spite of the legion definitions of "all that," there is one bottom line. There are rules, and the girl who thinks she's all that breaks them. They are the rules of femininity: girls must be modest, self-abnegating, and demure; girls must be nice and put others before themselves; girls get power by who likes them, who approves, who they know, but not by their own hand. Break these rules, and "all that" looms on the horizon.

Here is the common denominator for "all that," the one that never changes: The girl who thinks she's all that is the girl who expresses or projects an aura of assertiveness or self-confidence. She may assert her sexuality, her independence, her body, or her speech. She has appetite and desire. The girl who thinks she's all that is generally the one who resists the self-sacrifice and restraint that define "good girls." Her speech and body, even her clothes, suggest others are not foremost on her mind.

The "all that" label flummoxes girls. On the one hand, they know it's not cool to be conceited, to think you're better than others. On the other hand, they sometimes find themselves jealous of the ones who do. "It's bad if you think you're skinny because then you're full of yourself. But if you're fat? Then you're bad," said Sarah, a Marymount eighth grader.

Our culture has girls playing a perverse game of Twister, pushing and tangling themselves into increasingly strained, unnatural positions. We are telling girls to be bold and timid, voracious and slight, sexual and demure. We are telling them to hurry up and wait. But in the game of Twister, players eventually wind up in impossible positions and collapse.

Game over. In a culture that cannot decide who it wants them to be, girls are being asked to become the sum of our confusion. Girls make sense of our mixed messages by deciding to behave indirectly, deducing that manipulation—the sum of power and passivity—is the best route to power. The media reinforces this culture of indirection, prompting duplicity and evasion in girls.

The culture of indirection reflects a desire to have it both ways— to give girls the world but keep them on a leash. It is *yes, but: yes,* you may be anything you want, *but* only if you don't stray beyond the parameters of what is acceptable. *Yes,* girls can compete and win, *but* only while being modest, self-abnegating, and demure. Go too far, tip the scales, even without meaning to or knowing it, and you may be the next girl who thinks she's all that.

The culture of indirection permeates every corner of girls' lives. Deceit is eroticized in the media, where we are titillated by the prospect of a prim facade concealing a truer, dangerous passion. Think of the mousy librarian who tucks up her hair and conceals breasts, hips, and eyes beneath dowdy dresses and chunky glasses. This is the girl who "works it," who appears sweet while suggesting the boil of sin beneath the surface. The sexually indirect girl milks the good girl/bad girl dichotomy to the bone.

The sexiest among us, writes Elizabeth Wurtzel, is "the small town sweetheart who drips sugar and saccharine for all the world to see but is in fact full of lust and evil . . . and malice and bad thoughts."[50] The erotic value of this girl emanates directly from the layer of truth hidden beneath her false exterior. It is the very fact of her lie that arouses us. As the tagline for the film *Sorority* drawls, "When they're bad, they're very, very good."

Manipulation, especially when it's sexual, is often shown to girls as the path to power. This woman can't get what she wants by earning it, so instead she deceives and manipulates everyone around her. The classic female villainess, Wurtzel argues, "rarely holds up a bank, and she gets to be seductive and sweet until that creepy moment when, suddenly, she just isn't. She is conniving and manipulative and tempting and treacherous."

Glorifying female duplicity is not limited to Hollywood. A multi-billion-dollar market that has sprung up to cater to girls has also cashed in on the appeal of duplicity. In a July 2000 issue of *Teen* magazine, two photographs of the same young teenager were displayed: on the left, she was pierced and in leather, wearing heavy red and black makeup and a black tank top with lace bra. Her hands were clasped over her breasts, lips parted suggestively. On the right, the same girl was chastely clad in a cardigan, demurely hugging her schoolbooks, a Shirley Temple smile on her face. Above the racy photograph: "3:00—THE MALL." Above the other one: "3:15—FOR MOM." The product? Jane Cosmetics' makeup remover, promising to "clean up your act."

Other advertisements portray indirection as a form of beauty. These images suggest that the ideal girl should be indirect or duplicitous. The ads help reinforce the culture's message that being too assertive is unattractive in girls. Some feminists have argued that the image of the sexual temptress is a sign of empowerment, since it allows women to call the shots by saying when and where they'll become intimate. However, the temptress suggests that female power is palatable only when it's used for sex, and even then when it's defined by insincere or manipulative acts.

jealousy and competition

The culture of indirection places a massive psychological burden on the girls who internalize it. When girls call each other "all that," they are showing us the friction produced by a culture that is confused, a world that at once prohibits and promotes a language of body and voice in which girls can be confident.

Fifteen-year-old Tasha Keller told me about an attractive classmate who triggered her clique's anger because of her forthright behavior with boys. "You see her go up to the guys and it scares [the girls]. . . . [In a movie] you see this girl going up to a guy and you've never been with a guy before. It's not like that. It never happens like that.

"They say you're supposed to get the guy and stuff, but the one who's closest to getting it is the one who's actually trying. And you're not supposed to try.

"Now that it's all about girls taking initiative and power and stuff, you get all these mixed messages. The media says girls should take control, like Nike ads," she continued. "The people on TV, they show you these scenarios, but they never show you how life is."

And how is life? I asked her. "It's this whole competition," she replied wistfully. "At school you don't have this perfect world around you.... There's so much jealousy. There's so much insecurity."

Two steps forward, one step back. It's not that we've done a bad job in teaching girls to reach for the stars. If they're privileged enough to enjoy a girl-positive school, American girls are overrun with a pastiche of powerful images past and present: Amelia Earhart, Sojourner Truth, Rigoberta Menchu, Lisa Leslie. They know women outnumber men in law school and college, that they are on the road to evening the scales in other fields. They ask, "Who will be the first woman president in my lifetime?"

The problem is with the means to get there. So fiercely have we focused on winning girls the right to dream that we have overlooked the cruder reality of what it will take to get them from point A to B and make their dreams come true. We have, in effect, put the cart before the horse.

What do I mean by this? The fear of being called "all that" and the demonization of girls who appear assertive or self-satisfied force underground the very behaviors girls need to become successful. Confidence and competition are critical tools for success, yet they break the rules of femininity. Openly competitive behavior undermines the "good girl" personality. Consider, for example, how competitive people aren't "nice" and oriented to others. Competition suggests a desire to be better than others. Competition and winning are about denying others what you wish to take for yourself.

As a result, being competitive, a sixth grader told me, becomes "a silent battle between the two girls. They don't say to their friends,

'I'm better' or 'I am competing with so-and-so,' but they kind of challenge each other, like 'beat this' through looks and actions.... They do it all in front of their competitor. That way the other person will see how great they are." Do you want to pinpoint the popular girls at school? The ones who shrug, "There is no popular group," or insist that "everybody's friends with each other" are your popular girls. As with aggression, as with conceit, competition violates the terms of femininity and so must be carefully shielded from others.[51]

The same goes for jealousy. To be jealous is to desire more than we have been given, to wish to take rather than to give. Jealousy is unbridled desire. Jealousy transforms friends into mere objects, as girls obsess over whatever part of them—body, hair, boyfriend, skin—they want for themselves. A group of ninth graders talked to me about sitting around comparing bodies during free time at school. "If we're not doing anything," one said, "we're like, 'I want her legs,' and 'I like her height' and 'I love her hair.'"

Girls are loosely aware of the way feeling jealous violates the expectation that they must be both perfect and self-sacrificing. One-on-one jealousy "bothers us," a Ridgewood ninth grader told me. "If we're jealous of somebody, I think it's because they're admirable, and maybe they have physical features that we like or something like that, and we don't want people to think that we don't accept ourselves." For some girls, jealousy is selfish, a refusal to embrace the caregiving qualities of a grown woman. "Well, I feel immature [when I'm jealous]," a ninth grader told me. "You feel like a little— you're not supposed to feel like that. You're acting like a baby."

As with aggression, girls learn to mute feelings of jealousy and competition. As with aggression, jealousy and competition do not disappear but instead morph into "acceptable" forms. And as with aggression, to remain steadfastly "good" and "nice," girls must resort to hidden codes. They learn, in other words, to express competition and jealousy indirectly.

"All that" is the hub of a hidden code that allows girls to displace feelings of competition, jealousy, anger, and desire. "Sometimes," a ninth grader told me, "I'll get angry about some little thing, and then," she said, switching to a fake-crying voice, "I'm like, 'I'm just jealous of you!'" A classmate offered, "I mean, you don't go around saying, 'She's so pretty.' Instead you say something bad to make you feel better."

speaking in code

Code words, I found, are scattered all over girls' lives. They are often used to set standards of behavior. "All that," for example, inscribes a border around girls' assertiveness. It is a social red zone used to telegraph to girls they have drifted beyond what is acceptably feminine, a vehicle allowing girls to police each other into passivity when they become too much of something—when, in other words, they become too assertive.

The remarks that earn you the title "all that" are often not even explicit: "You like my shoes?" can be perceived by the listener as bragging. "I don't know which party to go to this weekend!" is heard as conceit. "Do you like my hair?" or "Are my nails okay?"— even frequent checks of makeup or hair combing are taken as signs the girl thinks she's thin or pretty. There are cruder signs, too: the girl who thinks she's all that may dare to suggest she thinks she's pretty. She may not speak to and smile at everyone throughout the day. She may attract and flirt with boys, even the ones already spoken for.

All of this is not to say the "all that" girls aren't actually conceited. Plenty of them may be. But "all that" is less a fixed identity than it is a hidden repository in which girls can store uncomfortable feelings of anger, jealousy, and competitiveness. Quite often the distance between "all that" and jealousy is really a matter of degrees.

Indeed, the girls who get ostracized are usually the ones who have what most girls are expected to want: looks, the guy, money, and cool clothes. When I ask girls what they get jealous of, a Mississippi freshman summed it up: "Who they go out with, what they wear, how much money they have, who likes them, who hangs out with them, and in some cases the grades they get." What is "all that," really, but *acting like* you've got some or all of these things instead of just quietly owning them, in an aw-shucks sort of way.

Jacqueline, a sophomore, explained that a girl who thinks she's all that "flaunts everything. Like if she's smart, you know, she always has the answers around the teachers. She knows she always gets praise or whatever." When I asked why it bothers girls so much, she said, "Because if you have a lot of stuff, you have it.... My mother always told me nobody's better than anybody." I pressed harder. Why does it make girls so insecure? "Because we want that and we don't like the fact that she has it. We want to be like that.... You don't have to show the whole world you have good grades. That makes other people feel bad."

Another code word between girls is "flirt." You might think girls aspire to be attractive to guys, but calling someone a flirt is rarely a compliment. Many girls think flirting with a guy is tantamount to being physically intimate with him, and if a girl happens to be seen flirting with a guy who's already spoken for, her social life may be in danger.

The trouble is that no one can say for sure exactly what flirting is. Like "all that," just about anything qualifies, as long as it's with a guy. As Stephanie discovered, a girl could be talking to a guy, looking at him, working with him, responding to him, writing him a note, instant messaging with him, playing around—or she could be seen doing any of these things. The definition of flirting depends not on the doer, but the viewer. A ninth grader illustrated the murkiness of "flirt" in a story she told.

"This girl in our school, she was liking this boy. He was always coming up and talking to me. I didn't like him like that. He was my friend. One day I was talking to him and he grabbed my waist and pushed me back and pulled me and I'm screaming and she was thinking that I was flirting with him and then the next day at school she put White-Out in my hair. I asked her why she did that and she said, 'Because you're flirting with my dude.' I was like, 'No.' She went and asked him and he was like, 'No, we're just friends.' And then she apologized."

Needless to say, it is a short walk from "flirt" to "slut." Although most adults believe a slut is a promiscuous girl, often the opposite is true. The accused girl is often only assertive, not active; because she wears tight-fitting clothes and approaches boys fearlessly, she is labeled a slut. It is not her sexual behavior that earns ire, but her departure from the norms of feminine sexual modesty.

A girl who refuses to be "nice" all the time and to everyone may also get called a slut. She may flirt with a guy who is dating someone else or have a crush on a boy who is already spoken for. As Lyn Mikel Brown observed in her study of girls' anger, "a 'slut' is not someone who is sexually active per se, but rather someone who is disconnected from her partner or from other girls."[52] Psychologist Deborah Tolman writes that "the fact of girls' sexual activity is explained in terms of relationships: girls have sex in the service of relationships."[53] When a girl's sexuality becomes indiscriminate, performed to entertain or pleasure only herself, it has broken the rules.

In Mississippi, girls often used the word "skank" in a similar way. Like a slut, a skank is sexually brash, but she's also conceited. "[A skank] talks about [herself] more than anything else," a ninth grader said, imitating her: "'Well, I can do this. I can get any person.'" A skank may sit with her legs open, wearing baggy, skater clothes, or she may wear wear skintight, "slutty" clothes. She may talk in slang, not use proper language, or get into fights; or she might be excessively sexual with her boyfriend in public.

Some code words have multiple meanings. "I'm so fat" is a common lament with at least three separate translations. When I first started meeting with girls, middle-class students complained constantly of peers who overused the phrase. In fact, in a study called "Fat Talk," researchers noted that most girls who said "I'm so fat" weren't fat at all.[54]

First, "I'm so fat" is used as a tool of indirect one-upping. "Girls ask each other if they are fat, and that is a way of competing with each other," an eighth grader explained to me. "If they are skinny and ask themselves if they are fat, what does that say about me? It's a passive aggressive way of saying the other person's not skinny." In

"Fat Talk," girls described "how their friends practically 'accused' them of being thin, 'as if it were my fault or something.'"

"I'm so fat" is also used as a roundabout way to seek positive reinforcement from a peer. "'I'm so fat' is fishing for compliments," thirteen-year-old Nicole said. "[Girls] want attention." The researchers confirmed that "for many girls, the motivation in saying 'I'm so fat' is to gauge what other people think about them. Girls are really competitive but they don't make it seem that way," Mary Duke explained. "Like, 'I'm so fat.' When they say that it's because they want attention."

Finally, girls use "I'm so fat" to short-circuit the possibility of getting labeled "all that." The researchers found that if a girl didn't say she thought she was fat, she would imply that she was perfect. "In other words, saying she doesn't need to diet would be an admission that she didn't need to work on herself—that she was satisfied." Instead, they found, the "good girl" must put herself down, and so wind her way to the compliment she is seeking.

Another code word is the accusation of "copying." At Marymount, an eighth-grade girl threw out her shorts in tears after Lisa, a popular girl, was enraged by her wearing the same pair that Lisa had purchased at a special outlet. After alliances were built and the whole grade was talking, the "copier" wrote Lisa an anguished note and barricaded herself in the guidance counselor's office. I am astonished by the fever-pitch rage that flies across cliques when one girl is copying the look or behavior of another. Whether they're eight or in the eighth grade, the response is clearly disproportionate, suggesting "copying" has a hidden meaning.

Like "all that," "copying" is an accusation in which girls sometimes hide competition and jealousy. Often girls will say they detest copiers because they want to have their own unique style. Press a little harder, and you hear this: "If she copied me, people would think she looked better than me." A sixth grader explained over e-mail that "it feels like they're stealing my ideas. . . . I guess because we kind of compete with each other." The copying accusation takes a girl from being on the defensive, feeling discomfort about jealousy and competition, and changes the terms of the conflict. Now, right-eously indignant, the copied one can deflect attention from the messier feelings fueling her reaction, directing her anger toward someone else.

What about the popular girl who gets angry that a wanna-be is dressing like her? The copying accusation is extremely effective. "Copying" gives the popular girl a concrete fault to attack. It deflects attention from the real issue: the wanna-be's attempt to get into the popular clique. Because being accused of copying can be such a heavy blow to a girl's social status, the popular girl manages to defuse the threat entirely and isolate the wanna-be from the group.

girl passive

Girls are expected to be passive and powerful at the same time. I never understood this more clearly than during an afternoon I spent at a leadership workshop for girls. The twenty-eight girls were between thirteen and seventeen; one quarter were nonwhite. Standing before a pad perched on a wooden easel, watched by fourteen pairs of eyes, I began.

"Caroline"—I pointed over to a younger counselor—"is going to be Vanna White." They giggled. "I want you guys to call out the qualities you think the ideal or perfect girl has. Then I want you to tell me who the anti-girl is—the girl no one wants to be. Think of a girl you know, or one you see represented in the media." I nodded at Caroline, who uncapped a red marker. And here is what they said (boldface added):

IDEAL GIRL	ANTI-GIRL
Very thin	**Mean**
Pretty	Ugly
Blond	Excessively cheerful
Fake	Athletic
Stupid	**Brainy**

Tall	**Opinionated**
Blue eyes	**Pushy**
Big boobs	Dark features
Fit	Not skinny
Expensive clothes	Imperfections
Unproportional	Promiscuity (slut)
Naked	**Professional**
Trendy	Insecure
Popular	Dorky
Boyfriends	Unhappy/depressed
Smiling	**Masculine**
Happy	**Serious**
Helpless	**Strong**
Talking on phone	**Independent**
(has friends)	Gay/lesbian
Superficial conflicts	Artsy
(solved easily)	**PMSish**
Looks older	**Unrestrained**
Girlie	**Egocentric**
Dependent	Not social
Impractical clothes	Hard to get along with
Manipulative	**Bookish**
Sex = power	
Rich	
Good teeth/clear skin	
Smart	
Perfect	
Romantically attached to	
someone with status	

What I noticed first was how the ideal girl was *physically* perfect, a Caucasian Barbie doll: bone thin, tall, pretty, blond, blue eyes, big boobs, good teeth, clear skin—in other words, what you'd expect. Moments later, I realized that what these girls also find perfect is not

just a flawless body, but also an indirect, middle-of-the-road character. For them, the ideal girl's true perfection was her ability to hold
herself back from the world, expressing herself through manipulation.

Look again at the lists. The ideal girl is stupid, yet manipulative.
She is dependent and helpless, yet she uses sex and romantic attach-
ments to get power. She is popular yet superficial. She is fit, but not
athletic, or strong. She is happy, but not excessively cheerful. She is
fake. She is tiptoeing around the lines that will trigger the alarm of
"all that."

The anti-girl, on the other hand, lacks the ideal girl's sophisticated
indirection. She is the polar opposite of the "nice," other-oriented,
relational girl. The non-ideal girl is mean, opinionated, and pushy.
She is egocentric and selfish. She is not the sweet girl everyone wants
to be around; she is unhappy and insecure. She is not social. She is
not in control of her emotions. She is moody and hard to get along
with.

The anti-girl doesn't blend in. She doesn't agree and she doesn't
get along. Yet persistence, maverick thinking, and a fighting spirit are
precisely the qualities girls are taught to embrace in the heroines they
grow up to admire. The competing messages translate into conflict-
ing visions of the women they are supposed to become. That day, I
was confused and disheartened.

American culture is built on dual pillars of independence and competition, values that run directly counter to the passionate intimacy,
care, and friendship between girls. Giving girls a chance at success
means giving them full, equal access to the tools of the game: to the
acts of competition and desire required to excel and to the knowledge that relationships can survive them. When competition and desire cannot be enacted in healthy ways and when girls are expected to
give priority to care and relationship, resentment, confusion, and retribution follow shortly behind.

For the past twenty-five years, a growing number of psychologists
have celebrated different cultures of play and work among boys and

girls. Their portrayals carry the legacy of science's refusal to explore female aggression, and they end up idealizing female relationships. Where boys "stress position and hierarchy...girls emphasize the construction of intimacy and connection. Girls affirm solidarity and commonality, expressing what has been called an 'egalitarian ethos.'" Sadly, this work has reinforced the image of girls' lives as idyllic, free of impulses toward unrestrained competition and desire.

It's not just girls who must learn to be comfortable with competition. Our culture stigmatizes assertive, professional women, casting them as cold, frigid bitches doomed to failure in their personal lives. I want to emphasize how this particular stereotype communicates to girls their worst fear: that to become assertive in any way will terminate their relationships and disqualify them from the primary social currency in their lives, tenderness and nurturing.

As we push girls harder and expect more, girlhood's codes will continue to divide them from one another. These codes have confused, shifting meanings. They are built on a second layer of truth hidden beneath a deceptive exterior. They leave girls ever suspicious of what is really being said and who will be branded next, leaving deep fissures of trust between them. "Someone can be a really good friend," an eighth grader told me, "but she won't be happy for you. She'll be jealous. It's not spoken, but you can feel it." Friendships are corroded in the silence that is a weak substitute for what must be expressed, for what is real and human and yet feels so sinful. Girlhood's stigma against competition and desire can never allow girls a healthy outlet for their feelings or the kind of straightforward truth telling to which every human being is entitled.

It would be nice to think we live in a time of cultural transition, of flux, of a world that is learning to give its girls equality in the ways it finds hardest. But by not socializing girls into healthy, supported acts of competition and desire, we consign them to a culture that refuses to put its money on the table and wager who and what it wants girls to be. We ask them to suffer the "tension when the ideals of womanhood and femininity are those of 'selflessness,' and the ideals of maturity and adulthood are those of separation and independence."[55] Do we want to give girls the freedoms boys enjoy or don't we? If we as a culture haven't yet decided, girls most certainly have not. And if girls can never be sure who they are supposed to be, they will play out their (and our) anxieties on each other, policing themselves into the ground, punishing and bullying and fighting to know the answer for themselves.

the bully
in the mirror

Popularity, like trigonometry, was something I never quite grasped. It was like reaching under my bed to grab an errant shoe, willing my fingers to stretch out of their joints, feeling my fingertips closing in, and yet always coming up short. Sure, I had plenty of access, could count the popular girls as friends, sat at lunch and passed notes, went to parties. But there was something that separated us. It was unnamable, invisible, and yet utterly obvious. The knowledge sat in me like a sandbag. It followed me wherever I went. I was an addendum, an extra. What I wouldn't have given or done to be on the inside.

When Anne and I met one evening for drinks in Washington, I hadn't planned to talk about the day I stopped speaking to her over a decade before. Anne had been my best friend in the fifth grade, and our love for each other was irrepressible. We were frequent visitors to Mrs. Katz's time-out chair, where we nearly fainted choking silently on our laughter, squawking "Dead dogs! Dead dogs!" to get control. We named each other the Booger Twins, after the animated Wonder Twins. We passed notes marked with skull and crossbones, labeled "BBL" for "Booger Breath Lives."

Anne lived in Washington's Cleveland Park, and because of her I got to ride the subway for the first time. We spent nights in her huge bed listening to the Top Ten at Ten on the radio and days making bracelets with beaded safety pins bound with elastic. For a while that year she was like me, gingerly toeing the borders of the popular clique. Then, one day, without ceremony, she was swallowed inside.

By ninth grade, Anne, Rebecca, Sandy, and Julie were the powerful four. They were the usual: best dressed, prettiest, got the most guys. I hung out with them, as I had for the last four years. Rebecca and Anne both liked Geoffrey, a freckled, ginger-haired sophomore. One day, before the last bell, someone passed me a note. "Omigod!" it said. "Rebecca dumped Anne!"

That day, Rebecca had decided she didn't want to be friends with Anne anymore and over sandwiches and juice boxes had told her as much. Within minutes, the popular clique stopped speaking to Anne. And so did I.

I remember very little beyond that day. For a while Anne floated through the hallways, sallow and empty-eyed. Eventually, we saw her eating lunch or on the bus with other girls, unpopular, of course. By year's end, she and Rebecca had reconciled, but the lines connecting us were torn. The last time I saw her, she was cleaning out her locker. She never returned to school the next fall. Three years later, during my first week of college, I bumped into her seeking shade beneath a maple tree. It took years before we were able to talk for more than a few strained moments. Each time I saw her, I felt something curdle inside me. I remembered what happened the way I might wake from a dream in the night, in pieces that didn't fit together but still left me uneasy. Shortly after college, we both took jobs in politics and became friends. With enormous relief, I felt sure I had earned the right to let go of what I had done.

Now as adults, twenty-five years old, we were sipping drinks in an elegant D.C. lounge. So removed had I become, so fiercely had I clung to our present friendship, that I cheerfully summed up my project on girls and bullying without a single thought to our past.

Anne played absently with the ashtray. "Remember ninth grade?" she asked. I froze in my chair. As she began talking, I pulled out my tape recorder. She nodded as I placed it on the table. I listened. Toward the end of her remembering, she said, "I just spent that whole year like a *wounded animal*. Like I just didn't know how to collect myself. It was so . . . God. You just feel like you have no way to protect yourself. You feel like there's nobody there to help you. You feel like naked in a room filled with people pointing and laughing at you and nobody will hand you a blanket to cover yourself with. It's that feeling all the time, all this vulnerability. You don't have the tools at that age to pick yourself up and wipe yourself off."

There was a long silence. "You were part of it, too. You witnessed it," she said. She took a sip of her water and looked at me. "What do *you* think it was?"

It felt like someone had dropped an anchor in my stomach. How could I have done this? How could I, always the outsider, once a target—how could I have done this?

Easily.

When I pulled into the horseshoe-shaped driveway at Linden, Megan was hanging out with her friends. She waved and hopped in the back seat, followed by another girl, who slid in next to me. "Hey, I'm Taylor," she said. "Can I come, too? Cool music," she added, nodding to my Jill Scott CD.

We headed to Starbucks and grabbed a table. While they scoped out the other girls there, I got us a snack. Then Megan began to tell me her story.

In fifth grade, at her small Catholic school, Megan got into an exclusive clique for the first time. Though she loved being popular, it was hardly the paradise people made it out to be. It was work. "I always worried that they would do something without me," she said. "That I'd be left out. I wasn't like one of the main people. I wasn't the one that all the guys liked." She strove for the attention of Jackie, the queen of the grade. If she liked you, you would be safe. Apparently it had always been that way.

Megan paused. I knew she was here to talk with me about being a bully; she'd told me as much over e-mail. I stared at my coffee so she wouldn't feel self-conscious, wondering if like so many girls, Megan would clam up, deny what she had done, claim she'd forgotten, play dumb. "I was kind of like, the nice person, kind of. I wasn't really anything special," she said, beginning to backpedal.

"There was this one girl named Liane Chapin," she said, exhaling. The group had always thought she was kind of weird, and in fifth grade, Liane started acting like she was friends with their clique. "She was *such* a follower," Megan said. "She tried to be like us in every way." Liane copied them. It was annoying.

One day, hanging out after school, someone had an idea. What if they invented a rock band to see if Liane would act like she knew it, to see if she'd copy them to the point of lying? "So we were like, 'Liane, have you ever heard of Jawbreaker?' And she's like, 'Yeah!' And we were like, 'Really!'" It went from there. The girls wrote lyrics to songs, sang them in front of her, and snickered when Liane tried singing along. "She'd be like, 'Yeah, I heard that on the radio yesterday,' and we'd be like, 'Really?'"

It was a joke that never lost steam, and a genuine opportunity for Megan. She applied herself diligently, composing several songs. Jackie loved them. By year's end, Jawbreaker had an album's worth of material and a half-choreographed video. Megan was the closest she'd been to the inner circle. "It kind of made me feel like I had a more secure place in the group," Megan explained. "It made me feel like—when I would write the songs, they'd be like, 'Yeah, that's so funny!' It made me feel like, 'Wow, I can be mean, too, kind of.'"

It all felt easy, like the transition from ice skates to Rollerblades. People say you'll be good at it, but you never quite understand why until you feel yourself rolling forward. That's how being mean was. Plus, the girls never said an unkind word to Liane. To the contrary: "We acted nice to her. Like, we acted nice to her face, but we totally just like talked about her so much behind her back. We totally like destroyed her." It was easy to keep Liane hanging around because she had considered Megan a really good friend since the previous summer when they had gone to camp together, long before Megan had gotten really popular.

One day, for no good reason, Megan felt something within her catch as abruptly as a sweater on a nail. At her old school, Megan told me, her best friend, Anna, had used her as bait for the popular clique, abandoning and insulting her publicly. As she told me this, Megan was trying intently to fish ice out of her plastic cup with her straw. "It was so bad," she remembered quietly. She gave up on the ice and started chewing a cuticle. "It was horrible. I didn't have any friends. I would look in the mirror and, 'Oh, I'm just like an ugly person, inside and outside. I'm just disgusting.' Like nothing was shining." After recalling her own victimization, Megan said that being mean to Liane felt easy and hard at the same time. "We would be laughing at her, in her face, and, like, I'd be thinking this is exactly what Anna did to me, and I'm doing it to her right now."

But Jackie was the sun, and the other girls orbited around her, each maneuvering to move closer in. In the girls' bathroom, Megan and Jackie were fixing their hair. Megan glanced compulsively under the stalls and saw platforms belonging to Jenny, the second most popular, just as Jackie started berating her. Megan nodded and uh-huhed, glancing furtively at the platforms that stood still as stone. "I didn't make her stop," Megan explained, "because I knew Jenny was listening."

As Megan had predicted, the conversation triggered a six-month war between the girls, and the hostility never dissipated. Megan's silence led to a tectonic shift in their social universe. "Everyone was like, 'What happened?' And I was like, 'Oh, my God.' I could exaggerate however much I wanted. I was in the bathroom with Jackie and Jenny who were the most popular girls. That was really big." People Megan didn't even know approached her for information. "If you're involved in something," she told me, "you know what's going on and you're a part of it." Simple as that.

But the betrayals Megan witnessed and experienced have filled her with social anxiety. "I still feel this way," she said. "I'll get kind of like panic attacks. My personal thing is that everyone's talking about me, so when I see two people whispering, I'll just be like, I'll kind of read their lips and catch part of their conversation. People are talking about me. I hate it when people do things without me, and I'm like, 'Oh, I'm going to miss all these inside jokes, or they'll be talking about me.' We have another best friend, and whenever I miss going somewhere, I'm even like, 'Shit, I'm going to miss all these inside jokes.'"

Taylor, who was nodding gently throughout her friend's interview, described the surprise party she and Monica threw Megan last month. Taylor had been stealthy in the planning, and the day before the party, she'd tried to plot details with Monica during soccer practice. When Megan approached, the two girls stopped talking. Megan stood frozen watching them, then ran to the locker room, got her things, and went home. "I was sobbing. I had a panic attack. I was like, 'Oh my God, I don't have any friends.'" Taylor smiled sheepishly at her friend and rolled her eyes.

In a social world where anger explodes unannounced, anxiety is the norm and security a luxury. For Megan, the sudden, inexplicable abandonment of her best friend taught her that people and feelings are not always what they seem. Never knowing for sure if she was truly liked by others made the need to exclude someone else a fact of life. "I guess I wanted someone else to feel bad," she said simply.

It's often said that one girl alone is rarely a problem, but get two or three together and they're different creatures entirely. Because girls often aggress as a group, exclusion and its cruel trappings can be a perversely good opportunity for secure companionship. An odd girl out is undeniably so; her exclusion is made possible by the banding together of many. When it happens, all bets are off and the borders are unpatrolled. Anyone with guts can make a run for status and acceptance by attacking the designated target. For Megan, writing songs and positioning herself in the middle of a fight were chances to stand out. They were a way in and a step up. They may have been fleeting opportunities, but they felt very real and very safe.

But if the gratification is as temporary as it is cruel, it begs the question: What takes someone over when she surrenders to these impulses? What did I stand to gain when I turned my back on Anne and left her to wither?

If I had to name one trait many girl bullies and targets share, I'd say that both draw a potent mix of power and security from the close relationships in their lives. And they are terrified of being alone. When the dark cloud of relational instability dominates girls' *everyday* social worlds, the threat of isolation hangs over them. For some, it is a gripping fear; for others, an emotional white noise. It's true that popularity is a gravitational force, inexorably pulling girls into behaviors that in a normal world would seem outrageous. But in some cases, the ambition for popularity may be secondary, even beside the point. The girls I met described an equally powerful drive to avoid the desolation of solitude.

Solitude, after all, undermines the essence of the girl identity. Girls know we expect them to be sociable creatures, to be in nurturing relationships, especially with other girls. The constant sense that isolation is imminent and the ground unsettled can make girls feel desperate. Without the luxury of social security, a girl will do anything to survive at school—whatever will get her through the homeroom, the lunch hour, the hallway. Acts of exclusion in these instances assure a girl that she is acting as part of a group and won't be the one left behind.

Indeed, some girls describe a kind of exhilaration derived from excluding one of their own, which bears a disturbing similarity to the joy of close friendship. Michelle, profiled in chapter three, described the mesmerizing hold Erin had on her when they first met. Erin was like "a drug almost. . . . She says everything that you want her to say and she acts like she's such a good friend and acts like you're the best thing ever to happen to her, and you're kind of excited because you're like insecure and you're her everything. That's what people generally want to be. They want to be important to somebody else."

Later, Michelle explained her clique's retaliation against Erin in nearly identical terms. "It was amazing to be able to let it go when everybody else was, so you weren't by yourself. It was like you had control over her, which was just like the best feeling." She added, "I know that it had to do with having a sense of power that I'd never felt before.... I think it was mostly just like, nobody can get mad at me for something. I was the good friend. I wasn't the problem.... I have everything that she thought she had. It was just like a sense of empowerment. I didn't need anybody, like I had everything I needed."

Both of Michelle's accounts emphasize the rush she felt when her connections to others seemed unbreakable, when the specter of isolation was at bay. In these moments, friendship feels pure, unthreatened, and free of insecurity.

musical chairs

Lisa was early, in time to watch me spill coffee on myself jiggering the key in the door to the room where we'd planned to meet. Athletic and dark-eyed, with a ponytail of raven hair that curled and frayed at the ends, she watched me quietly from beneath a thick arc of bangs. As we sat down to chat in a parlor on her college campus, her words were as spare and sharp as her looks.

Lisa spent her first three years in school as the girl everyone pretended not to see. From the first days of kindergarten at a small Catholic school in New Jersey, she was alone on the playground. At recess she would tarry behind a large metal box and stare at her reflection, holding her coat at different angles. "If my coat touched the ground," she recalled to me, "I would be a princess, but if it didn't, I wasn't. That was my whole world. I was either a princess or nothing." Through the end of second grade, Lisa would go home after school and cry in her room. She performed poorly in class, and teachers warned her parents of possible developmental delays.

Lisa convinced her parents to transfer her to a public school, where she got straight A's and found social respite. Two years later, she moved on to a large middle school, a feeder for several area public elementaries. Barely a day passed before Lisa's stomach tightened in that familiar knot. "I saw the same stuff happening. Girls being

mean to other girls. But this time," she said evenly, eyes fixed on me,
"I was going to be the one to be mean."

Lisa met Karen the second week, when she successfully faked
needing a tissue to pass Karen a note from Jason. Karen smiled grate-
fully and passed her a note. It said, "Thanks! What school are you
from?" with a smiley face and bubble letters. When the girls sat together that day at lunch, it was clear Karen had been popular at her
old school. You couldn't deny the special electricity she gave off. Lisa
felt an uncomfortable sense of—what was it? luck? guilty pleasure?—
whenever they were together.

"I always thought she was cooler than me, and being mean was
something we did together," Lisa told me. "It made us better than
everyone else." The girls filled their lunches and study halls with
notes, gossip, giggling, and furtive glances at other girls. They
started the We All Hate Vicki Club, drafted a petition, and convinced the whole school to sign it. The chubby girl in chorus was
next; they wrote a song about how she was fat and unloved, called
her a prostitute, wouldn't look at her while she sang. The girl didn't
come back to school after spring break.

For Lisa, meanness was as much a part of middle school as meals
and morning announcements, as basic and oppressive as the stale air
and annoying tick of classroom clocks. Yet Lisa clung to Karen by gossamer threads at best. She could bet everything that others were talking about her, too. The constant hum of under-the-breath remarks
and whispers and notes and nasty looks swirled together and filled the
air around them. Even if she stopped being mean, it was clear there
would always be someone to slide into her place. As Lisa explained,
"Maybe there were twenty girls in the class, and all of them would be
talking about each other behind their backs. Because you sort of felt
like everyone was your friend, but if everyone else was like you, they
were talking about you because you were talking about them. It was
just terrible. I remember feeling terrible all the time. Because I knew
my friends were talking about me, and I was talking about them."

The constant manipulation and ganging up, the uneasy sense that
no one was who she seemed or said she was, was dizzying. In her

frenzy of betrayal and insincerity, Lisa constantly wondered who her real friends were and at times, if she had any at all.

Meanness was Lisa's social amulet. Still, she said, "the only thing I wanted was for somebody to be my friend. Someone I could depend on. And there wasn't anyone like that." In spite of her efforts, her relationships felt increasingly unsteady. "It was a time," she explained, "when I didn't really feel like I had anybody except the girls that I was being mean to someone else with." She couldn't win. No matter what, "I always thought there was something wrong with me. I felt like a bad person. I was either a dork for being the target or a mean, horrible bitch for being the bully." And anyone could beat up the dork. Her mother had begged her not to be the girl who bullied. "But I couldn't do that," she said simply. "I didn't want to be the dork."

When she graduated eighth grade, Lisa felt worn and beaten. She was convinced she was, as she put it, "a dork and a loser and a bitch." As a joke, her class voted her most likely to become a nun, but she was crushed by the prude label.

Two years later it all began again. When she'd turned down some boys who asked her out, they called her a lesbian. News spread, and Lisa felt her sorrow relapse. She found solace in writing poetry and was asked that spring to read an original piece at assembly. The next day, she was pegged a feminist, at her school the equivalent of being a lesbian. It was the last poem she wrote.

Today, Lisa describes herself as "really defensive. It's made me not willing to share myself with other people. It's made me hard to become friends with." Her first year at college, most people called her "Ice Queen" because she never told anyone anything about herself. At the end of freshman year, she met someone who encouraged her to trust others: her boyfriend. "I hate to say that," she told me. "It isn't true that it was him who saved me. It was me that saved me. He loved me for who I am and it didn't matter that in school I was a bitch or a dork. I am who I am now."

———

There is a kind of musical-chairs quality to Lisa's middle-school experience. Winners and losers are easily interchangeable, and for no compelling reason. Some women and girls I spoke with described weeks when they were the odd girl out, only to be on top the following week when it was someone else's turn. "It was all about having somebody be 'out,'" Maggie recalled. "If there were three of you hanging out, two of you would make a plan to 'go off' and just have inside jokes and tease the other person and just make them feel bad." Just who rotates into the odd-girl position is arbitrary. As one guidance counselor remarked to me, "The same girls who are ostensibly the doers will be in here crying about what others are doing to them."

Lisa's story is about the intense hunger for retaliation. The desire to take an eye for an eye is a common fantasy for many victimized girls. "For all the times I'd been excluded and cried, I wanted her to know what it felt like to cry," Emily, a ninth grader, told me. "I was so angry at this person. I got joy from seeing her upset because she had gotten joy from seeing me upset." Said sixth-grader Jessica: "I want to get back at them. I want them to experience what it's like not being wanted." Again, the punishment envisioned is isolation and the loss of human connection.

Research indicates that girls who are victimized are significantly more likely to become bullies themselves.[56] Indeed, memories of being the odd girl out figured prominently in the stories of girls willing to identify themselves to me as bullies or mean.[57] Like Lisa, these girls framed their behavior in terms of avoiding injury and maximizing security. In other words, they bullied because they felt threatened, because in their minds there was no other choice.

memories of betrayal

It was Thursday, and Kathy Liu had forgotten about our interview. Again. Clearly she had me on her to-do list between "alphabetize canned foods" and "start stamp collection." I took this as a good sign.

When she finally answered the door to her Washington home, she was clutching tissues and wearing flannels. Aha, I thought. Too sick to ditch me. Kathy let me in, smiling and apologizing. A senior at Georgetown University, she was living in what can best be described as a girl frat house. Indie movie posters plastered the walls. I'd like to say the carpet was once green, but I wouldn't bet the farm on it. It was furry, an inadvertent shag, closer to brown now. The kitchen was gnarled with hanging rusted pots and piles of bottles and dishes and spice jars. An errant Hoyas sweatshirt was draped on an easy chair that was leaking stuffing. "Sorry about the mess," she said sheepishly. "Oh no!" I told her, remembering my apartment in college, "I feel right at home."

A first-generation Korean American, Kathy was twenty-three. "So," she said, raising an eyebrow. "Do I get to quit school if I make it into your book? Make lots of money?" We laughed. She pulled out a cigarette.

Kathy grew up in South Carolina. Her parents, Korean-born, emigrated to New York following their wedding. Kathy's father was accepted to study engineering in South Carolina and upon graduation was hired locally.

Theirs was the only Asian family in the small community, and they were among the first Asians many there had ever seen. At age three and four in the grocery store with her mother, Kathy noticed the pointing fingers, eyes pulling back, nudging elbows, and whispering. By middle school, people saw no problem with making "chink" jokes in her presence. She was even nicknamed Suzy Wan at school. In the hallways, she was often trailed by high-pitched "ching chong" noises. Most people, including her friends, thought this was hilarious.

Kathy did not. Fitting in meant everything to her. She felt something was wrong with her, that she looked funny and wasn't normal. She loved going over to friends' houses and begged her mom not to cook Korean food when her friends were around. They thought the kitchen smelled funny, that the food looked weird. She hated it. Kathy was stylish and cute, able to wear, as she put it, the "right brands." She spent a great deal of time on her hair and makeup (no

small expenditure in the late-1980s South). She was second-tier popular, B-level: a hair's breadth from the top. In other words, she had
potential.

By eighth grade, Kathy had been best friends with Nancy for
three years. They were passionately close and spent class time writing
long notes to each other, folding them in funky shapes and squeezing them in each other's lockers throughout the day.

One afternoon, Nancy wrote a letter about one of the popular
girls being snotty. "I agree," Kathy started to scribble, then stopped
midsentence, pen in the air. "I realized," she told me, "that wait, I
could win favor with the popular kids if I told them what Nancy had
said." Kathy gave them Nancy's notes. The popular girls promised
not to tell.

The next morning, in the auditorium where everyone hung out
before the bell, Nancy walked in holding a few wrinkled pieces of
paper. Her face was red, her eyes swollen. Kathy asked what was
wrong, "even though," she told me, "I knew exactly what was
wrong, why she would be crying, why she would be upset." Nancy
looked at her with blank, defeated eyes.

"How did they get these?" she asked.

"I don't know."

"How did they get these?" she repeated.

Over the thin sound of her own voice, Kathy suddenly felt the
weight of the damage she had caused. "I couldn't bear to assume
that responsibility," she told me, curling her legs under her, sucking
hard on her second cigarette. "I couldn't bear to say, 'I did this to
you. This is what I did.'" All day long, people bombarded her in the
hallways, pumping her for information. She pleaded ignorance. "I
kept trying to get the blame off me, to create this phantom third
party so I could get out of it," she said, blowing her nose.

Their friendship was over, of course. "It was a complete betrayal."
Kathy sighed. "It's almost unimaginable why the desire to be popular and accepted would make me do something that's so malicious.
To betray someone so close to me." She cleared her throat, her voice
deeper. "I was—I'm sure that—I'm sure that it has significantly

scarred her." Kathy said she wants to forget what happened. "But you can't forget when you've caused so much hurt to someone."

She grew quiet. Her cigarette smoke hung in the air before us. "It is a little hard to talk about." She flicked her ash into a chipped bowl overflowing with butts. This was the second time she had ever spoken of what happened. I asked her why popularity was so important.

"I guess I thought that it kind of represented acceptance and belonging and desirability," she said. "I was feeling degraded from other instances of being bullied. If I were to be accepted by them, it would be to kind of get myself out of the degraded position. It wasn't really so much that I wanted to be friends with them. I felt like, then it wouldn't matter that I was Asian."

Nancy was one of several girls Kathy bullied. In one instance, she demeaned a close friend constantly out of jealousy over the attention she was getting. "I remember thinking, 'Why can't I stop this? Why can't I just sit back and let her have her time in the spotlight?'" Looking back at that time, she said, "I felt like there were so many people above me, to know that there was someone below me was comforting."

Kathy asked me again if I would definitely change her name in the book, and I said, yes, of course. "Well," she muttered, "if somebody can learn from my experience..."

"What would you like them to learn?" I asked.

"I guess to make them understand the impact that they're having potentially on another person's life," Kathy replied. "I can tell them for years and years I couldn't be friends with that person anymore. I was questioning my own loyalties to people. I was kind of like, 'Wow, if I'm capable of doing this, I'm capable of completely betraying somebody close to me for the possible favor of someone that doesn't really care about me at all.' I basically sold her out. You're giving up what's real for something that you see as more desirable, a higher social status or something."

The knowledge that she could so coldly hurt her friend, in spite of her values, was "very disturbing. I was old enough to know what's right and wrong. It was almost like I felt I wasn't really in control," she said.

"I can barely explain how much guilt I feel from this one situation," Kathy continued. "I don't know where to begin to make up for what I did. I always hoped that maybe my feelings of guilt would subside as time went on, but I don't feel like they have. I feel like on some level I can identify with soldiers that go back to villages that twenty years ago they had completely destroyed and ransacked, those soldiers that go back and apologize to the people they harmed, their kids and grandkids. And maybe in the future I will do something like that and talk to her about it."

A few months after we spoke, she did. Nancy was surprised to hear from her. Kathy e-mailed me:

> I lost the friendship and trust of the one person who meant the most to me. We are now friends again, but we lost the level of trust that we once had, in addition to the time that we weren't friends. What I lost through the thoughtlessness of my actions can never be regained, and if I could have understood that the state of our relationship today is the consequence of my actions, I think things would have been different. I never realized that I could potentially destroy my friendship with my best friend, and if I could have realized that, I would never have imagined that it would bear this much influence on my life these years later.

Kathy believes the experience has made her more compassionate and empathetic. Nevertheless, the memory of her betrayal has never faded. "What good does it do to say I'm sorry?" she asked me.

in control

Like Samantha, whose relationship with Annie is described in chapter two, some girls may be unaware of their cruel behavior. When I first started interviewing people for my book, I began speaking with my friends. Roma, whom I met in college, told me about being abused by one of her best childhood friends. Jane's aggression ranged from telling Roma she hoped she died in a fire to forming elaborate clubs that Roma wasn't allowed to join. Jane prank-called her, called her clothes cheap and her mother a hippie, frequently exercised her ability to turn her other friends against her, and ridiculed Roma's intense affection for friends. At the same time, Roma remembered, "She was a charmer. That was the other part of her. When you were in her favor, it was so great. She was fun and silly and just really sweet." The torment lasted eight years. It was ninth grade when the two finally let go of each other.

When Roma was twenty-three, Jane's mom called Roma's mom, Ellen, searching for Roma's number. Jane wanted to talk to Roma. Ellen explained that her daughter was not interested. "What do you mean?" Jane's mom asked incredulously. "They were such good friends." When Ellen told Jane's mother about her daughter's behavior, she was astonished.

Shortly afterward, Roma and her best friend Sally were home for the holidays and hanging out in a café when Jane came in. Roma remembered, "She started talking to Sally like I wasn't there, saying things like, 'I live in San Francisco now. Doesn't your best friend live in San Francisco?'" Finally, Roma asked Jane if she had something to say. Jane turned to Roma and said, "Why did you tell your mother that we were never friends?" She began to weep. "If we were never friends," Jane cried, "how do I know that you like to sleep with your feet above the blanket and that you don't like peanut butter?" Jane ran through a list of personal facts about Roma as Roma listened stiffly. The two women recalled such vastly different stories of their friendship that Roma didn't know how to respond.

Danielle, a sophomore at Linden, met me over lunch to tell me about how controlling she was of two girlfriends between third and seventh grade. She struggled to describe her behavior. "I don't know how to . . . explain it," she said haltingly. "I wanted to control them and who they hung out with. I wanted to make sure they were never closer to the other girls than I was. And that they never did stuff with them when I wasn't there."

Danielle wanted to be the girls' only friend, although she allowed herself as many friends as she wanted. She was afraid the other girls would be more liked than she was. "I think that's basically why I did it," she said, remembering Jessica in a low, strained voice that sounded far older than her fifteen years. "She was really nice and everyone loved her. I guess I wanted to have control over that."

Later on in our interview, which was filled with increasingly long periods of awkward silence, Danielle admitted that Emma also made her jealous. "I remember when we'd just be hanging out and people would be like, 'Oh my God, I love your hair.' I was so jealous. And I used to be like, 'That's so annoying.'"

Mostly, however, Danielle remembered her need for control. "I never wanted her to do things. I wanted to be with her doing things, like going out. I didn't want her to have a sleepover somewhere and me not be there. That's the main thing," she said. That way, she explained, "I would have someone to fall back on, who would always be there for me and never be like, 'Oh, I'm doing something with someone else.'"

Danielle lived with her parents, both professionals, in an affluent Northeastern community. Her mother and father were invested in her social life, and her dad was especially interested. She told me, "I always feel like he wants me to live through him and be more—I'm definitely more outgoing than both of my parents. So I guess they feel like, um, they always make sure that I have tons of friends and that I'm happy."

After a long pause, she added, "I don't tell my dad when I'm having problems with friends because I think he would be disappointed in me. I'm just afraid he's going to look down on me, like why are you having problems? Or if I'm not friends with someone anymore."

I had never known Danielle, normally exuberant, to be this quiet. "I look back on it now and I realize it was so mean and cruel," she said. And then, somewhere after sixth grade, she said her personality did a "complete change." It was as simple as understanding that control isn't the right way to make friends. "I should gain my friends by being nice rather than..." She didn't finish. She could hardly imagine herself behaving in those ways today, and it was hard to remember the other times.

Listening to Danielle, we are returned again to the centrality of relationship and connection in girls' lives. As the fear of isolation has fueled some girls' decisions to stay in bad friendships, here it inspired Danielle's controlling behavior. Adrienne Rich has written that a person who does not tell the truth "lives in fear of losing control. She cannot even desire a relationship without manipulation, since to be vulnerable to another person means for her the loss of control."[58] A fear of isolation or abandonment, then, may be key to understanding some alternative aggressions.

the wages of repression

"When my parents divorced, I was mad a lot," said Molly, who was sitting opposite me on the yellowed grass in the sun outside her junior high. Pale and lanky, she had a mop of brown hair, green eyes, braces, and the awkward, slightly stretched features of a girl on the cusp of a growth spurt. "I was mad at my friends," she explained, "because, you know, everybody has two parents and I don't."

Molly was in eighth grade and living in Ridgewood with her mother, who has a degenerative disease. Although her mother was not wheelchair bound, her walking was impaired and she was in chronic pain. Molly's father, whom Molly saw every other weekend, lived in another town. Her mother's illness made her father's absence even more difficult.

Molly thought her friends often bragged about their nuclear families. They talked about going to the mall with their mothers, a trip Molly's mom had never been well enough to make. Recently, a friend had a birthday party and invited all the girls and their mothers to shop together. Molly couldn't go. When her friends asked why Molly's mother did not volunteer at church, or mother-daughter activities, Molly felt embarrassed and left out. "I'm like, 'Well, that's kind of hard for me,' and they're like, 'Well, I can't help it,' and I'm like, 'Well, I can't either.'" Molly looked at me. "It's not fair. It's like they're laughin' at you or something."

I asked Molly if they have laughed about it to her face.

"I don't think they exactly laugh at me," she said slowly, thinking. "I'm sure most people feel sorry for me. I just think that maybe when I say stuff like that, they kind of look at each other, look around, just try to get off the subject or something. And that really hurts my feelings."

When she gets angry, Molly said, she tries to ignore it and stop thinking about it. "I try to look on the bright side," she said, "and think, at least I have a mother, some people don't have a mother." She listed a few things that could be worse. But sometimes, when she can't ignore the anger, she feels it inside all day "till it drives me crazy." Then she cries. During those times, she said, her father is not around when she needs him, so she may get angry at her friends or their parents. "It's not their fault," she said, "but the anger has to go somewhere so it goes to whoever I'm around."

She had "blown up" only once at her mother for the ways her disease constrains Molly's life, and especially for not having a boyfriend. "I didn't mean to," Molly said, twisting a clump of grass into rope. "Now I'm just kind of sorry I did." After Molly yelled, her mother was silent for a long time. "She goes, 'Well, I can't help it. I'm disabled. Nobody wants me, you know.'" Surely there was someone out there, Molly pleaded. "And she just sort of looked at me funny." The conflict "sort of blew away," she said, because they never spoke of the subject, or the fight, again.

In general, Molly tried to keep her mother at arm's length. Molly was always having to take down posters in her room when they offended her mother's fervent Baptist beliefs, even the Backstreet Boys pictures. Her mother wouldn't buy her rock-and-roll music and preferred to hear Christian music in their home. Out with her friends once, Molly mentioned her mother didn't like her browsing through the rock posters. "They look at me like I'm crazy. And that makes me mad because I'm like, y'all, it's just the way she is, I can't say anything about it."

Molly said she has made fun of girls over the years: "Their clothes, hair, just anything that came to mind." Afterward she'd feel bad and try unsuccessfully to be friends. Other times she's gotten in fights. "I was so mad," she explained, "and I wanted to start a fight." She threatened a girl, so they went outside, but nothing happened. Like the conflict with her mother, "it sort of blew off."

I asked Molly what it feels like to be angry. "You feel hatred toward somebody and you try not to, but it's like they've been pulling on you and it's kind of hard to stop yourself when someone's pulling," she said. "You keep thinking about it and the more you think about it, the worse it makes you feel." When she finally decides to act, "Going after somebody, you have the intention to tear into them. You build all these emotions up into this steam like you want to run that person over. And you feel hateful, you feel hate towards them, and a lot of times you want to go at them. A lot of times you can't stop yourself. You want to but you can't stop yourself. It's hard to stop yourself once you start." Like the aggression Anne Campbell observed in women, Molly's aggression emerges only unpredictably, when she no longer has the strength to resist it.

Molly cherished her best friend, but lately there had been a lot of tension between them. "She gets mad at me and I'll do anything to be her friend again. I'll do anything," she said urgently. But Kate has rarely said why she was angry at Molly, so Molly has asked, waited patiently, written "nice letters." Then, she explained, "just one day, the next day, she'll start talking to me, and we'll start talking, and it just all goes away. I don't think about it anymore."

"I can't say anything about it": these words, Molly's own, were the story of her life. On her plate were more restriction, more stress, than most reasonable adults could handle. Divorce, disability, economic hardship, religious restrictions—the list went on and on. Molly was, against the odds, trying to be a "good girl," to "look at the bright side," to care for her ailing mother, to swallow life without an attentive father, to be understanding of the disease that debilitated her mother and bridled her own life, a disease that made even things like car pooling and play dates and clothes shopping embarrassing.

Like so many girls, Molly lets go only when she can't stop herself, when the anger pops, although most times, as she said, the conflict "blows away." Her passive tone belies the truth she feels: that in fact she is not entitled to conflict, to anger, to expressing her intense emotions. Her mother, who asks Molly to empathize and nurture, cannot bear the burden of her frustration. Nor can her father, whose rare company must be treasured, whom she must please. Under these circumstances, aggression will seep through only the most permeable wall, and it is likely Molly feels most herself, and least restricted, when she is with her friends.

Molly is as passionate and fierce as graffiti, telling me hurriedly that she wants to be better than others, to be the best student, the prettiest, and "all that stuff." She has run for class president and homecoming queen (this last one is frustrating; she never wins because she isn't popular at all). Even as she told me of her penchant to cut people down who compete with her, to make fun of girls' families and friends, to spread rumors and talk behind people's backs, she told me, "I try to be nice to everyone. I just want to be everyone's friend. I want everyone to like me, and if I do anything to hurt somebody's feelings I want them to know that I didn't mean to do it or anything."

Perhaps more than anyone else I interviewed, Molly exemplifies the girl who has been taught not to know aggression, and yet is incapable of *not* knowing it. That she is clearly not a conventional bully makes her story a powerful example of how keeping girls away from natural feelings of anger can lead them to cruel or inappropriate acts. For Molly, anger is both foreign and central to her self, and the combination leaves her at once blinded and submerged by it.

When I asked women and girls to talk about times they had bullied or been mean to other girls, they were suddenly indisposed. There were closets to be cleaned, homework to get done, cavities to be filled. After reading some of my interview questions, one girl blocked me from e-mailing her ever again.

At first I thought my inability to track down girl bullies would be a fatal flaw in my research, but it turned out to be the research itself. If girls were going to such great lengths to hide their aggression, they'd hardly be breaking down my door to talk about it. Girls think being "mean"—conveying open, individual expressions of negative feelings—is just as bad as being fat, ugly, or uncool. So, for that matter, do most women. "Mean" undermines the core of the feminine identity: to be nice, to nurture, to say yes. As it turned out, I was coming up against the same problems as the first aggression researchers, who took women at their word when they refused to be aggressive under the microscope.

I can see things more clearly now. I can remember girls widely acknowledged to be bullies, girls whose multiple targets had interviewed individually with me for hours, who assure me that, "When I get angry, I'll read my Bible" or "When I'm mad, I'll get sad. It doesn't feel good to be angry." I waited for a disclosure that would never come.

The same thing had happened the first time I asked a group of mostly white, middle-class girls to volunteer stories of being mean. They'd looked at me as though I'd asked them to swallow live goldfish. The next time, I took the hint. I asked the girls to role-play a hypothetical situation with girl bullies and targets they didn't know. The floodgates opened. As long as they didn't have to personally identify as mean, they had plenty to say.

The weirdest thing was, I had done the same thing. When I first started hanging out with girls, I never identified myself as a former mean girl. My victimization in third grade was a trump card that had embedded itself comfortably into my life's narrative. People nodded gravely when they heard why I was writing the book. "Oh, of course," they said, their eyes serious and sympathetic. The truth is, I approached writing this chapter the same way I'd sauntered into that

Washington lounge to meet Anne: without a thought to my own capacity for cruelty. That wasn't me, I thought; *I* did what I had to do.
I was merely an accomplice, an enabler. I was different than Abby,
than Rebecca: *they* were demons. *They* were evil.

Then, after writing up the stories of Kathy, Megan, and the others, something felt wrong to me. I couldn't put my finger on it, but
eventually I knew: I couldn't deliver the demon. There was no evil
child here, no bad apple. These girls were good people who had
done bad things, and for understandable, if not good, reasons. They
were not the cold, cunning creatures girl bullies are so often made
out to be.

The belief that we are only targets or only bullies has caricatured
the memories and discussions of girls' meanness. It has also helped
many of us dismiss the complexity of our own behavior. The upshot
is that it's transformed "us against them" into "us against us."

By washing our hands of our own capacity to injure, we perpetuate the stereotype that females are nonaggressive. We become ac-
complices in the culture's repression of assertive women and girls by
making aggression pathological, private, and hidden. We also help silence the public discussion of the ways and reasons girls are mean to
each other. Most disturbingly, we become strangers to each other. By
leaving these episodes in the private, emotional realm, by continuing
to imagine those who have bullied us living in the gutter and falling
off cliffs—and trust me, I have—we deprive alternative aggressions
of a fair hearing and ourselves of a more honest sisterhood, because
to put it out there would mean we have to admit to ourselves that inside we are all mean, that inside we are all aggressive. And girlfriends,
we *are*.

"Oh, yeah," I'd hear in cafés, at parties, on grocery lines. "It happened to me." Nearly everyone I met had a story to tell, a wretched
moment to remember. But meanness, anger, impulsive, thoughtless
behavior—it's in each of us. Even my conscience cannot throw itself
fast enough before the speeding train of my meanness: I have indulged
in the knowledge of a shared secret, in eyes locking exclusively with

someone else's or rolling in furtive annoyance. I have said I wasn't angry when I was, then degraded people behind their backs. I have gossiped. I have relished that rush of inclusion at the expense of an odd girl out. Have you?

The question bears answering.

It is time to own our own feelings—to own up, as author Rosalind Wiseman would say.[59] It is time, in all seriousness, to get in touch with our inner bully.

When we hide natural feelings of competition, jealousy, anger, and resentment, we lie to each other and ourselves. Our friendships, as so many of us know, pay the price. When I started living with my close friend and college roommate Jenny, our first big fight swelled rotten and quiet inside our small apartment until one day it cracked wide open. "You make me feel badly because I wake up at eleven in the morning!" she said. "Your boyfriend's too loud when he comes in at night," I shot back. We went back and forth, beckoning each other toward the edge, where we finally teetered perilously. I seesawed between rage and panic. I knew I was being defensive, even irrational, but I could hardly contain my anger. "I'm just not sure if this is going to work out," she said quietly. She sounded resigned and sad. "I just don't know if we can do this."

My head felt gummy. I was holding my breath, tingling with fear. "What is it?" I finally shouted. "What is so bad here that we have to end our friendship?"

Then, abruptly, she asked, "Don't you think you're arrogant?" I froze. Was this a trick question?

"Yes?" I half asked, mental fingers crossed.

"Good," she said. "Because if you hadn't said that, I wouldn't be able to trust you."

Now we said it: I was jealous. I was jealous of her beautiful body and her irresistible sexual allure. I was jealous of her spiritual enlightenment, the ease with which she loved and was loved. Jenny was jealous, too: of my steely self-discipline, my grasp of current events. She envied my social life and my regular gym schedule.

Here we were, two young women standing tremulous before the Great and Powerful Oz. The curtain had been pulled back, and jealousy, expelled between us on the black couch, was laid bare. Now that we had confessed it, face to face, now that it had been yanked from its hiding place, jealousy was nothing special, nothing insurmountable. In fact, as we looked at each other, still sitting there intact, jealousy felt like nothing much, not even half of what we thought it would be.

Thinking back to that day, I remember the summer I learned to kayak. The guide instructed me to lean into the rush of the river's current, but when I began to lean in that first time I jerked back, muscles taut. No way: I was going to capsize. My body's instinct was to lean *against* the weight of the water to create balance. If you do that, the instructor warned, you're going to flip over.

Jealousy feels this way: that it must be sequestered, that it will be the end of our friendships if we show it the light of day. But what saved Jenny and me that day was that the jealousy and anger became ours—not mine, not hers, not inside of us as it was, silent as a tumor, corroding us from within. When we acknowledged it, when we named it, it lost its dark, baleful hugeness. We gave it a place inside our relationship, made it a part of us, for better or for worse. And we were released.

How close I came to saying I wasn't arrogant but instead humble and sweet, ever respectful of others. How easy it was to forget Anne, to let my betrayal fade away from my consciousness. Our culture has made truth telling and anger, indeed, everything that is "not nice," feel very wrong to girls. We have been taught that the right answer is the one that hurts the least. As Brown and Gilligan have shown us, it is critical that girls learn how to expose their most uncomfortable feelings to "the air and the light of relationship."[60] For at the core of us are natural feelings of anger and desire, the messy, uncomfortable truths that make us, our relationships, our friends and lovers, imperfect.

Denying those feelings locks us away from ourselves and so from

ODD
girl
OUT

authentic relationships with others. Denying those feelings doesn't make them go away but somewhere else, leaving the people around us unsure of what we mean, who we are, and how we feel. Denying them takes us to a place others sense but do not see. It is a place no girl deserves to be.

popular

I have been invited to hang out at a birthday sleepover. The girls, who are all students at an exclusive same-sex school in the Northeast, barely notice my entrance. They are scattered like flower petals across the birthday girl's bedroom floor. Each has dutifully brought a makeup bag that spills over with glittering gels, lipsticks, shadows, and glosses. Some sit contentedly in front of friends as their hair is braided and smeared with sparkly goo. They have yet to eat dinner, but a few have already changed into pajamas. Soft cotton tank tops with short bottoms that furl up seem to dominate. Hair is long and blown dry, nails manicured and polished.

After a light dinner, the girls move to the living room, where they spontaneously begin painting toenails. The television flickers and hums. Foam toe separators have been supplied by the host. As images of Marc Anthony and Christina Aguilera flash through the room, a girl chirps, "Oh, he is soooo hot!" "Totally!" a few voices rise up from the couch. An ad for a film with Matt Damon appears. "I'm *so* excited he's single again!" coos a girl who has momentarily stopped buffing.

Almost as soon as her toes are done, one girl, willowy as a reed, hops on the stationary bike and shouts, "I'm going to work off my dinner!" A few others jump up and begin clamoring for a turn. For the next hour, the girls climb on and off the bike, making sure to announce the number of calories they are burning with the regularity of train conductors.

They are nine years old.

Researchers have nailed down some broad ideas about what makes girls popular, but they remind me of my mom out to dinner without her reading glasses: She knows what restaurant we're at, but she can't read the menu. When a prominent research team observed students at an Ohio public elementary school, they witnessed the most pronounced sex differences in popularity politics. For girls, they concluded, success was having money, good looks, and "social development," which they defined as the "early attainment of adult social characteristics."[61] Which most mothers could have told them without the trouble of a formal study.

As parents with a pulse know, popular girls get maximum access to the booty of womanhood. The cool girls are the first to discover makeup and boys. They get the parents born without genes for party supervision, bedtime setting, and credit card control. They look and act like they just stepped off the pages of a Delia's catalog. They do just about everything and anything to simulate womanhood.

But here is the truth about girls and popularity: It is a cutthroat contest into which girls pour boundless energy and anxiety. It is an addiction, a siren call, a prize for which some would pay any price. Popularity changes girls, causes a great many of them to lie and cheat and steal. They lie to be accepted, cheat their friends by using them, steal people's secrets to resell at a higher social price. It is an accepted fact of life, an eleven-year-old advised me, that "if girls have a chance to be popular, they will take it, and they wouldn't really care who they were hurting."

Women have long relied upon their affiliations with others to enhance social status, and at its core, popularity is a mean and merciless competition for relationships. When women lacked earning power and equality, they were especially inclined to "marry up: to marry men who are taller, richer, older, stronger, with at least the promise of more social clout."[62] Despite the advent of girl power, many girls today cut their friendships from the same cloth. Lexie remembers the thrill of having a popular friend. "It meant so much for me and my self-esteem," she told me. "I used to drop her name in conversation with friends or write her name in my schoolbooks because I wanted people to know that Susan K., one of the cool girls, liked *me*!" Jessie Johnston, a sixth grader, explained, "It's pressure you put on yourself. I wish she was my best friend because she's really popular and that would make me popular, too." A high-school junior put it more bluntly: "You use people to advance up the hierarchy."

With scientific precision, girls track their bearings on the relational landscape. They chart alliances in professional-looking graphs, monitoring the balance of power. One sixth-grade graph I saw positioned peers along an axis that began with *A* ("Acquaintance") and ended at *BF* ("Best Friend"). In the diary of seventh grade she lent me, Lily Carter's story of her life is always told in terms of relationships. "It is really hard for me to write about my life," she begins, "but I'll try."

Today Arlyn was talking about Asia and how she didn't have her own personality. It got me thinking about myself. Julia has stopped talking to me since her Bat Mitzvah. It really bothers me. Liz is nice to me except she never calls me, I call her. It makes me feel inferior or something. Anyway I was thinking that maybe Liz has stopped being as nice to me as she was at the beginning of the year.

With relationships in constant flux, girls pressure peers to evaluate their friendships, their looks, their personalities. Emily's friend presided over a weekly ritual in which she seated their clique in a secret circle and gave each girl a grade out of one hundred. Such events are anything but frivolous. In the uncertain world of girls' relationships, the need to know anything for certain is urgent. The number may be the one thing you can hold on to.

"People ask, who do you like more as a best friend, me or so-and-so?" Ashley Vernon said, just after telling me shyly that she is the most popular girl in her grade. When she told her friend that she likes people equally, the girl replied, "Well, you gotta like one of us more. You gotta have a really, really good friend." Once, when the girl learned she was liked more than someone else in their clique, she left a gloating note in the "less liked" girl's locker. Ashley's friends compete to sit next to her, often making her pick a number; the closest guesser gets the lucky seat. "They think it's a privilege to be there or something," she said sheepishly.

In the race for popularity, girls take on as many friends as they can, trying to balance them like so many saucers stacked and swaying on a tray. America Online hit the jackpot with its Instant Messenger technology, which allows girls to exchange cybermessages with their peers in real time—actually, about as many online buddies as can fit on a single screen. Girls can have a hundred people or more on their buddy lists. They can exchange messages with five people at once, have someone over at their house, and still be on the phone, thus managing multiple relationships at once. "It's like being able to be on the phone but with six individual conversations!" crowed eighth-grader Shelley McCullough. "It's a way to extend your friendships." IM, as it's called, is dominated by girls, no doubt because it's a girl gizmo that fits their social specs to a tee. Perhaps that's why one junior chortled to me cheerfully, "IM is God's gift to teenagers!"

Lily's diary tracks shifting alliances with growing panic. "Today was awful," she writes in January 1998. "Julia hasn't been nice to me all this week and I don't know why. Julia is taking over Liz and the two of them are completely excluding me. The same thing is happening to Asia with Arlyn and Julia." At soccer practice, she notes anxiously that Liz and Arlyn are mysteriously sitting in another row. "Neither Liz nor Arlyn waited for me or Asia after the game....Arlyn turned her back on me the WHOLE PRACTICE! AAAAAHHHHH!"

Girls' fierce attachment to their friends illustrates the powerful influence relationship exerts over their lives. As they grow more socially sophisticated, the love between girls takes them into new, enchanting territory. But for girls on the popularity treadmill, friendship is rarely just friendship; it's a ticket, a tool, an opportunity—or a deadweight. You can own everything Abercrombie ever made, but if you don't have the right friends, you're nobody.

In the 1989 film *Heathers,* it is the threat and promise of relationships that drive the characters' jockeying to become "Heather #1," the most popular girl in school. Jason Dean is the dark new student who seduces the protagonist Veronica, helping her weave her repressed anger toward her friends into vengeful acts of violence. He forces one of the Heathers into his service by waving around an old photograph of her with Martha "Dumptruck," the biggest loser in school. Heather gasps. A long-expired relationship with a "lesser" person would be enough to bring her down, and she knows it.

After Veronica embarrasses Heather Chandler by throwing up at a college party, the ringleader corners her and snarls, "You were nothing before you met me. You were playing Barbies with Betty Finn. You were a Bluebird. You were a Brownie. You were a Girl Scout cookie." Without me, she crows, "Monday morning you're history. I'll tell everyone about tonight."

Relationships are the Rosetta stone of girls' social status. Not surprisingly, they often inspire suspicion: *Why is she my friend? Why did she buy her that gift? What does she want from me? Or I from her?* The popularity contest leaves many girls dubious of their peers' intentions. Daniella mused, "When you're separately with your friends, they're like, 'Oh, you're so much better than [the others], the way you do that is so great.' You get all these compliments but they're not always meaningful. Or, like, [they say] you have better hair, or you're *so* much better than they are. But what they're saying to you is meaningless. . . . it's to make you think you should go to them."

At Marymount, Emily listed some of the relational calculations she and her friends have made. "She's going to be invited to the next party, so I'll be friends with her, or I'll be friends with her because she's rich." The strategy also works in reverse. A fifth grader in

Mississippi explained, "They can act like you're the most important person and then they'll leave you. When you need them the most, they dump you....When they're popular enough, they just move on." Jessie Johnston said, "I'd rather just go around 'cause if you're in the popular group and something happened, suddenly no one really likes you. With their influence you can just plummet to the bottom."

Authentic connections between girls are the first to go in the race for popularity. Getting popular requires strategy and calculation, that affection be shown selectively, that some be left behind, that others be attended to in private, and that the rules change from day to day. "It's not a contest," warned the ad for *Popular,* the WB's hit television show. "It's a war."

friends, sometimes

The sudden loss of a close friend to popularity is one of the most wrenching and common experiences I observed. The course of things is simple enough: one girl's window to popularity opens and she jumps through it, leaving her close or best friend behind. The abandoned find themselves alone with the knowledge they don't have what it takes to be cool.

The aftermath of the change is far more complicated. The break is often not clean but gradual, and there are a variety of scenarios. Some girls are mean in public and nice in private. Others are the reverse. Some girls simply behave as though their friends no longer exist.

But when the ditched girls cling to broken pieces of friendship with those who have only partially abandoned them, they suffer well beyond the moment of initial loss. By staying friends with these girls, they learn that they will be cared for at times and under circumstances beyond their control. There is no language to articulate this behavior, and especially the confusion and sadness that result. As they lose control of their relationships, girls feel privately responsible for their loss.

As any witnessing parent knows, these are not simply part-time friendships. They are abusive. They are a training ground in which vulnerability and disempowerment are learned and the ability to identify abuse is lost. One girl described the situation this way: "It's kind of like a new friendship begins and then it ends three hours later. And then it begins the next week and it ends three hours later." But there can be little self-respect when a girl learns to be loved on someone else's terms. The willingness to give oneself over to another's omnipotence in a friendship bears disturbing similarities to the willingness of a target to remain in a violent relationship. I worry that if we do not teach girls early on to know and resist these dynamics, we may be permitting the groundwork to be laid for violence in their adult lives.

For children, there is something almost profane about being abandoned by a close friend. It undermines the few assumptions they are old enough to make—that friends are nice, that love and care will be reciprocated in kind—at a critical developmental moment. The impact of such a loss should not be underestimated.

Lucia and Haley had been best friends at Sackler since third grade, and this year, in fifth grade, they'd been placed in the same class with the lion's share of the popular girls. During the second week of school, Haley got the uneasy feeling that Lucia was ignoring her. She decided to check and asked Lucia a few times to play at recess. Sure enough, Lucia apologized and refused, telling Haley she was playing with someone else. It was always one of the cooler girls. In no time it was clear that Lucia was getting popular, playing soccer at lunchtime and being partners with new girls during class.

Haley and I were rocking gently on a damp wooden swing outside her house in the balmy April air. As she dipped her sneaker down to kick up chips of mud, I swung my legs around and leaned back against the armrest. I noticed the contrast her pale skin made against the tiny freckles pooling under her eyes. Haley's coffee-colored hair was broomstick straight, and her eyes were serious behind wire-rim glasses as she watched the mud. She reminded me of Harriet the Spy. I asked Haley how she was feeling.

"I feel hurt," she said, her words slow and measured. "I feel she's got other things to do and that I'm not as important as other people. Sometimes I just try and brush it off, but I really can't, and I have that feeling that you know, it's gonna end soon, our friendship. We never had a fight, and then all of a sudden, she's in another crowd, she doesn't care about me anymore. We stopped talking, it's finished."

I asked the obvious question. "Did you talk to Lucia about it?" Haley's eyes widened and she thrust her chin forward, indignant at the stupidity of the question. Of course she had. Lucia denied anything had changed in their friendship.

"So . . . who's right?" I asked hesitantly, bracing for another reprimand. Haley's voice tightened with frustration.

"Sometimes I know that I'm right because I know who's hurting me. But I mean, then who is? I would know who's hurting my feelings! I say, 'You're hurting my feelings,' and people go back and say, 'What are you talking about? I'm not doing anything.' That's what I get a lot of: 'No I'm not!'"

For a brief moment there was nothing but the muted creak of the damp swing. "I think that maybe I'm not sure about my feelings," she said more evenly. "I don't know! I question my feelings. I'm like, 'Is she really saying this?' Because I was really sure that yesterday she was *ignoring* me, or yesterday she wouldn't talk to me at recess or something like that. And I really question the fact."

Haley echoed the remarks of so many girls: the feeling of "being crazy," of not being able to know for sure the realness of one's own feelings or version of events in the world. Haley knew she was being ignored, yet the girl she loved and trusted was telling her otherwise. For Haley, it was as though Lucia said the sky was brown with as much certainty as Haley felt when she saw it as blue, yet Haley could not decide who was right. Lucia was pulling Haley away from what Haley knew was true about herself, her feelings, and her life, and into a place where she would doubt the worth of all of these, offering them up to Lucia for definition. Lucia had managed to hurt Haley while assuring her that, in fact, she was not hurt at all, that she was imagining all of this.

Anyway, Haley told me, kicking her legs up and swinging us forward, Lucia was still a good friend.

"When?" Did I miss something?

"Sometimes, every Thursday after school, I stay till five and have dance class till six. So I stay for an hour and thirty minutes. Then we're friends." I sat quietly, unsure what to say, listening to us swing.

"Look," she said. "You have to make very sure you're not going to yell at them for no reason, and make a mistake."

"Why?" I asked.

And here was the real reason Haley was afraid to press the case. It was the thread of fear that runs through so many girls' relationships: the fear that conflict of any kind will result in relational loss. "Because then you would lose—they would be like, 'No, why are you doing this to me? Maybe I shouldn't be your friend.' So you could lose somebody."

"They can break you down," she explained, "until you're like, 'Oh, I shouldn't speak to anyone else. I should just curl up in the corner during recess and just not talk to anybody anymore.' Sometimes it makes you think you've got no friends even if you do. And it makes you hurt other people sometimes."

As Haley saw it, she had two choices: put up with the best she can get or speak up and lose everything. Hold on to the tatters of a relationship because it was preferable to no relationship at all. At ten, with her best friend Lucia, Haley was learning to settle for much, much less, and so to feel disposable and used. She was learning, as many girls do, to carve a tiny space for herself in this relationship— in this case ninety minutes a week during dance class—where she would tell herself that she was happy, that indeed this may be the most she deserves. And she would come to blame herself for the way she was being treated.

Haley would draw the line, she said, when Lucia was no longer nice in private. "I mean, I know she's always going to be a good friend to me and that I can talk to her. It's just the fact that when we're in class or . . ." She trailed off. "I don't know. I don't know."

Haley was still unsure. She veered between what she knew was true and what Lucia wanted her to believe. "Maybe she feels she spends too much time with me, and she needs to spend time with other people. I just don't wanna—I'm just—I'm just afraid—I don't want to try it—try risking a friendship outside. I'm just going to leave it because I've got other friends." She exhaled loudly, spluttering with frustration.

Like Haley, many girls describe their feelings in part-time friendships as simply "bad." There is a hint of resignation in their voices, a somber recognition that this is the way of their world. As Jessica told me, "Even though you feel like girls only want to be your friends for a few hours, they have to [do what it takes to] be popular."

the price of popularity

Some girls can't get popular unless they pay for it. Call it a dowry or hazing, a cover charge or a sacrificial offering of loyalty: however you look at it, sometimes a girl has to squash a friend to rise above the mortals. Girls told me two versions of this story: in the first, the supplicant, as I'll call her, publicly bullies her friend while she is nice to her in private. In the illustration to this story, I see the bully blowing on a single dandelion, her friend. Some wisps of friendship cling to the stem while others flutter to the ground, leaving parts of the core bald, bare, and struggling, yet still alive. In the second story, the target is offered up as booty to the popular clique, and the shroud of friendship falls away completely.

Now in her forties and living with her partner in the Northwest, Janet says her mind wanders often to the memory of Cheryl, her best and often only friend from third through eighth grade. Every day after school, the two girls talked on the phone or played together. They spent nights holding elaborate dance contests at each other's homes, which were only two blocks apart. In the winter, they ice-skated and drew maps of the sinewy streams that ran through their southern Illinois college town.

But when the homeroom bell rang, Janet never knew if Cheryl would be her friend. Cheryl wanted to be in the popular group, and Janet, short and awkward with thick glasses, was a liability. Cheryl was bigger and taller than Janet, a lightning-fast runner. At school, she always looked right in her clothes. Around the cool kids, Cheryl called Janet names and told her to get away. She nicknamed her "Bottle Eyes" and ordered the other girls to steal her glasses. She laughed the loudest while Janet, frightened and blinded, felt her way on bended knee along the black tar playground, searching for the school door. Whenever the cooler girls left Cheryl out, she would run back to Janet, who never protested.

Janet found comfort in academic success and relied on it to distract her through the rough days. Often the only one to raise her hand in class, Janet remembers a powerful intent to be good and do the right thing. Despite her success, Janet confided that "my doing better in school didn't count in my eyes that way. She dominated me. She wanted to be in control." When Cheryl asked Janet why she'd gotten a better grade on a test, Janet answered, "I think I'm more focused than you are." Cheryl teased her mercilessly about using the word "focused." In her junior high yearbook, Cheryl wrote, "To one of the dumbest people I know. Oh well, maybe you'll grow out of it. Your friend, Cheryl." Janet was crushed but remained silent.

Eventually, Cheryl's attacks moved beyond the perimeter of the school. Little was visible to others as she hollowed out the center of their friendship and filled it with meanness and hate. To anyone looking from the kitchen window into the backyard the girls were the picture of loving friendship, while outside on the grass Cheryl dominated Janet, demanding that she obey her every wish. The murmur behind Janet's door was the familiar hum of chattering girls, while on the rug Cheryl snarled that Janet's shoes were stupid and pushed her to wear her first bra, pantyhose, and other "cool" accessories. Janet was broken and quiet, attached to and abused by her only friend.

Today, in counseling, Janet feels certain that resolving her feelings about Cheryl will help her cope with lifelong feelings of low self-esteem. Not surprisingly, the hardest part has been renaming the friendship as the abuse that it truly was. "I'm still struggling to know that it was abusive," she told me. "At the time I thought there was something wrong with me, that I deserved this treatment. I thought of her as a real friend. I thought this is what friendship was. I'm still working on extracting myself from that point of view.

"I don't remember ever thinking she shouldn't be treating me like this, that this is not what a friend does. I really didn't know that," she said. "I took whatever friend was willing to play with me. When she was mean to me I thought I deserved it because somewhere down in there I believed I was a bad person who hurt people, so if someone was angry at me or hurting me, that was what I deserved."

As a child, Janet was sexually abused. Now, looking back, she sees shadows of her friendship with Cheryl in her experience as a survivor of sexual abuse. Both episodes, she told me, deprived her of power and control. "Someone has the right to do whatever they want to me and it doesn't occur to me to say no. There is the feeling that it must be right for this to happen to me just because someone else is doing it," she said.

Janet cannot explain why she endured Cheryl's treatment in the first place. "That's still a mystery to me." Thinking of Cheryl today, she remembers "a very vivid image of her looking at me, her eyes hard and slitted." Yet she also remembers a best friend that she loved.

Janet surrendered her version of reality to her tormentor. Her need to remain in the relationship became destructive as she steeled

herself at the greatest costs to know this relationship as friendly. The
impulse of some girls to cling to a damaged relationship at any cost
demands our attention. Its link to the trials of bullying remains
largely unexplored.

Elizabeth had no trouble telling me that Deirdre was no friend, that she ruined fifth and sixth grade. Elizabeth e-mailed me that she'd like to talk, so I called her one day in Indiana, where she was in graduate school for psychology. Elizabeth said she became an outcast in third grade, though it was really only the popular girls who disliked her. Although she had always been well-liked at summer camp and during afterschool activities, she became the main target at school. Every September, Elizabeth prayed for a new girl to come to school. "It was my only hope," she said, laughing ruefully. "Anytime there was a new girl in school I would try my damnedest to sit next to her and talk to her and get to her before they did, because then I might be able to prove that I was worthy of being her friend before she found out I wasn't cool to be friends with."

In sixth grade Elizabeth had her chance with Deirdre, who slid behind a desk next to Elizabeth on the first day. It was friends at first sight, and they had a blissful month of busy sleepovers and lunchtimes and recesses. On the day of the Oktoberfest festival, Deirdre signed up to sit at a table during lunch selling baked goods with two popular girls, and their friendship was over as quickly as it started.

"She must have realized she was jeopardizing any chance she had of being popular by hanging out with me," Elizabeth told me. "She found out it just wasn't cool. She began to realize this would not bode well for her future. All of a sudden, she just switched, like night and day, and she was in with the popular girls and torturing me. She became the ringleader of the girls who did this."

Deirdre carried out flashy demonstrations of cruelty to show off to her new friends. She pointed and laughed from the lunch table and insulted Elizabeth at recess, often using what she knew intimately of Elizabeth to sharpen her barbs. The popular girls circled Deirdre like the petals on a single flower, and Elizabeth watched, stunned and silent. She steeled herself at school, refusing to let the girls see her break down, and collapsed on the couch at home to cry to her mother every night. "I had no self-esteem. I didn't trust anybody. I cried myself to sleep most nights," she said.

Once she was safely ensconced in the folds of the clique, Deirdre let up, but their group's disdain vibrated around them like a forcefield. By the time Elizabeth graduated eighth grade, she said, "I had a wall a mile thick around me. I was the most defensive little ball, no one could get into me. Everyone had hurt me. Everyone I had trusted had abandoned me and made me feel like shit. I would trust people and think they were my friends, and then they would turn around and stab me in the back." Elizabeth began viewing herself as her own twin, inventing stories about her other life to new kids in the neighborhood. "I thought that maybe if I didn't tell them anything about who I really was, they might like me."

Like many women I spoke with, Elizabeth is certain the experience permanently altered her development as a person. "I had always been mellow and easygoing and all of a sudden I was hostile and sarcastic and bitter," she said. I can almost see her shrugging resignedly through the phone. "I had never been that before." Today Elizabeth studies psychology in part to understand how she was changed and how, as she put it, "could someone do this? It's just so wrong. It just didn't work in my head. It didn't compute."

In high school, Elizabeth's sudden popularity shocked her. She was amazed that people could like her just for who she was. Nevertheless, she said drily, "I'm still reaping the benefits of all this." She has only now, in her late twenties, begun to reconnect with women. Elizabeth felt safer around guys because, as she put it—echoing countless women I spoke with—"there was no bullshit, there was no cattiness, there was no competitiveness, there was nothing." She attended a women's college to avoid fraternities, only then realizing how fearful she still was of other women. "I put myself at a distance. I wouldn't trust them right off the bat. I always felt like there was a hidden agenda." Even now she can never shake the feeling of being an "outsider, feeling like I will never truly belong and also feeling like not wanting to."

secrets and lies

The popularity race shines a harsh, relentless spotlight on its contenders, raising the stakes on everything they say and do, making every utterance and outfit subject to peer punishment, reward, or worse, indifference. A girl at Linden explained, "Girls are judging me every second, examining me and thinking if they want to be my friend or not." A classmate added, "You don't see girls for who they are. You see girls for what they wear, who they hang out with. It's a package." The feeling of constant scrutiny creates an unpredictable social landscape that frequently causes sudden changes in behavior, so that many girls become different people depending on who they're with.

Chloe Kaplan, a fifth grader at Sackler Day School, and I were hanging out one afternoon on her tall twin canopy bed, white ruffles and stuffed animals spilling out beneath us. The wall above her desk was plastered with gummy, curling magazine cutouts of *NSYNC and Backstreet Boys, and a wicker dresser was scattered with tubes of glitter cream and disks of lip gloss. We sat cross-legged, shoes off, facing each other and unwrapping sticks of bubble gum.

For a ten-year-old, Chloe had an astonishing grasp of the politics of popularity and betrayal. She learned the hard way. In the first weeks of third grade, Alisa had approached and asked to be best friends. Delighted, Chloe said yes. At the time, she told me, "I didn't have the most friends in the third grade and I was making as many friends as I could." Chloe and Alisa played and spent recess together every day, chatting, playing jacks, trading stickers, and—their favorite—having upside-down contests on the monkey bars.

Some months later, Chloe found out that Alisa had been making up lies about her and telling her secrets to the popular girls. Chloe said she felt "really bad. It was like if you write in a diary, and someone reads it and they tell their friends what was in it and they tell their friends." When you've trusted someone that way, it hurts a lot. Chloe was afraid to say anything about it, she said, because "most of the friends I had came from her. If I lost her, I lost the rest."

Two years later, Chloe was still sad and perplexed that someone who seemed to care for her so much could also coldly violate her trust. But in the time she'd had to think about it, she'd figured out a couple of things.

For one thing, Chloe said, she notices now that some girls can change themselves depending on whom they're with. When her mom, who's president of the PTA, takes her to ice-cream socials, there are popular girls there who "act totally different—like they've been friends with you for a long time," and when they see her at school, "act like they don't know you and don't care about you." She told me about a popular classmate who's cruel and critical in school, but at sleepaway camp becomes a "whole different person . . . so much more nicer there."

The other thing, Chloe told me, is that she knows now that everything she did and said was being assessed and reported by Alisa. That it was, above all, currency to be traded with more popular girls. This year, she could sense the feeling of being judged following her around like a shadow, and it made her uncomfortable. The other girls watch and talk about everything: what she eats and wears, whom she plays with. "They care about everything but your person-ality," she said glumly. I asked what she meant. Well, she said, there was a girl in her class who wore capri pants with hearts and a match-ing shirt. "Everyone's gonna remember that," she explained, "be-cause that's like baby and everything. Everyone will know that came from Kids 'R' Us. Everyone popular will be embarrassed to be her friend because they wear the updated clothes."

Chloe told me that fifth grade was a minefield: one misstep and you were done for. "If you do one stupid thing," she explained, "people will never forget that. Then they know you could not *ever* be a cool person. If you change, they don't realize it because they think of that stupid thing you did before." It's not worth it.

I asked her for an example of a "stupid thing."

"Like if you say a dumb comment," she said, blowing a bubble.

"Such as?"

"Such as if we're out telling jokes in school and everything, and you make a stupid joke, like why did the chicken cross the road, when they're making mean jokes. Or we're all in music [class], and the teacher leaves the room, and everyone's like, 'Oh, that's a really stupid song,' and you're like, 'Some parts of it are nice,' and they're like, 'Well, we're all saying it's stupid and you're talking about it being nice.' And everyone will say that together.

"It's just weird," she explained, squeezing a Beanie Baby, "because the quieter you are, the better off you are, because no one's going to find out or have rumors about you or anything. And the quieter you are, no one's gonna find out who you like and everything. And then you're better off because you're quiet and no one's going to find anything out about you. You don't tell. So no rumors about you and they only think of you as a quiet, nice person."

She placed her palms in back of her and dropped her head back, staring at the ceiling. "It's like each girl has a file, and everything you wear—if you wear like one off thing—goes in it," she said. "They don't even care about you anymore. And they throw the file away."

Chloe told me that her best friend's duplicity had changed everything for her. At the moment her capacity for emotional intimacy was deepening, as she shared the first quiet feelings of her heart, she was betrayed. What she shared with Alisa was laid bare to be dissected and mocked by everyone else. She could no longer completely trust that a friend was a friend, even if she appeared that way.

There is a movement within feminism that believes the female orientation to relationship and connection—to nurturing and caregiving—gives women a uniquely wise approach to their world. Popularity, however, turns this phenomenon on its head. In the race to be cool, some girls transform friendship into a series of deals and calculations, using relationship as much to destroy as to build. Relationship is no longer simply an end; it is also a means.

If popularity is a competition for relationships, getting ahead socially means new relationships must be targeted and formed, old ones dismissed and shed. Juliet, a ninth grader from Linden, explained why she and her two best friends used code names to describe the peers they ridiculed in fifth grade. "We wanted to be with our friends. We didn't want anybody to get in the way. We didn't want other people we didn't like hanging out with us. There were three of us and we knew so much about each other, and we didn't want that to break up or something. We didn't get pleasure out of making people feel bad. But we had to protect ourselves."

If girls' relationships are distinguished by secret telling and intimacy, the popularity seeker—or in girlspeak, the "wanna-be"—will use the accoutrements of relationship to her advantage. In a relational race, the winner will use intimacy as the mortar to wedge herself most tightly among the "right" people. She will communicate in words or actions that she can be depended on and trusted. To signal her loyalty, she may appear to abandon other relationships in her life; hence the mean-in-public, nice-in-private behavior. To shore up her position or edge out another girl, the wanna-be may have to minimize, even eliminate, the relationships of someone else; hence the tormenting and secret telling in the presence of popular girls. In the typically tangled parlance of a teenager, a Mississippi ninth grader explained, "A lot of people may really like Melissa, but maybe the person [a girl is] talking to doesn't like [her]. To keep friends with both of them, she talks bad to the one who doesn't like [Melissa]."

In friendship, girls share secrets to grow closer. Relational competitions corrupt this process, transforming secrets into social currency and, later, ammunition. These girls spread gossip: they tell other people's secrets. They spread rumors: they invent other people's secrets. They gain calculated access to each other using intimate information.

Despite their dreams of glory, plenty of wanna-bes still fear direct conflict. A girl who, like Plunkett of Tammany Hall, "seen her opportunities and took 'em" is equally likely to abandon her lower-status friends without explanation. Rather than face an uncomfortable conflict where she has to announce her intention to move up and on, the wanna-be may assure her old friends that nothing at all is wrong; hence, Lucia's repeated assurances and Haley's feeling of craziness.

Girls bullied by their best or close friends often find themselves in these situations. Many parents have asked me to decipher the power these girls exercise over their daughters. The only answer I have is the one the girls give me: the bully controls her target by controlling her version of events. For instance, when Michelle protested Erin's behavior, Michelle was told that she was almost always wrong, that it really happened this way, or not at all. "She would always get mad," Michelle recalled. "If you were mad at her about something, she would turn it around so that it was your fault. It would always be my fault, my fault, my fault."

When I suggested to Natalie that she confront Reese, Natalie retorted, "When you talk to her, she'll tell you a different story, and she's going to have all these explanations that make sense to you!" For these girls, it feels easier to believe someone else's story rather than their own. If they can know themselves as at fault and in need of forgiveness, they can continue to believe in the relationship rather than feel that they have been cast out of the circle of friendship.

the truth about popularity

It may come as a surprise, but once a girl gets her coveted status, popularity is no walk in the park. Competition and insecurity are rampant. When popular girls talk about their social lives, many of them talk about losing themselves. Their feelings closely mirror the symptoms psychologists associate with girls' loss of self-esteem.

Corinna, a sixth grader, was devastated when she lost one of her close friends to the popular clique. The girl and her new friends would "talk and walk very close together, and if one of their other good friends said hi, they won't, they don't, they can't hear," she remembered. Corinna set out to be included in the popular group and eventually won her way in. Once she was the one excluding her other friends from the popular crowd, Corinna felt dislocated and strange. "I know that I am kind of excluding [my other less popular friends] and I don't want to do that. But I feel like it's literally a bubble or something, and you get sucked in and then when you go out and stuff, it's just like so weird." She paused. "It's like, you go in, it's like, all of this talk and I don't know what else. They talk about boys and all these things. They have inside jokes that I don't really get."

I asked what it felt like inside the bubble.

"It kind of feels good because I'm like included, but then again I know these aren't the best friends for me," she explained. Here Corinna echoes the observations of Lyn Mikel Brown and Carol Gilligan: she has sacrificed her connection to her true feelings in order to remain in less authentic relationships with others.[63] In the process, she becomes disconnected from herself.

"I belong but I don't belong," she continued. "I fit into a lot of groups but I'm not part of any group. I'm walking around alone at recess. Sometimes I feel like I have so many friends but sometimes I feel like I have none, and everyone likes me or maybe they're just being nice." And sometimes, she said later, "sometimes I'll get sad and go into a shell even though I'm a happy-go-lucky person."

At Linden, Alexis, an extremely popular freshman, confided how hard it can be to keep up with other girls. "You don't trust anyone. You're totally insecure. To everyone you look fine, but it's very fake." Her friend Sarah agreed. "Are you my friend because of me or because I know this guy? False friendships are kept up for image all the time."

Now a sophomore, Lily Carter told me, "It takes so much more effort to be a part of that group than not to because when you're in that group it's so intense. It's like every second of every day you have to be perfect. You need to be perfect, your makeup needs to be perfect, you need to be wearing the perfect clothes. Your whole presence needs to be perfect, the way people look at you, the way you look at yourself. You know, I mean, what you say, everything you say, how the guys treat you, everything has to *be perfect....*[The hardest part] is that you're not perfect. That you're not doing everything perfectly. And that one day, you're going to wake up and you're just not going to be popular. And you're not going to have those friends anymore."

The closer they edge toward the center of the clique, the more some girls are urged to silence their own authentic voices. A few spoke to me wistfully of wanting to appear less "hyper," while some mentioned friends who warned that boisterous play was inappropriate and unattractive. These girls feel like they are no longer entitled to "be myself."

Heathers was the first in a string of movies depicting the clandestine politics of popular girl cliques. By the late 1990s, however, something had changed. A new fairy tale was being spun, and this time the prince was beside the point. In films like *She's All That* and *Cruel Intentions,* the romance was with popularity, the transformation of the girl from school geek to clique goddess. Popularity became so popular that it got its own show on the WB channel. In the film *Jawbreaker,* Courtney is part fairy godmother and mostly witch as she offers Fern the chance of a lifetime: "You're nothing. We're everything. You're the shadow, we're the sun. But I'm here to offer you something you never dared dream of. Something you were never meant to be. We're going to make you one of us. Beautiful and popular."

For better or worse, popularity is accepted by researchers and schools alike as a tool children use to group themselves socially. But the sheer volume of incidents of aggression spawned by the race for popularity deserves a closer investigation. Why is it so many of us are well trained to spot destructive images portraying girls as thin and beautiful, but we overlook the subtext of the race for popularity: that girls must be liked, even worshiped by their peers, often at the expense of authentic relationships? If some girls who want to be skinny starve themselves, some girls trying to be popular destroy one another. This makes popularity, and the race for it, as dangerous an issue for girls as weight, appearance, or sexuality.

When the politics of popularity devastate girls' relationships, the loss is multilayered. A girl is abandoned by someone she loves and trusts. The loss signals her low social value, an event that shrinks her self-esteem and for which she blames herself. She learns a new, dark understanding of relationship as a tool. And where the abandonment is public and followed by cruelty, there is public scorn and shame. For the newly popular girl, there is the danger of losing herself as she moves on and up into the "bubble."

The rules of popularity require that the girl who has arrived police herself as harshly as others do to maintain her status. The myth that popular girls are blissfully content couldn't be more wrong. The closer you get to the epicenter of popularity, the more perilous it gets. "Even though it looks secure, it's the most insecure thing in the world," Erin told me. "Everything changes in there. You compete with those five people every day: who does things first, who looks the best. It's hard and competitive. There's so much insecurity and fighting because you're selfish."

Lounging in a circle, sixteen eighth-grade girls were speaking informally with me about the feeling of being judged by others. Leslie, lying on her back, head propped up under clasped hands, had had it with me. I could tell. If her brown eyes rolled any higher they would disappear. She rocked her body up, exasperated. "Look, we can't stop talking about each other, okay?" she said. "We're addicted! As soon as we walk out of this room we're going to talk about what everyone said."

Bronwyn, a popular girl who had been sitting quietly for thirty minutes, finally raised her hand. "I just wish that people wouldn't judge each other, saying this person's not good enough. I hang around some people who just sit there and make fun of what people wear. I sit there and listen to it because I consider them my friends, but it bothers me. If they talk about other people, what are they saying about me?"

No one answered. They were thinking.

resistance

For some girls, silence and indirection are neither attractive nor an option. They are instead signs of weakness. I found this to be true especially among the girls I met whose lives were marked by oppression. For them, assertiveness and anger were tools of spiritual strength. These young women might encounter the misogyny of families and neighbors, the racism of teachers, and threats of violence in their neighborhoods. Where economic struggle and disenfranchisement prevail, self-assertion and aggression become as much a part of the social landscape as playgrounds and ice-cream trucks. In this world, silence can mean invisibility and danger.

Lyn Mikel Brown and Carol Gilligan have found that girls on the margins of their school communities, whether because of race or class, "were more likely to stay in touch with their thoughts and feelings and to have close, confiding relationships."[64] Researchers studying the self-esteem and emotional health of some working-class girls and girls of color report findings that run directly counter to the signs of loss so epidemic in white, middle-class girls.

Indeed, the now-famous American Association of University Women's 1990 report on girls found that black girls scored highest on self-esteem measures throughout adolescence.[65] In interviews with urban adolescents, psychologist Niobe Way discovered a unique tendency to "speak one's mind" in relationships. The girls she interviewed, who came from predominantly working-class African American families, described relationships empowered, not dissolved, by conflict.[66]

These girls are exceptional. The heart of their resistance appears to be an ease with truth telling, a willingness to know and voice their negative emotions. When girls make a choice to value their emotions, they value themselves. They tell the truth because their survival may depend on raising their voices in a hostile culture.

How might the face of girls' anger take on a different appearance, and why? Not all girls resort to alternative aggressions as a primary means of releasing negative feelings. In this chapter, I explore the use and origins of truth telling as a means of resisting silence and oppression. I conclude with the story of a target of bullying, whose despair prompted her to fight back.

My own white, middle-class background made me especially aware of my difference when I spoke with girls in less-privileged communities. At times, I was positively floored by some girls' courage and outspokenness, which felt so different from my own. In spite of this, I repeated to myself—and now share with you, the reader—the words of bell hooks, who cautions us to avoid romanticizing the truth telling of African American girls. Truth telling and assertiveness, she argues, are "not necessarily traits associated with building self-esteem. An outspoken girl might still feel worthless because her skin was not light enough or the right texture."

hooks urges us to remember that "[t]here is no one story of black girlhood."[67] Indeed, now that the white, middle-class experience is being dislodged as the exclusive model for research, it is especially important to heed hooks's words. To imagine a universal minority female experience would be to repeat exclusive patterns of research. Girls from all walks of life have different experiences. Not all white, middle-class girls avoid conflict, and not all other girls embrace it. Every child is her own person, with her own unique set of life circumstances.

Indeed, dominant middle-class notions of femininity are foreign to the experience of many white girls. "I know where I come from," writes author and essayist Dorothy Allison, "and it is not that part of the world."[68] Research confirms that some working-class white children are socialized by their parents to use physical aggression to protect themselves from peers. After spending a year in the working-class Maine town of Mansfield, Lyn Mikel Brown noticed how the girls she studied resisted some aspects of the middle-class model of femininity while embracing others.

> Although these girls are care-givers and nurturers, they reveal, often with pride, that part of themselves that is outspoken and direct, that knows and expresses deep, passionate anger, even that part of themselves prone to uncontrollable rage....While their experience of themselves and their perception of relationships contest the selflessness and purity typically associated with white middle-class notions of motherhood and femininity, care-taking, nurturance, and responsiveness hold a central place in their lives.

Although Brown would find, as I did, many working-class girls who were unwilling to bring anger into their close relationships, she concludes that "they do so, not because anger is a culturally inappropriate emotion, but because they need their friends."[69] The Mansfield girls at once appreciate and elude anger, presenting an alternative picture of girls' relationship to aggression.

getting physical

The e-mail came a few days after the 2000 New Year. "I am a Caucasian female who often experienced physical confrontations by African American and Mexican American females. *I was not the aggressor.* I protected myself and my two sisters were always looking out for me. We did not tolerate any crap, we knocked the shit out of these girls. Do not get me wrong, though, I never looked for, or wanted to fight."

Bonnie was twenty-eight and studying at a midwestern university for her master's in social work. "I was in so many fights," she wrote in her e-mail, "that I was expelled from the entire county school district. Basically my high school education was ruined. I finally graduated with a GED from the Job Corps in 1989." The youngest of three girls and a boy, she grew up in rural Southern California. Shortly after her brother died, the family moved to a working-class neighborhood in San Jose, "a suburb-city," she noted, "but it certainly didn't seem like [a suburb] to me."

The family was raised by Bonnie's mother, a survivor of multiple violent relationships with men, including a husband who beat Bonnie and her sisters. When Bonnie began her freshman year, her two sisters were already upperclassmen. They were everything to her. If anything truly anchored Bonnie during this stormy time, it was the almost religious devotion the sisters had to one another. "If there was some sort of crisis," she explained, "we would always know about it and be right there for each other. . . . We were very tight. No matter how angry we were." She recalls one sister as a guardian angel. "She would appear at these strange moments when I was in trouble."

Bonnie's new school was a confusing patchwork of the cliques and fervent musical subcultures that marked 1980s America. African American students were embracing hip-hop, while Bonnie was swept up in the culture of Lita Ford–style rock and roll. Pictures show Bonnie's hair blond and feathered back, her Levi's tight and tapered down the leg. She struggled through her first year, and by January was failing nearly all of her classes. She was cutting school more than she attended it.

Bonnie clashed often with her African American peers. Nasty looks were exchanged in the halls, insults were traded about clothing and style. Remembering the hostility, Bonnie was unrepentant about her own role in the conflicts, refusing to take responsibility for provoking anyone's anger. "I never considered myself to be a bully," she insisted, "or someone that would harass or assault anybody, although if someone assaulted me, I was going to protect myself and what I perceived as my own honor."

Bonnie does concede that her social skills weren't great, but she is quick to point out that she prized friendship above all else. "That was one of the things we prided ourselves on—making friends. Being accepting of others," she said. "I wasn't lacking in the fact that I knew how to treat people, and that you don't hit people unless you expect to be hit back."

One day, along the south side of the school, the rock-and-roll and heavy-metal crowd mingled on their part of the block, colonizing their patch of curb. An acquaintance of Bonnie's ran up, breathless. She had turned away an interested African American boy, and another girl who had been interested in him, also African American, was angry.

Twenty minutes later, the girls saw a crowd of African American girls coming toward them up Elm Street. "White trash!" they shouted. One of the girls came dangerously close to Bonnie. She told me she still can't remember who grabbed who first. "I think it was us—we grabbed her and threw her on the ground and jumped on top of her." A melee ensued. Bonnie looked up and saw one of her sisters surrounded by three girls, one of whom began swinging.

Once again, she couldn't remember what came next. "I went blank. I must have flipped out," she told me. "My friend said I threw the girls up against fences and went crazy."

Bonnie was expelled and sent to another high school. She could return to her old school if she went without a fight for six months. At the new school, determined as she was to return to her sisters, there were more fights. Bonnie was sent to yet another school for troubled youth, or, as Bonnie put it, "where all the fuckups went." Bonnie grew angrier and skipped even more school.

Cat had been Bonnie's best friend for two years. Pugnacious, rowdy, and an inveterate rule breaker, Cat inspired suspicion in everyone around her. Bonnie was no exception, not least when she finally got her first serious boyfriend. "I said, 'You can do anything you want. You can have anyone you want, but don't fuck with me and don't fuck my boyfriend.' . . . I said, 'Listen to me. You sleep with my boyfriend, I will kick your ass. I will do this to you.'"

When she heard that Cat had hooked up with her boyfriend, Bonnie marched up to Cat in the hallway at school. "I didn't want to," Bonnie told me, "but people had known that I said that, and I had a reputation to protect. I was forced to. I had no choice but to put my hands on her. I said, 'What the fuck do you think you're doing? I don't even want to kick your ass and now I have to.'" Bonnie led her off school property to avoid further disciplinary action.

"I knew if I didn't, people were going to lose respect for me," she said, "and that opened me to more potential threats, disrespect. I told her straight out, over and over again, 'Don't do this or these will be the consequences.' I guess," she added, probably for my sake, "I was being a bully but in a way I was showing consequence to her."

Bonnie knew if she didn't fight Cat, she would disgrace her sisters' reputation, something she could not live with. "We had a real reputation for not taking anyone's shit," she explained. "If I would have backed down, everyone would have felt free to walk all over us." Bonnie stood opposite Cat, having repeated for the last time the terms of the deal. Cat had broken the rule. Bonnie grabbed Cat and punched her in the chest. Cat didn't move. Bonnie punched her four or five times, in the arm, in the stomach. Cat fell limply on the ground and lay there silent, refusing to fight.

"Don't you get it?" Bonnie yelled. "You do this, and this is what happens. I *told* you."

Cat didn't answer.

"I didn't want to hurt her," Bonnie said, "but I felt like I was in too deep."

Where many white, middle-class girls dispense justice in covert

ways, Bonnie described a world in which anger and vengeance are in-
scribed deeply into the school culture. Here, aggression is not ignored or avoided but is a tool used to confer or maintain social
status. Moreover, conflict for Bonnie and her sisters was an essential
part of preserving their dignity.

Bonnie's comfort with physical aggression was the product of a life
of struggle, including a childhood spent in a home marked by family
violence. Her defiance of feminine social norms was not a matter of
conscious, political resistance. Her ferocity was balanced by a cautious, at times socially avoidant, personality. She told me, "It's hard
when someone's not there for you, when you hardly ever need
anybody. I'm very independent-minded, strong. Very much do-it-
myself. I won't introduce myself to you. I won't show you who I am
and I won't be honest. . . . I see people very clearly sometimes. I see
people the way I do because I've been conditioned. I've lived in a
hostile environment and I can recognize potential threats."

Bonnie's self-imposed isolation has been observed in some
working-class girls and girls of color, especially those who feel showing emotion or vulnerability is a sign of weakness. "Even among
those who feel more free to express their anger, power, or sexual interest," write Jill McLean Taylor and her colleagues, "the overriding
move is to 'stay to myself,' 'not talk to anybody,' 'keep my feelings
bottled up,' and 'not tell anybody about anything.'"[70] Long-term
isolation can impede cognitive and emotional development.

keeping it real

Waiting outside Ridgewood Junior High for my next interview, I
noticed a tall, thin African American girl sitting bone straight on a
stone bench by the main doors. She was so still I could hardly see
her breathing. It was twenty minutes after the last yellow bus had
pulled out of the parking lot. A white pickup truck approached,
stopping in front of the main doors and raising orbs of milky brown
dust. An elderly African American woman emerged. She was stately

and gray, regal looking. She strode toward the girl on the slab, rais-ing a thick arm.

"I *told* you, girl, whenever anyone hits you, you hit 'em back! You should have took off your sneaker and hit her in the face!" The girl stared straight ahead as her grandmother swished past through the school's main doors. The passenger door of the truck swung open and another girl hopped out. She ran toward the first girl, shouting, "I'm gonna get her! I'm gonna get her!"

"You're going to get me *expelled*!" the tall girl cried, suddenly standing. "Is that what you want?"

"Then after school," she replied, winded, "when it's nobody's business."

The tall girl sat back down on the bench, mouth pursed in defi-ance, tapping her sneaker. The girls' soccer team was trickling into the parking lot, and I barely noticed the assistant principal, Pam Bank, suddenly standing next to me. She apologized for being late and jerked her head over at the sisters, now silent. "She tried to beat up the sister of the boy who was pickin' on her brother. She got the shit beat out of her, and she wants to fight again. I told her, girl, you got your shirt torn off!"

The front door swung open and the principal, pale and wispy as his combover, moseyed out, followed by Keisha, a frequent contrib-utor to my freshman group discussions. Buxom and strong, Keisha was dressed stylishly in black capris and a purple button-down shirt with matching sandals, one of which she was carrying in her hand. She was walking the way my grandmother always tells me to, chest forward, shoulders back.

"That's the girl who beat her up," Pam whispered.

Keisha followed the principal to a sedan and opened the passenger door as though she had done it before.

Pam sighed. "He's taking her home."

I met Keisha during my first week at Ridgewood. She seemed to love our group discussions, and she filled the room with laughter and stories. Her group, a random mix of girls from driver's education and study hall, was mostly African American. In response to the question, "When you are mad at someone, do you tell them about it?" she did not hesitate. "I do," she said. "I do let her know. If I'm sad, I'm going to act sad. I'm not going to put on a fake smile and walk around like everything's perfect every day. If I'm sad, don't talk to me. Be warned."

"Yeah, you better not!" her friend Brittney confirmed, snickering and pretending to cower.

"Yeah, if I'm mad at you, I'll tell you what you did," Keisha continued. "I'm not going to keep it back. That would be childish, just to sit there and be mad at someone and not even—I mean, I don't know." Many of the girls nodded. When I asked them where they learned to confront the people that upset them, nearly all of them responded, "My mother."

African American mothers are renowned for their determination "to mold their daughters into whole and self-actualizing persons in a society that devalues black women." Research indicates that many parents socialize their daughters to use independence and self-confidence as a means to resist the oppression likely to touch their lives. Scholar Janie Ward observed that "parents provide their children with ways of thinking, seeing, and doing," a "psychological script" that is transmitted intergenerationally and intended to empower offspring. Girls learn to expect to work and use education to attain power.[71]

These mothers "know that if daughters fit too well into the limited opportunities offered black women, they become willing participants in their own subordination." Like some working-class girls, black girls may learn to walk a fine line between fitting in and speaking up. Ward also found that significant numbers of African American parents used personal experiences and feelings to introduce their progeny to the problems of racism. In one example, a parent told a researcher, "I don't teach it's an even playing field, all men are created equal, do what's right and you will be treated fairly."[72]

African American families typically enjoy extended kin networks; some children have "othermothers," women who share in child-rearing responsibilities. These women live out a "more generalized ethic of care where black women feel accountable to all the black community's children."[73] When a freshman at Clara Barton told me about trying to ignore a problem with a girl who was bothering her, her cousin Tanya wouldn't have it. "My cousin will be like, '*Tell her!*' You'll be like, 'No, I don't want to, I don't want to.' She'll be like, 'Tell her.' Then your cousin will come up and say, 'If you don't tell her, I'm gonna beat your behind.'"

The older women in her life, she explained, "tell you you're supposed to do it like this, do it like that. They just trying to teach you because out here it's like a game. It's just a big game. You got to play. You got players in the game. And the game is a player's game."

Such marked differences in parenting practices distinguish the socialization of some black girls in at least two important ways from many of their white, middle-class counterparts. First, psychologists have linked the withering of girls' self-esteem to an avoidance of authentic relationships and feelings. Many African American parents, however, are apparently blunt about the pain and anger they have felt as black citizens. As a result, their daughters are in some senses shielded from the "idealized relationships" that signal the onset of a girl's alienation from her true self. Instead, many girls are urged to confront the realities of human behavior, especially aggression.

Second, the everyday threats of racism and oppression make it unsafe for some girls of color to put relationships first and be "nice" to everyone. The African American girls I met, from the middle and working class, used their own language to set boundaries between themselves and others and so resisted creating the social conditions that end up damaging many girls' friendships. In groups and private interviews, they differentiated between "friends," peers they trusted and were committed to, and "associates," or acquaintances. They used the words to demarcate clearly who was deemed trustworthy and who wasn't. On the other hand, like Brown and Gilligan, I heard white, middle-class girls "distinguish between 'real, real good' friends, those they could trust not to whisper or talk about them behind their backs, and 'just' friends"—those who might.[74]

The concept of "associates" clarifies the status of those girls who have yet to prove themselves as true friends. It rejects the expectation that a girl must be everyone's friend, that she ought to be nice and accept everyone she meets. "Associates" empowers a girl by allowing the choice, rather than the assumption, of a relationship.

African American girls made further distinctions between associates and girls who are two-faced, that is, those who lie or are otherwise duplicitous. For some girls, being exposed as two-faced can be grounds for a confrontation. Where white girls often felt resigned about the frequency of behind-the-back whispering—"As soon as we walk out of this room we're going to talk about what everyone said!"—many African American girls spoke in unequivocal terms about avoiding relationships with such individuals and about having been raised by their mothers to do so.

When I talked with Danielle, a freshman at Clara Barton, she told me it's important to confront someone who is talking behind your back. "I learned that from the streets. I was raised in . . . two projects. In both places you got to learn how to stick up for yourself. You can't let people push you down. Supposed to tell people how you feel." A black fifth grader in Ridgewood told me when she hears someone is talking about her, "I'll say, 'If you have something to say, say it to my face.'"

Other girls referred to two-faced behavior as a deal breaker in a friendship, or a red flag. Tamika, a sixth grader, said, "If you have to act two different ways to be yourself, then your friends aren't your friends." Evelyn, her classmate, agreed. "I don't want to be her friend anymore." Chanel, a Ridgewood freshman, remarked, "When a girl goes behind another girl's back, that other girl don't know what the other girl is saying about her. When a girl goes behind another girl's back, I think it's to steal her boyfriend or do something to hurt her real bad."

Finally, African American girls from different class backgrounds commonly referred to trustworthy, true friends as "real." Someone who is real will never be two-faced but will always bring a problem directly to you for resolution.

Many of the African American girls I met demonstrated the effectiveness of developing a vocabulary for girls' relationships. They provided a glimpse of an alternative scenario for girls, one in which relationship may be chosen and the need for aggression acknowledged. A shared language anchored the girls as they negotiated their increasingly complex relationships, giving voice to the betrayals that are so often swept under the rug. In addition to the cultural permission that enabled them to express overt aggression, language acted as an additional buffer to the social pressure that would move these girls into false, conflict-free connections with others. Language helped girls stay with their feelings simply by providing a means to communicate them.

In some urban Hispanic and black communities, the language of relationship is common. Losing or avoiding a conflict can brand a girl a "punk," leaving her exposed to further violence. "Punking out" means choosing not to fight back when attacked, which is "staying hit," a cardinal sin in some households. "I believe if a girl hits me," Nydia, a Puerto Rican sophomore, told me, "I'm not going to stay hit. If I do stay hit, everybody's going to think that they could tease me." Lauren, a black sixth grader at Ridgewood, explained, "Sometimes people will call you, they'll say, 'Oh, you're so ugly.' You can't just say, 'Well, thank you very much.' You have to say, 'Okay, your mom's so fat she can't fit in the doorway of her car!'"

Fifteen-year-old Jacqueline Ruiz, a Puerto Rican freshman at Sojourner Truth, said a punk "don't speak up for herself. She doesn't think. She doesn't stick up for herself. Somebody's yelling at her or cursing at her, she'll just stay really quiet all the time." Although Jacqueline sometimes felt the impulse to avoid confrontation, she had concluded she was better off being direct in the long run. "What

I learned through experience," Jacqueline explained, "is that you have to say it, and there are ways of saying it. If you attack the problem when it starts, you can avoid future problems. By not saying anything, people call you a punk or you feel like a punk because you don't never say anything to that person and she continues doing what she does. That just makes everything worse."

when cultures collide

An awareness of their feelings, the ability to distinguish between levels of relationship, and a willingness to speak out do not necessarily insulate black, urban, or working-class girls from losing self-esteem at adolescence. Nor do they refrain from alternative aggressions. Researchers point out that "[b]eing able to speak out in some situations, however, did not necessarily suggest a confidence or willingness to speak out in all relationships."[75] For instance, high-achieving African American girls can dissociate psychologically and become silent as they move deeper into mainstream white academic culture, attempting to avoid raising the ire of others who might resent their success. Other black girls may resort to a self-destructive form of resistance, in which a girl's outspoken behavior endangers herself and her future.[76]

The middle-class African American girls I met reported difficulties thriving in a white social universe. With uncanny regularity, girls confided frustration when their attempts at truth telling were rebuffed and even punished. "I'm trying to tell the truth," Michelle explained to me in one such instance, "but they think I'm a bitch." These girls struggle in a social desert between "nice," where no anger is shared, and "bitch"; they inhabit female identities of assertiveness and truth telling, identities that the culture, and consequently most girls, pathologize as "mean," "bitchy," or "skanky."

Some of the urban Latina girls I met expressed a willingness to engage in conflict that would be considered problematic in certain

Hispanic communities. The socialization of Latina girls most re-sembles that of their white, middle-class counterparts. Latin American culture is family centered, and parents socialize children along traditional gender lines. Wives and daughters are expected to be nonaggressive and honor the authority of men. Women are "traditionally idealized as pure and self-sacrificing, like the Virgin Mary," and rules of behavior for girls can be extremely restrictive.[77]

The Dominican and Puerto Rican girls I met were mostly working class or poor first-generation Americans. They came from homes where parents spoke little or no English, where the girls had to translate notes and report cards sent home. These girls live in two worlds: the one more traditional and sheltered, and the other a contrary world of youthful license and temptation. Their personalities reflect the convergence of different cultural forces: the legacy of obedience imposed by their community, alongside the self-protective armor necessary to survive in lower-income communities.

Thirteen-year-old Jasmine found herself in a world of privilege that contrasted sharply with her working-class upbringing. When I came to Arden Country Day, where she was on full scholarship, Jasmine sat close to me, raising her hand often, eager to participate. We met a few weeks after school let out for the summer at a pizza joint near school. Jasmine had long, black kinky hair and a full beautiful face, which she made up expertly every day. After seven years as the only Latina in an all-black public school in her neighborhood, Jasmine transferred to Arden to begin seventh grade.

Jasmine's mother is an immigrant from the Dominican Republic. "I can describe my family," Jasmine told me plaintively, "as loose strings held together by a knot. That knot was my grandmother." The family congregated at her grandmother's small apartment every weekend for meals and conversation. When she died, Jasmine said, "all these strings went every which way. They disintegrated. The whole family." Jasmine had been growing closer with her grandmother at the time of her death, and the loss weighed heavily on her.

Jasmine's grief felt especially keen, since she had seen so much of herself reflected in her grandmother's stewardship of the family. Jasmine's own mother, she told me, could be "weak-minded." The contrast between this and her own strength made Jasmine uneasy. "She's always been the kind of person that listens to what other people tell her a lot." Jasmine perceived her mother as inconsistent, allowing Jasmine something once and then forbidding it without explanation. When mother and daughter argued, Jasmine was sometimes told she didn't deserve what was being lobbied for. Jasmine vehemently disagreed.

"I feel that I do [deserve] a lot. I wake up at five in the morning to get to school. I get home at 6:30. I do my homework. Iron my clothes, take a shower, go to sleep. I end up going to sleep at one or two, and I get up at five." Jasmine complained that her mother wanted her to clean the apartment too much on the weekends. "She forgets that I just turned thirteen. She's so used to me having like an older mentality that she kind of thinks I can take more things and responsibility."

Her mother's inability to make her own decisions frustrated her, especially when there seemed to be so many to make right at the time. Perhaps because of this, Jasmine told me that "my mother doesn't know me as much as my friends do."

In one sense, Jasmine's complaints have the texture of typical adolescent angst—my mother doesn't get me; she makes me do too much. Jasmine's frustration, however, ran deeper, and her anger pointed to a gulf between herself and her mother that paralleled the two worlds she was living in. Her mother didn't speak English, and her mind, Jasmine said gingerly, "is kind of set back to the culture in DR (Dominican Republic). She doesn't understand the way things are now." The values Jasmine was learning at school—of competition, ambition, and individual success—conflicted with her mother's attempts to socialize her into interdependence. To survive the confusion, Jasmine turned to herself, holding fast to her own voice.

From the first days at the new private school, Jasmine told me she steeled herself to remember certain things. "I came in with a certain attitude. That this is me. You like me, that's it; you don't like me, that's it, too. I'm not going to try and change myself because someone doesn't like me." She was surprised to attract more friends than she could handle, but some girls viewed her with animosity. "I'm not going to be trying to impress people because I want them to like me. I think that kind of intimidates people that I'm sort of more assertive and more aggressive in what I do. In my thinking I'm not weakminded. I consider myself a very strong person. That scares them because they're not like that."

Jasmine described public school as a place where "you can't show weakness," and private school as a hotbed for emotions. Yet she was confused and insecure about the duplicity she noticed in some of her new peers. "A lot of people are hypocritical," she told me. "They pretend to be your good friend. They pretend nothing's changed. That's just worse." When she tried to tell people how she felt, they often thought she was being "mean." They were offended by her directness. "Can't you just take what I'm saying as coming to you?" Jasmine remarked. "Don't try and change it. I'm just saying, this is it."

Jasmine struggled with the unexplained abandonment and silences from the girls she loved most, and the friction in her group of friends had Jasmine questioning herself. Bewildered and sad, having tried fiercely to keep her relationships intact, she remembered thinking, "What is it that I do that pushes people away? Why is it that so many of my friendships are failures? What do I keep on doing wrong? When you see a pattern in your life, you look to yourself for the problem." Eventually, however, she realized that trying and hoping and wanting would not be enough. "There's only so much you can do in a friendship," she said simply. "You can't give 110 percent and another person gives 5 percent." Eventually, she told me, some of the friends who had stopped speaking to her confessed they had been jealous.

Jasmine resented it. "I have had to work really hard for everything I have in my life. Nothing's been handed to me. A lot of girls in this school have. It's a really expensive school. I'm on scholarship. I'm not paying for anything for this school. And it's like they don't grasp the fact that you have to work for things. You're not always going to be given things in your hand." She later told me, "I've been through a lot in my life and I've learned that in certain situations you have to be more aggressive because, if not, people are going to take advantage of you."

Jasmine's marked self-reliance complicated her relationships with her friends. She found competition with other girls so jarring that she preferred friendships with boys. She balked at the disdain she felt emanating from girls who seemed to resent her academic success. "I have to keep my grades up!" she said in protest. "It's a must or I won't be attending [the school] or any school like that. They just don't understand that."

Jasmine was perplexed by the need of her girlfriends to rely on each other so much, especially their endless barrage of questions about how they looked and what they should do. "It's not like, 'Oh, my God, I hang on the opinions of my friends all the time.' I do depend on opinions. I always ask, What do you think? But it's not like I'm going to change something about myself because someone doesn't like it. If I really feel I should do it, I'm going to do it."

Whether at her old public school or Arden, Jasmine had always been a minority, and she found particular comfort in her identity at her mostly white school. Yet she found that "people kind of forget who they are and they start acting a certain way." At school, minorities rarely attended gatherings for students of color. "Like you know?" she asked. "They're forgetting their heritage. They kind of get lost in all that. My friend Ray is a Dominican. It's so sad. He doesn't speak Spanish." She told me she was ashamed that she could write only a little Spanish. "What are you trying to be?" she asked no one in particular. "Don't forget who you are."

She noticed her white peers trying on "ghetto" fashions like bandannas, imitating Jasmine's Spanish slang and Dominican inflection. One classmate shared her address with the caveat that she "lives in the ghetto," and Jasmine silently imagined her coming to visit her neighborhood sometime. There, Jasmine said, she can't wear a bandanna because it signals gang affiliations.

When I asked Jasmine who she turns to for help, she echoed many urban girls observed by researchers. "Mostly I don't talk to anyone. Sometimes I'll talk about stuff. Most of the stuff I deal with on my own."

As a working-class Latina, Jasmine's transition into white, middle-class culture had left her a stranger in both worlds. She was caught in the space between, and to adapt, to avoid the overload and confusion of mixed messages, Jasmine was digging in her heels and holding fast to the memory of her grandmother. Where the messages of her world collided, she chose to rely on herself and her own voice, the only sound she could hear clearly.

Parents' attempts to empower their children were evident in my discussions with urban girls. I was struck by the extent to which many of them were socialized to defend themselves physically. In some instances, girls reported being struck by their parents for returning home beaten. One urban African American girl who lost a fistfight was given some credit by her mother. "My mother says at least you tried. My mother doesn't want me to be no sucker, nobody's fool." It is important to emphasize that these girls are not expected to be aggressive generally, but to defend themselves when they have been provoked. Their comments confirm the observations of researchers who found parents training their children to expect affronts on their dignity.[78]

Martin Luther King Elementary's students are predominantly African American, Puerto Rican, and Dominican. Twice a week, when I arrived for our group discussions, the open expanse of the first floor hovered over a cliff of afterschool chaos, thick-skinned maroon balls crashing out of the gym and into lockers, children's voices raised in laughter and shouts as they moved toward their activities.

Ntozake, the head of the afterschool program, had chosen a mix of known bullies and targets to speak with me. These fifth- and sixth-grade girls were assembled around a conference table used by teachers. In the dim, smoky light flowing through crisp venetian blinds, the girls fidgeted in too-large chairs, looking apprehensively at Ntozake.

At this school, Ntozake said, shaking her head in wonder, the girls fight as often as and sometimes more than the boys. Standing at the front of the room on our first day together, she asked a simple question. She said she wanted to know the answer as much as I did, and I was grateful for the comforting effect her presence clearly had on the girls. "Why," she asked pointedly, eyes narrowing, "is there so much fighting?"

"The reason why we fight so much is because when they spread rumors, and you tell them to come to your face, they change it around and talk about your mother and dead family members," Rosa said.

"We have fights because sometimes we say to say it to our face to show that if you want to talk, talk to my face!" Marisol added. "My sister told me, 'If someone calls you a word, you say it back. If they say something, don't take it because it's not true.'"

"My mother says to bust 'em up if someone hits you," Tiffany volunteered.

"You can't stay hit," Latoya explained. "If you don't hit, they gon' say, 'Oh, why don't you hit, you a punk?'"

Rosa gestured at Ntozake. "Even though you tell us not to fight, our parents tell us not to stay hit."

"In third grade," Jessica began, "I used to be a punk. There was a boy. He hit me and I wouldn't do nothing. I'd go home crying. My mother would be like, 'What happened?' One time he punched me in the mouth. My mother said, 'If you don't hurt him, I'm gonna hit you.'" The girls erupted in cheers and shared similar rules from their homes.

Later, after the discussion had ended and only a few students lingered, Rosa approached. "I don't want to be in fights," she said, "but I feel like I have to. My dad says, 'Beat their behind up.' But I don't want to. I'd come home with bruises and my father would yell at me. So I had to fight."

Some physical fights between girls bear a powerful likeness to nonviolent alliance building, explored in chapter three. Tiffany, an African American ninth grader in Mississippi, explained that fistfights between girls are often prolonged by the need to get other girls involved in a supportive backup, not unlike the way girls build alliances.

"They gotta go get their clique," she explained. "They gotta take all their time. The girls have to get their clique because ... they're likely to jump in and just have your back, just like that." Notably, although girls in the Northeast and Mississippi described girls standing behind a friend to back her up, they said it was extremely rare for witnesses to enter the fracas themselves.

Nevertheless, Tiffany explained, their presence "tells you who your real friends are," adding that "you feel much stronger" with them by your side. Tiffany alluded to R & B singer Jill Scott's video "Gettin' in the Way," in which Scott decides she must resort to physical violence to convince her boyfriend's ex to stop trying to sabotage his new relationship. Scott charges up the scorned woman's front steps, trailed by her closest friends (and most of the neighborhood), and tears off the woman's wig, to the delight of the crowd.

Jacqueline explained, "If you have your friends there, it's kind of a threat. If you're just talking to the girl, she probably won't be as nervous to say what she has to say. Or she probably won't get as loud. But if you have another friend there, you're dominating her because it's two of you." Like the middle-class girls who use emotional alliances, these girls make pacts to defend each other physically.

Fourteen-year-old Amanda shared intriguing insights when I asked her about her observations of boys fighting in her Puerto Rican neighborhood. Amanda had watched boys move up the social ladder when they won a fight one-on-one. "If he would win, he's stronger than that boy. . . . They're like, 'Oh, I beat him up. He knows the next time not to say nothing.'" The rules of masculinity demand displays of individual strength. Girlfights, she tells me, have different goals.

Girls "continue arguing. Usually when girls do that . . . she's beat up, she'll be scared of her, or she'll bring more people into the fight. Boys, they'll fight, they won, and leave it alone. If girls fight, it's just constant." Girls who lose fights often wait for the next moment they will be able to fight again. "It's like back and forth."

As with Jenny in chapter one who waited years to retaliate against her bully, feuds can last for years between girls as they seek opportunities to avenge their loss. Tiffany explained, "After a fistfight, girls feel like they need to get that girl back. Whoever beat that other girl up is going to have to watch her back all the time."

Similar to alliance building, in which middlegirls may have a stake in causing a fight, girls who fight physically also describe those who instigate. "Somebody'll pump it up. They're gonna say, 'Oh, she said this about you.' They're gonna come back in your face, and then, you know, they don't want to hear what you got to say."

Keisha explained, "They get stuff started. That's how it all happens."

unbidden resistance

Inner strength reveals itself at unlikely moments, often when we are at the end of our rope. For some girls, rock bottom points the way up and out. A fusillade of bullying can batter someone into hopelessness, and yet the same extreme situation can lay the groundwork for extraordinary acts of personal strength, like when a stunned father hoists a car off a trapped child.

The girls who decide to fight back seem to confront moments like these. Like girls living under economic and social stress, the girls who resist find themselves with few other choices. These girls, however, are not usually prepared for it the way their counterparts are. Rather, they come into an instinct to defend themselves and preserve their integrity, one that is only semiconscious, born more of desperation than desire.

Where they may have once drawn self-esteem and strength from their friends, solitude augurs new perspective and self-awareness. As my friend Astrid recalled, "Having it happen stripped me of all external sources of confidence, and I had only what I had internally to draw on. I realized I had a lot of strength and integrity." Shelley McCullough learned about her own limits, and especially the things she needs in her relationships with others. That insight has been critical to her friendships today. "I know how I react to things. I know more about myself. I learned more how to deal with stuff."

Alizah moved from California to live with her father in New Jersey when it was clear that the cruel campaign of the popular girls would not let up. The last straw came when one of the girls stole her sneaker and refused to return it. Alizah confronted her, the girl still refused, and when Alizah pushed her up against the lockers, the girl claimed Alizah had pulled a knife. When she was suspended, Alizah was furious, ready to go anywhere, even three thousand miles away.

In New Jersey, Alizah resolved to remake her image. She spent hours assembling a wardrobe that would fit in, and when she spoke to me, nearly fifteen years later, she could describe the first-day outfit down to the angle of her shirt collar. As she stood in line at the cafeteria, the cool girls swarmed. "What's up with the shoes? My father wears those shoes. You can't afford socks? Why does she have a triangle on her ass? What the hell is Guess? Why do you have a horse on your shirt?"

At that point, Alizah said, "I can't do anything else. I can't try any harder. I'm not even getting a chance here. I thought, screw you. I'm going to do what I want to do, and I'm going to wear what I want to wear." The next day Alizah wore the camouflage print pants she loved, with a tight black sleeveless top. She spiked her hair. "The girls said I had fishing lures in my ears and I glared at them."

Alizah befriended a girl who looked like her in the cafeteria. "Everyone said she was drinking bleach out of her thermos because she wanted to die. I sat down, introduced myself, and that was it. I thought, she's as much of an outcast as I am and we're going to get along just fine. We were best friends and are close to this day."

As I tried to understand what made the difference, Alizah explained, "I think I just didn't care anymore. I thought, I'm not going to try and be your friend. If you want to hang out with me, that's cool, but I'm not going to overextend myself and tell you my secrets and put myself out on the line."

Alizah had tried so hard to make people like her in California that she had been involved in few school activities. Her world revolved around trying to win others' affection. So she made changes. She started making her own clothes in high school and joined journalism, yearbook, and theater clubs. She became the first junior to edit the school newspaper.

"I became my own person. I was determined that I wasn't going to fall into it again. I didn't want the pain. I thought, even if I don't have a lot of friends, I'm going to keep myself busy and do the things I like to do. And I made friends that way, through my activities, as opposed to following everyone around and doing what everyone else was doing."

For some girls, being cast out is a blessing in disguise, as many are guided into a more centered, authentic self-awareness. Being the odd girl out helped Naomi off a treadmill of want and disappointment. "I felt like nothing, like no matter what I did it wasn't going to be okay, because nobody cared. I didn't have to live up to the standard other people had to live up to. I looked at these popular girls and they had these boyfriends that were like those cafeteria boyfriends. I felt like there was—these people, they had to be pretty, beautiful but not too sexy. They had to be desirable but not slutty, they had to be an ideal but always an unreachable ideal. Whereas I felt that as nothing, I had the freedom to be what I really was because nobody was looking to me for anything."

For twelve-year-old Alix, being bullied empowered her to demand respect in her relationships for who she is and to settle for nothing less. "It taught me to always be myself. I want people to respect me for who I am, not who I'm pretending to be." Ruth, now in her twenties, said, "My communication style became fiercer because I had to fight to earn it." And, she added, "It taught me compassion and independence. I can be alone and not feel insecure."

Girls who survive bullying can emerge from the experience with new strength. They can grow into women who learn to choose the right relationships and avoid abusive ones. They incorporate from their experience the ability to recognize harmful people long before harm can find them. If girls can go through their pain in a culture that validates it, more and more girls will get to walk away with silver linings.

When it is expressed, the overt aggression of girls is pathologized as unfeminine or worse. Minority and low-income girls are often stereotyped as aggressive, loud, and disruptive, and therefore "at risk." "Those loud black girls" is a term used to demean the brassy presence of African American female youth. When Jill McLean Taylor and her colleagues asked urban girls to fill out a questionnaire, they found that over half answered the question "What gets me into trouble?" with "my mouth" or "my big mouth." The girls spoke "as if repeating a mantra given them by some higher authority."[79]

Scuffles between boys, though met with swift punishment, are nevertheless seen as a predictable side effect of male adolescence. Yet when girls fight physically, their aggression is seen as a sign of deviant behavior. This double standard has grave consequences, suggesting to girls that their aggression will be more acceptable if only they keep it indirect or covert. Moreover, physically aggressive girls appear to be disproportionately working-class girls and girls of color; when they are punished disproportionately, officials perpetuate stereotypes about them, suggesting it is only they who break the rules. Not surprisingly, when girls of color are studied, it's often to identify high-risk behavior, individual deviancy, or social problems.

Our culture has long pathologized the black female as a willful matriarch. Black mothers are portrayed as domineering disciplinarians who promote disobedience in their children. The culture's anger toward the black female can be traced, in large part, to her mouth. The black woman crystallizes the culture's discomfort with female strength, voice, and aggression: her willingness to raise her voice and defend herself publicly, to provide for her family irrespective of the presence of a man, and to speak her heart and mind—all of these disrupt the social and sexual order of society.

What little we know about girls' relationships is based mostly on studies of white, middle-class girls. Indeed, most of the stories in this book come from that part of society. The rich diversity of female relationships found among other races, ethnicities, and class backgrounds has often been overlooked.

That the girls who engage in direct conflict may have little real social power is a sad irony, to say the least. The assertiveness shown by some minority girls may reflect not self-confidence but their vulnerability in the larger society. Their voices indeed challenge the picture of indirect aggression painted in other chapters of this book. Yet in many instances their forthrightness stems from the girls' sense that they can make themselves heard only by using physical force or dangerous speech. Because it is linked to their marginalization, their directness cannot serve as a model for overcoming girls' sense of powerlessness.

Dealing effectively with that feeling of powerlessness is essential to fighting the loss of girls' authentic selves. What we can learn about assertive girls would be undeniably useful in developing concrete strategies to fight the loss of girls' authentic selves. The more we know about these girls, the more we honor their voices, the closer we will get to developing concrete strategies to combat female bullying in all its forms.

CHAPTER *nine*

parents speak

Suzanne Cohen was preparing for an emergency conference with her six-year-old daughter's teacher when she was suddenly uneasy. Standing before the classroom's closed door, poised to discuss the abusive behavior of her daughter's classmate, "I realized that I was about to describe this child [as] extremely manipulative, competitive, and underhanded. And to say that about a six-year-old girl—you sound like a lunatic!"

She is right. A system that refuses to classify these behaviors as genuine aggression will look askance at complaints of indirect, social, and relational aggression. As a result, parents who confront girl bullying face an experience that, in its own way, can be as upsetting as their daughters'. In the absence of a public language to talk about bullying, it's hard to avoid inflammatory words like "liar," "sneaky," or "manipulator." As their daughters fear going public and facing retaliation, parents are afraid of being designated "hysterical" or "overinvested" by the school. And where girls must overcome the embarrassment of low social status, parents may quietly worry over the role their errors might have played in their daughter's experience.

The attempt of parents to tone down their demands on teachers is one of the most powerful subtexts in this chapter of the story of girl bullying. Sitting with four mothers who meet regularly to chat at a Washington coffee shop, I asked them to explain.

"As a parent, you're aware of the incredible amount of power the teacher has over your child's life," Ellen said. "You don't want to jeopardize that relationship in any way." Her friends nodded. Added Christine, "I think parents worry that teachers will take things out on their children because of how a parent acts." Because complaining about alternative aggressions is often perceived as overreacting to everyday school behavior, many mothers harbor a fear of becoming the classroom's "hysterical mother." The need to remain calm and dispassionate, they emphasized, is key.

Perhaps more than any other event in a child's life, bullying forces the question every parent struggles with: How much should I intercede on my child's behalf? While the answer to this question should depend on the child—is she ready to fend for herself? is she being prematurely exposed to danger?—too often the answer is determined by the anticipated response. Will other parents take offense? Will the school be responsive, or worse, punitive? With most schools strapped to accomplish the most basic extracurricular objectives, getting somewhere with a busy teacher can be an uphill battle.

Parents seeking justice for their daughters face cultural and personal obstacles. Most daunting is the fact that alternative aggressions are ignored or rarely considered a legitimate social problem. More often, school officials downplay the problem or blame the target. Many parents described daughters being sent to psychological counseling for treatment when there was nothing wrong with them, encouraged to get costly social skills training when it was the aggressor who in fact needed the help, or ignored because the aggressor was stealthy and it came down to a case of she-said, she-said. Not surprisingly, plenty of parents opt for silence.

Shame is also a reality. The discovery that your daughter struggles socially is painful; finding out she's not to blame is hardly a consolation. Every family handles it differently. It took no small courage for

Linda to confide the shame that felt to her both searing and ridiculous. "There was this nagging piece, and I never went to this place," she told me. "This is even hard to say but I thought it sometimes. As much as everything I said to [my daughter] did not reflect this, deep down I thought, 'My kid isn't *popular*? She isn't one of the cool kids?' Even though I know that's not what I really want. But you want your kid to be wonderful." It took Suzanne Cohen great courage to overcome her instinct to block the whole incident out. As she waited for the teacher, she recalled, "I secretly harbored this fantasy that someone would turn around and say, 'Why can't Hannah stand up for herself? Why don't you teach her how to stand up for herself? Why is she letting this happen?'" Although these feelings are common to anyone coping with a child's misfortune, shame weighs more heavily when most people regard the problem as a trivial phase in child development.

When a child is found to be learning disabled, there is a specialist. The child's parent suspects the problem, often using accessible literature, and expresses her concern to a knowledgeable official. The parent is reassured her child's situation is neither her fault nor that unusual. In time, her child may receive specialized attention to provide her with tools to accommodate her different needs and perform to the best of her abilities.

When a child is the target of alternative aggressions, there is often nobody to help. Without rules to refer to or a language to narrate a child's pain, parents know the cards are stacked against them from the get-go. As Suzanne explained, "If I made too much of a fuss about her social issues, you know, it would be like, 'Well what's wrong with your kid if she can't deal with her issues? Why doesn't she just walk away and get over this?' And I was embarrassed—I was embarrassed to appear the way I felt."

Silence is a second skin for American families. We put our best foot forward and draw the curtains in times of trouble. From across the yard we quietly blame parents for their children's plight. Middle-class families in particular are committed to keeping children's social, emotional, and learning problems secret, especially psychological pain. One mother, confiding the pressure to stay silent about her daughter's problems, put it simply: "We're afraid our kids aren't perfect. And that it reflects our mothering abilities. That we're home too much or not home enough. It reflects on us."

With ever more opportunities to showcase children, parents compete vigorously to project an image of social bliss and indomitable health. They stack trophies and throw glamorous birthday parties. Sharing the experience of despair engendered by girl bullying is for many parents impossible. Margaret Kaplan explained, "If I go to this person and tell them this is what's happening, who are they going to tell? How many people are going to know? How distorted will it become? Will it be, 'Oh, the Kaplans: *They're* having problems. *We're* not. *We're* all perfect. We have this idyllic lifestyle.'" Despite her deft organizing of parents to demand extra art classes, Susan Sussman gave a bitter laugh when I suggested a group to combat alternative aggressions. "There is no way I am going to organize a group around my daughter's experience of cruelty," she said.

Susan Patterson said the smallest incidents can become the subject of lunchtime conversations in Ridgewood. At forty-one, with her daughter bullied by a close friend, she was resolved to lock the town out of her private life. She closed down at even the thought of coming forward, brushing me off with a bitterness that seems to contain a lifetime of disappointments. "This town talks about everybody," she seethed. "They can't hardly wait to get up in the morning and find out who's getting divorced, who's sleeping with who. I mean, that's just the way life has been here forever." She pushed fiercely for her daughter to handle her bully on her own. "I wanted her to be an independent woman. I kept thinking, this is not as bad as it is. I didn't want to think it was as bad as it was. But it was really, really bad."

Parents are bit players in the national conversation on bullying. Our attention is fastened on the aggressors, their targets, and silent peers. Critics have faulted television and movies for stoking the culture of peer violence. The role of parents, however, is often reduced to bitter epilogues of disasters: parents who did too little, too late, or who did nothing at all.

In this chapter, I present five mothers talking about their girls' experiences with bullying and explore what teachers face in responding to them. Each parent has a unique story, and like her daughter, brings her own set of personal memories and beliefs to the episode. The stories illustrate parents' influence over their daughters' social choices. They reveal how a culture that silences and invalidates female aggression affects the way parents respond to their children's pain.

blame

Patricia runs a small child-care facility in Ridgewood. When I visited her at the end of the day, she was wearing a long, untucked collared shirt over rumpled khaki pants. Her tall sturdy frame suggested an ability to fix just about anything, from a shoelace to a lawn mower. Her voice was surprisingly gentle and low, and her eyes drifted across the playroom to where a lone child played quietly, awaiting her mother. We are both tall women, and as we plunked down to talk on tiny chairs at a round table, our knees popped halfway up to our chests. She grinned and shrugged, reddening slightly.

Patricia never expected that four years after moving here with Ben and their daughter, people in town would still treat them as though they'd just unloaded their truck. When Ben was hired as a senior pharmacist, an impressive promotion so early in his career, he had promptly moved the family to Ridgewood midway through Hope's third-grade year.

When Hope started school after the winter holidays, her sudden appearance troubled her peers. She was met with quick skepticism by the other girls and deemed a threat to existing cliques. What began as a brief shunning stretched into a yearlong hazing. Hope knew she was being challenged because she had not grown up in town, but the longer she lived in Ridgewood, the easier it became to blame herself.

By fifth grade Hope had fallen in with a group of girls from the church who attended choir and Sunday school. At school, the clique leader often asked Hope to go somewhere else for the day or made rude comments about Hope's looks or personality. When Patricia asked her daughter why she stayed friends with them, Hope insisted it was better when they were at church together.

One day in sixth grade, one of the girls informed Hope that the group did not want to be her friend anymore. For several weeks afterward, they refused to acknowledge her existence. "She was just left," Patricia said, her eyes filling with tears. "Every day after school, she'd come home crying. 'They don't like me today. They don't want to be my friend anymore. What do I do? Why don't they like me? What's wrong with me? Why can't I be friends? Why don't they want to be friends with me?' What do you say?" she asked pleadingly.

"What did you do?" I asked.

"Well, it was a very emotional time," Patricia said, clearing her throat, her shaken voice righting itself. She leaned back in the chair and stretched her long legs. "I'm sure a lot of it had to do with her growing up, you know, her period starting and all that stuff, a lot of emotions come with that, too." Listening to her, I wondered if Patricia was edging away from the center of her child's pain, ascribing it to the "legitimate" factors affecting child development.

Patricia asked her daughter if there was any truth to her clique's critical remarks. "I asked if there were some things within herself that she'd like to change." Hope tried to come up with a couple of ideas, then retorted that she didn't know what else she could do. I asked Patricia if she thought Hope should have changed herself.

"Hope has a very outgoing personality," Patricia explained, sounding almost apologetic. "She's very bubbly. And she can be silly. I guess I don't know the right word for her personality. But I think she could get on people's nerves. It might really rattle them. And they might get tired of it. She felt like she could calm down a little bit, you know, not be so boisterous or outspoken." In the absence of an explanation for her daughter's torment, Patricia could do little but suspect it was Hope's fault. She begged Hope to find other friends. Hope refused. She said they were her only friends.

Patricia tried to comfort her daughter by asking her to pray. "Even though it's very hard right now, we know that God can use this to bring good in your life somewhere. You may not see it today or tomorrow." She paused. "I'm trying not to cry."

We sat in silence.

"I wanted to go to those girls and say, 'Do you realize what you're doing!' I wanted to go and tell their mothers, you know, but then you stop and think, 'Okay, I'm hearing one side.' I trust Hope and I believe that she's honest with me, but you don't want always to think that my child will never do anything wrong.

"If it had turned into something where I thought Hope was really suffering or going into a depression, or you know, having really physical or health problems, I probably would have done things a little differently," Patricia said. "A lot of it I felt like, this is just part of life. You have to learn how to deal with people who don't always treat you fairly." And here, Patricia expressed society's approach to bullying through her parenting philosophy, even as she sat before me, shoulders slumped in a small chair, brushing tears away, questioning her own words.

When I asked what she would have done differently, she sighed and looked at me squarely. "I wish I had gone ahead and tried to get those mothers together and sat down with them for coffee or something," she said. "You know, in a nonthreatening way. I would never want them to think that I was saying my child is better. If we had worked though all that then, it might have helped them now. Their support system might have been stronger now."

Patricia's fear of angering other parents stifled her defense of Hope and helped her rationalize Hope's torment. For most mothers I spoke with, the fear of another parent's anger played an uncommonly large role in their response. The first unwritten rule of parenting, I learned, is that no one wants to be told how to raise their child; the second is that criticizing another person's child puts you in peril. Many people interpret criticism of their child's behavior as a veiled attack on their parenting, and they become defensive, sometimes irrationally so. Most parents of targets simply say they just "don't go there."

Mothers especially may harbor fears about engaging in direct con-flict. In smaller communities, the social costs of confrontation rise. Mothers may work together, volunteer at school or church, run into each other often, even be friends. Fathers might be current or hoped-for clients. It may be difficult to approach another parent without some aftershocks that reverberate beyond the girls' universe.

At times, bully-target dynamics can spring up between mothers of warring girls, kicking into gear a second tier of indirect aggression and anger. Parents of aggressors are naturally protective of their daughters, and especially when their girls aggress in total secret, often challenge the accusation. The approaching mother, already timid, can be silenced and bullied herself.

Jill's experience of bullying brought back a flood of memories for her mother, who was suddenly dropped by her best friends in jun-ior high. For Faye, watching what happened to Jill proved her the-ory that mean girls are universal and unavoidable. Jill had changed profoundly since being alternately ignored and attended to by her best friend. "She used to be the happiest kid," Faye told me. "She was so happy-go-lucky. She used to float and it was wonderful." Then around first grade, Jill became increasingly shy. When her first best friend dropped her "like a ton of bricks," her self-esteem shrank. Now that Jill's new best friend in fifth grade was treating her nicely only in private, Faye was not going to interfere. There was no sense, she'd concluded, in protecting your child from this. It's everywhere.

This time, the bully was the daughter of Faye's friend. This woman was, according to Faye, powerful, controlling, and socially connected. Because of that, her daughter had many friends. "We have had discussions [about the girls' friendship]," she said, "but you can't tell someone that your daughter is being a bitch." Since Jill had seen trouble in more than one friendship, Faye believed Jill's low self-esteem was to blame for her victimization. "If you don't feel good about yourself and people know it, and people know that this person doesn't like you, then no one else is going to like you."

When I asked her if she'd thought of pursuing her daughter's plight with the school, she balked. "Other mothers might have called the other mother and said, 'What's going on?' And it never occurred to me to do that. It never did. And now I say to myself, 'Should I have called?' Should I have, you know, found out what went on, you see, because my mom was really not involved at all. There were a lot of other issues in her life and this was not something she could clearly see as a problem. And then I think, you know, on a scale from one to ten you have people dying from cancer. This really is not a problem. You know, she will grow up and she will find her good friend. And she'll be okay."

After minutes of trying to minimize her daughter's ordeal, Faye abruptly gave herself over to hopelessness. "She'll have this for the rest of her life. We all do," she said simply.

fear

On an icy February morning, I was inching down a backed-up street in Washington, D.C., heading for a lunch interview with the wife of a friend I hadn't seen in many years. Trawling for parking in an underground garage, I remembered that Melissa was bringing along her mother, who was visiting from upstate New York.

When I entered the restaurant, Melissa was holding an armful of shopping bags and standing by the bar. She was about my age, with shiny, curly black hair, narrow shoulders, and a broad, pleasant smile. Barbara, who stood just behind her daughter, was stout and middle-aged, with long, curly salt-and-pepper hair. Both greeted me warmly, though as we were seated I noticed Barbara studying the menu intently.

After diet Cokes and salads were ordered, Melissa began.

"I have to admit that popularity was very important to me," she said, as though she were getting some shameful fact out of the way, confession-style. "I think I was always in the popular group. From the outside, people thought I was great friends with this group. I was always—*always*—thought of as being with that group." The reality, she was quick to add, was different.

Camille had always been her closest friend. She lived in the neighborhood, which made it easy for the girls to carpool to the many afterschool activities they shared. There was swimming, gymnastics, ballet, soccer, Hebrew school. Even when there was nothing to do, Melissa hung out at Camille's house after school.

Camille was cute and magnetic. She seemed to fill the rooms she entered, and though that meant lots of girls to play with, Melissa could not help but feel small in Camille's shadow. She was plagued by the constant hum of being too big, too homely, too uncool. Whenever Melissa liked a boy, the boy liked Camille. When Camille got around guys, she acted stupid and silly and ignored Melissa. At Hebrew school, Camille ditched Melissa if a more popular girl from another school was around. Melissa was often jealous and ashamed.

Camille was best friends with Nicola, who lived across the street, and whenever the two of them got together, they started to lie. They would pretend not to have plans, so that when Melissa asked Camille what she was doing that day, the answer would always be some variation on "Oh, I don't know what I'm doing yet." Undeterred, Melissa called Camille constantly. One time, riding her bike past Camille's house, she saw the two of them chalking the driveway. "Oh, we just got together!" Camille insisted. "We never knew you wanted to come over." Camille made you feel, Melissa told me, "like she would do these obnoxious, mean things so slyly that you couldn't really call her on it."

In seventh grade, Melissa's class was divided, and she was separated from all of her friends except Camille and Nicola. The shift would permanently alter the social chemistry. By October, the two girls had turned on her.

"They basically dropped me as a friend but very slyly," Melissa said, stirring her soda. "They would just not invite me. I was not invited to hang out after school, never included in plans. They were horrible. They made my life hell."

But the illusion of their friendship persisted, and so did Melissa. Only a sharp eye would have seen the truth. "Camille's instinct was to be nice to everyone and to never say a mean thing. She would just be very elusive, very sly." So Melissa still ate lunch with them, even though nobody talked to her. She would go to the bathroom with them, even though one time Camille whirled around and snapped, "Melissa, do you *ever* stop following us?" She would see them together at the movies and want to disappear under the seats.

"I was very social, very outgoing. It was traumatic. I would go home crying every night. But on the other hand, I felt compelled to be part of that group," Melissa remembered.

As she lingered among the girls who mostly ignored her, she recalled, "I got very good at listening to conversations. I remember spying, anything I could do to understand. I walked behind them to hear what they were saying. I got good at investigating."

"Um," Barbara said, clearing her throat. I looked over, for a moment having nearly forgotten she was there. She had been twisting her cocktail napkin into small pieces underneath her tall soda glass, staring at stringy lemon pulp floating near the bottom. Her face seemed frozen.

"Uh, I have to be honest," she said, eyes still downcast. "I encouraged Melissa to be friendly with Camille. I thought, you know, that it would be nice to have a Jewish girl to hang around with."

Melissa gave her mother a quick "that's nice" look. "I remember walking home by myself a lot. I felt very, very lonely. I felt insecure. I felt ugly. Disgusting. Depressed. I'd lay on my bed, thinking these awful thoughts, that people wouldn't even care if . . ." She trailed off.

"I thought I must be awful to have my friends hate me," she continued, shaking her head. "I must be pathetic. I don't have anything good to say. They think I'm annoying. I was the most annoying person this year. Everything you could think negative about yourself, I thought."

"You handled it very well," Barbara said. "When you talk about it, it makes me want to cry." And before I could move my head to see Melissa's reaction, Barbara was up and around the table, holding her sobbing daughter. Barbara's face was wet.

"I'm fine," Melissa sniffled, raising her palm slightly off the table. "I'm very in touch with my feelings. I have to say that the experience really made me such a better person. I learned such a lesson. I really learned what I'm looking for.

"I think it was just that having friends that were part of this cool group was the most important thing. I would have done anything, to some degree, to be friends with them. I don't know why."

Barbara returned to her seat. Our food had arrived and Melissa was wiping her eyes. I waited. I tried to seem casual. I did not want Melissa to feel embarrassed. Then Barbara exhaled loudly, half sigh, half raspy cough. This time, when she spoke, she looked straight at me. "When Melissa talks about this, it's very painful for me. I think I'm a little shut down on it. I can't really feel my feelings." She paused as the white noise of the restaurant rose in the background. "Because I feel I perpetrated this."

Barbara grew up an overweight child with few friends. She received the lion's share of girls' meanness. Even the memory of her large body hulking against a backdrop of delicate girls still made her cringe. She looked mournfully at her daughter. "I didn't want Melissa to know that pain." When Melissa was born, Barbara became determined that she would be popular. When Melissa was old enough, Barbara told me, "I encouraged her to be friendly with the kids in the neighborhood." She paused. "I pushed her toward these people."

I asked the inevitable, awkward question. Did she know what Melissa was going through?

"Yes," she said. I saw Melissa's head whip around to her mother. "I felt so inadequate as a person." Barbara's eyes were shining. "I felt so ugly and obese. When I had a child, it brought out all my old fears and insecurities. I had to keep saying, *Melissa is not me. Melissa is not me*. It brought back memories of my own childhood. And I did not want her to know my pain. I wanted her to be happy. I wanted her to be popular."

Barbara had met Camille's mother, Iris, at the community pool when their girls were young. With four attractive children, Iris exuded the easygoing confidence Barbara had always longed for. And yet, Barbara remembered, "Iris could also be very manipulative." But Barbara was in awe of how this woman managed to raise several well-adjusted children, and she wanted a piece of it. "If Melissa could hang out with Camille, then she'd have a good influence on Melissa," she reasoned. "Of course, Melissa didn't really need anyone to have a good influence on her."

I persisted. "Did you ever mention to Iris how Camille was treating Melissa?"

"I did try to talk to her," Barbara murmured. "I think that Iris could be very nice and yet then she could maybe talk behind your back." After a moment, she added, "I felt that I needed Iris to help me be a good mother. And if I had to do it again, if I was thirty today, it would have been different. I don't think I would have . . . pushed for Melissa to do all those things." Instead, Barbara went to see the school guidance counselor, who recommended Melissa see a therapist. The therapist told Barbara there was nothing wrong with her daughter.

"Part of it," Melissa said, "and I'm not blaming you at all, Mom, is that you would ask me, 'What are your plans? What are Camille and Nicola doing? What are your plans? Why aren't you playing with them?' You did that all the time." She turned to me. "I was getting it from my mom. I don't want you to feel bad," she said, looking back at Barbara, "but it's true."

"I can face it on my own," Barbara said.

"I don't blame you," Melissa insisted. "But as encouraging as you were, there were periods where I felt like I was being compared to them and not good enough." One time, Melissa recalled, she and her mother saw Camille with a new haircut at a café. "You took me to get my hair cut, and you wanted me to be like her," Melissa told her mother.

"You wanted the haircut," Barbara said.

"No," Melissa insisted, "it was right after we saw her."

Barbara and Melissa had never discussed their ordeal until our long lunch in Washington. Watching them, I knew immediately I had been given a great gift. So often when parents respond to a bullying situation, they instinctively focus their anger and blame on the bully. Despite the great difficulty of separating the feelings that surround these ordeals, Barbara's story underscores the need for parents to be mindful of their own role in their daughters' social choices.

Barbara and Melissa also helped me see the benefits of honest communication between parents and children. Through them, I realized that parents must be more than tear wipers and back patters. Barbara might have made a tremendous difference in her daughter's life had she been willing to share the vulnerability and pain that were causing her to pressure her child into popularity. From Melissa's standpoint, Barbara appeared invulnerable, which only reinforced Melissa's sense of fault.

Of course, Barbara's choice to make Melissa popular at any cost was conscious, and not all choices are. It is indeed a blessing and curse of human nature that we unwittingly create opportunities to repeat our own mistakes and to pass them on, like heirlooms, to the people we love the most.

generations

I met Donna and Tracy Wood through a college friend, and I spoke with mother and daughter in North Carolina separately by phone. Fifteen years after Tracy's ordeal, the two women narrated their stories with uncanny synchronicity, as well as generous openness.

Tracy spent her first years on a large farm near Raleigh, playing mostly with her brother or her ponies. After Tracy's parents divorced, Donna won custody and moved the children into town. She inherited a healing, protective network of brassy ya-ya ladies who warmed the new home and treasured Tracy. When Tracy visited her father he was physically and mentally abusive, his affection sporadic. At times, Tracy was the apple of his eye; at others, it was as though she didn't exist. Her unsupervised visitations were taxing.

In fourth grade, Tracy stunned her teachers by completing her math workbook during the first week of school. She was promptly skipped a grade into a class notorious for meanness. On the first day of fifth grade, the girls refused her at the lunch table, sniping that she wasn't really a fifth grader. They forced her to eat alone. After several days of solitude in the cafeteria, Tracy brought nail polish to entertain herself, and a monitor reprimanded her, consigning her to another silent lunch.

The lunchtime isolation quickly became a school-day pastime for the popular girls. They continued to ostracize Tracy throughout middle school, telling her she was stupid, that her jokes were bad, her clothes all wrong. They taunted her about not wearing a bra when she was ten and flat as a board. In the bathroom one day, she listened from inside the stall as the ringleader warned Tracy's only friend not to hang out with her. The girl was stone cold the next time Tracy saw her. One summer, she became best friends with a popular girl who rode horses at an area barn. In September, the girl pretended she didn't know her.

For years, Tracy suffered quietly. "I remember every day," Tracy told me. "It was just awful. Nobody liked me there. And I couldn't do anything right. Everything I did I got teased for. Nobody had the compassion or the maturity, including the teachers, to say this isn't cool, to say, stop it!"

Sitting on the sofa three years after she started fifth grade, talking with her mother about the concept of courage, Tracy looked up and said, "You don't know how much courage it takes me to go to school every day."

Donna asked her daughter what she meant. Tracy replied, "The girls don't want to let me sit with them." Donna was shocked. She had maintained contact with the school for years about her daughter's progress. "In this small private school," she told me, still seething nearly two decades later, "they couldn't bother to tell me that this child wasn't allowed to sit with anybody at recess or lunch. And I was appalled. I was absolutely undone."

Naturally, now that the secret was out, Donna assumed her daughter would be relieved to switch schools.

She was not.

The popular girls had tossed confusing signals of kindness into the mix of cruelty, ensnaring Tracy in a cycle in which she repeatedly tried to win her tormentors over. Some days there would be a glimmer of hope: a kind look, a day without comment or taunt, a shared laugh at the water fountain. To Tracy it felt like enough. She explained to me, "I just sort of thought that was how it was, and that it was incumbent upon me to change it. At some point, I was just sure I was going to triumph over the odds and make them like me and get all the things I wanted at that age." Fleeting moments and scraps of friendship sustained her, leaving Donna to struggle against a daughter who dug in her heels and refused to give up. Donna tried to coax her daughter's teachers without alienating them. She strained to listen to Tracy and accommodate her needs, even as she realized with horror that home was the only place where her daughter would feel respected.

But Tracy's resistance eventually slackened into a depression. Migraine headaches kept her out of school an average of three days a week, and she had to take shots of Demerol for the pain. One day, she found herself reading the same paragraph in her history book over and over again. For three months, her dog curled against her as she drifted in and out of consciousness.

Suddenly, it was Sunday night and she had to return to school full-time on Monday. "And I thought," Tracy said, "I'd just rather die than go back to school."

Tracy set her alarm for the middle of the night, awoke, and went downstairs. She got out some of the kitchen knives. "It just hurt," she said. "I sat down and fell asleep and woke up in the morning thinking I couldn't even do this right." Tracy went to her mother's bedroom, who assured her that she would not have to go to school. Tracy was hospitalized for several weeks. Nobody called.

Of her daughter deep in depression, Donna said, "I saw a huge sense of helplessness. Real discouragement. And really noticeable. She had an absolutely wicked and delicious sense of humor. A lot of that disappeared. I would think, what happened to my little girl? It was like she was disappearing. She was getting so depressed it was just not her anymore. She told me that even though I said loving and supportive things, I didn't really know the picture—that she wasn't smart, she wasn't pretty, she wasn't worthwhile." Donna felt waves of frustration as she tried vainly to sway her daughter. "There were times when I just wanted to shake her. She would just not be moved. She would become almost mute. You could just see her silent, thinking emotionally."

After several years of psychotherapy, Tracy understood that her steadfast refusal to leave the school was related to her relationship with her father. "I think my father's cycle of making me his favorite and then not having any interest in me created a cycle of wanting to win over people that didn't want to be won over," Tracy explained. "So it was like, if I could just be good enough or get the right pair of jeans, it was going to be okay again." Years later, Tracy remains awed by her own participation in her suffering. "I didn't have a sense of, my God, this is really messed up!" she told me, wonder palpable in her voice.

Although Donna was unaware of it at the time, she believes her own tolerance of bullying at the hands of an abusive husband helped communicate to Tracy that with enough effort, a person can adjust to anything, no matter how painful. "Here was Tracy caught in an abusive relationship that she refused to leave," Donna said. Having spent years recovering from a traumatic divorce in which she was abandoned by many of her friends, in which she struggled with two young children, little money, and alcoholism, Donna was realistic about why she didn't read between the lines. "I was still reeling from what had happened to me and what had happened to my children. I was dealing with my own issues," she said. She reacted to Tracy with the bottled rage, frustration, and anxiety that had been triggered by her own experience.

Sometimes families transmit dynamics of their relationships to girls. That girls identify with the caregiving practices of their mothers is often celebrated. Yet as we have seen, there can be great risk where relationship becomes the primary currency of one's life. The girls in this book who have remained in abusive friendships at any cost bear disturbing similarity to people like Donna, who are survivors of relationship violence. (The connections between bullying and relationship violence are further explored in the final chapter.) Just as daughters may learn to love like their mothers, they may also be learning not to terminate relationships that have become dangerous.

helplessness

Elaine was sitting with her daughter Joanna, and we were talking about Joanna's problems with Amy. "I have to tell you," Elaine said, leaning forward to rest an elbow on her knee, "that it is so much work the second time around. I was so betrayed by my best friend. She was really my very best friend. I know how [Joanna] feels and that there's not much I can do. It's bad enough experiencing it yourself, but when you experience your child feeling those feelings, it's the most painful thing in the world."

She gazed at her daughter, returning to the present. "With Joanna's [experience of bullying], I felt so defenseless and helpless, so hurt. I can't really say anything to make it better. At the very basic level, you want to protect your children from anything, do the best that you can. You keep them fed and you keep them sheltered and you give them love and all the things you think you can control, and from the moment you get a baby that is handed to you, it's the most incredible feeling and you love that child."

Not being able to help her daughter was devastating. "You're a mom, you're supposed to be able to fix everything," Elaine said, "even if you know that's not true intellectually. Emotionally, you want to. It may have been one of the first true moments when I realized that I wasn't able to protect her." Tears slid down her cheeks. Elaine told me about when Joanna got her vaccinations, about the involuntary tears that came at the sight of her daughter's pain. Thinking of Joanna's anguish over Amy, she could not help but wonder how her daughter was truly feeling inside. "These moments may define you," she said, her voice heavy with emotion.

Sorrow is a binding energy between mother and child, arguably the most visceral response a parent has when a child is hurt outside the home. But parents of victimized girls report feeling a range of emotions toward their daughters, including anger and frustration.

How is it, a mother wonders, that my child could endure such cruelty from her best friend all week and then skip cheerfully down the driveway to spend the night there on Friday? How could she have lain in my lap crying so hard she nearly tore my sweater gasping for breath, and now giggles on the computer as she instant messages and types her secrets into cyberspace? How could I have had my heart broken and stomped on as a witness to this pain, stayed up nights anxious in the dark, been inspired to cruel fantasies against another child, wanted even to wring her mother's neck, and today my child acts as though it is me who is crazy, unhinged, irrational, and unforgiving?

In particular, it's the girls hurt by their close friends who pull parents along on their emotional roller coaster. During the darker days, a parent is exhausted with the caregiving her daughter's sadness demands. Moments later, she rubs her eyes to ensure she sees correctly. Her child, full of smiles, behaves as though nothing is wrong. Understandably, her impulse is to seize the child by the collar and rattle some old-fashioned sense into her. But it's the daughter who often thinks her mother is crazy.

As girls grow older, moving with increasing self-reliance through the labyrinth of their social world, the gulf between mother and daughter widens. Mothers may struggle to understand the social choices of their daughters. The girls' tendency to return to their bullies, to tolerate the meanness—behaviors that strike their mothers as patently absurd—appear strangely logical to the girls. For some girls, anything is preferable to isolation, no matter how passionate their parents' entreaties.

What defies logic to a mother is unmistakably clear to her daughter. Thirteen-year-old Shelley practically punches the table, furious at her mother's cluelessness. "She doesn't understand that you don't just go and tell someone, 'I can't believe you've done something so mean to me.' It's just not how you handle a situation!" When Erin, profiled in chapter three, reconciled with her friends, her mother was dumbstruck. "I just really was worried. I was really angry at these kids. I didn't want them near her. I didn't trust them. I was afraid they would propel her back into this." She added, "People have said to me, 'You have to be forgiving.' People I respect! My reaction is, Wait, you weren't standing there! You didn't feel the hatred that their eyes were sending out and cutting the air with a knife!"

Of her daughter, Linda confided that "it was hard to live with her not taking my advice. I pushed too hard. She was passive. I wanted her to do something. It felt so awful that she wasn't doing anything. I knew someone was hurting her and she was not taking care of herself. But I couldn't do it for her anymore."

For some mothers, the sight of their daughter's surrender to abuse is an infuriating sign of weakness. One mother was astonished at her daughter's irrational behavior. Her two tormentors insisted they were born on the same day, in the same room. "Rebecca knew their birthdays were different but she *still* questioned her own belief!" she said. Especially when mothers have worked hard to model assertive behavior to their daughters, the frustration can be intense. Andrea, Maggie's mom, explained. "When I tried to push, she would just say helplessly, 'I can't, I can't.' There were times when I would feel angry at her because I'm such an outspoken person. It was hard for me to remember when I wasn't, so I would want her to speak up. I would give her the words and everything. Why couldn't she do it!" The weakening connection between mother and child during this difficult period makes approaching the crisis of bullying even harder.

fate

Stereotypes about females and aggression play a powerful role in the approach of some mothers to their daughter's ordeal. A girl who has a punishing experience can grow up to become a mother who is suspicious, anxious, and angry about her daughter's peers. These women watch their children's pain through the lens of their own suffering. Explaining her decision not to speak up when her daughter was victimized, Mary said, "I can't always jump in and pull her out of a bad situation. It doesn't change when you grow up. There are still adults who are just as backstabbing as little kids." She later became frustrated when I pressed her, and as her daughter looked on, she exploded. "I mean, girls are just—I don't have a lot of girl-friends! Because you have to know who to trust. And I don't think girls are as nice as boys in the long run. She has to learn how to choose her friends!"

One Sunday morning, Margaret led me through a swirl of children who raced around my waist, slid in socks across the foyer floor, and pounded up the stairs squealing. "It's a little crazy here," she said, rolling her eyes and smiling warmly, "but I hope we can find somewhere quiet." We headed into a room that looked like it was used about twice a year. Margaret had asked me here to talk about her daughter, Chloe (see chapter seven). Her face clouded as we sat down.

"I don't know what it is," she told me, hands clenched in her lap. "I look at her and I see sparkling water. It's a clean slate. Every day is just a wonderful thing. She sees the world, she loves people. And she's run into some very strange things with girls. . . . It's just this backbiting, this jealousy, this I don't know what it is."

Margaret was as awed as she was alienated by her daughter's beauty and brass. "I was in a different position," she said simply. Nearly thirty years ago, her clique chose a new girl to be picked on every week, and it was almost always Margaret. Sometimes they would pretend she didn't exist, and Margaret would hide and eat lunch in the library. Her feelings of hurt were still fresh today. "You really depend on your friends for acknowledgment and recognition and normality," she said. "Then they suddenly change how you trust people and whether you do trust people." Since then, she said, she had been hesitant to make new connections with people. She was less trusting. She gravitated to men because with women, "How can you know who's on your side and who's not?" Margaret said she is the most lonely in a crowd. Even when friends come to dinner at her home, she finds herself lingering over dishes, alone.

"So I was the dark one," she told me. "Distrusting. I was not happy. But I don't want to prejudice my child into thinking that everyone's terrible." It's hard. The rules of girlhood are, if anything, more elusive today. Chloe had been punished by her girlfriends because she played football at recess with the boys. "In two years," Margaret said, "it may be normal to play football. And then has she missed the boat? The rules are always changing. You never know what's right and what's not right. Who's in and who's not in. What's good and what's not good."

She felt less than optimistic about Chloe's impending physical maturity. "My daughter," she said, "is going to be a knockout. And I am amazed by her confidence. She walks around, shoulders up, head out, and she seems like she loves herself. I never had that," she added. Margaret felt certain Chloe's confidence and beauty would intimidate everyone around her. I asked why.

Margaret had only her experience of women today, informed so powerfully by her plight as a child, to guide her thoughts about her daughter's future. What came most often to mind was the unshakeable feeling of being judged by other women. "We're always comparing whose roots are longer: 'Oh, she needs to go have her hair done. Oh, she's getting heavy.' We're always judging because we're holding the mirror up to ourselves. Her roots are showing; are mine? If my roots are showing, are they all talking about it?"

It was the same thing with her daughter's social life, she told me. "Your kid has learning issues in school," she said, lowering her voice to a whisper. "It's a family secret. You're having trouble with the teachers. You're the only one who's having the trouble. You don't tell anyone." Later, she confessed, "We all know you'll be looking at the other person and judging them."

Margaret believed the women's movement failed to unite women and, as a stay-at-home mom, felt patronized by working mothers. She was often ashamed at social gatherings. She told me about a friend who asked her in amazement, "What do you *do* all day?" She grimaced. "We don't respect each other. Why can't we stop looking at each other's roots? We're all going through it together, and we should help each other out. If you're a working mom and I can help you, let me help you! We're still racing against men," she said. "Why do we have to race against each other?"

When I think about parents and bullying, I am reminded of the safety instructions you hear on a plane: if cabin pressure is lost, put on your own oxygen mask before helping your child. Currently, parents face unacceptable barriers to supporting their daughters through social crises. They need a new language to talk about girls' aggression. With a vocabulary to approach schools and speak the truths of girls' relationships, a parent can take back some of the control she needs. Empowered by the knowledge that so many of her peers share this experience, she can raise her own voice. Parents will raise stronger daughters who can know their own experiences as a shared, common chapter, and still grow up to cherish other women.

helping her through drama, bullying,
and everything in between

In this chapter, you'll get the best of what I've learned after a decade of teaching and working with thousands of girls, families, and educators. I have collected the wisdom and strategies of the most able professionals and seasoned parents, along with the voices of girls who have advised me on what works and what doesn't when they need help.

Some of what you'll read may seem obvious or intuitive. This is true enough, but keep in mind that when it's your own child who is suffering, rational thought can go out the window. When that happens, you may operate from a place of emotion and impulse, rather than reason and reflection. Consider this chapter an anchor to keep you grounded, a trusted voice of reason to bounce off your own feelings and ideas.

the first response: empathy

I asked every woman and girl I interviewed to rate her parents' response to her ordeal. Overwhelmingly, the most effective parents were the ones who actively listened. These mothers and fathers inquired every day about how school went. They held their daughters when they cried. They accommodated special requests, whether it was going to school later, being picked up within seconds of the last bell, or preparing a special meal. Elizabeth, from chapter seven, confided that "if it weren't for my Mom, I'd probably be demented. She respected my need not to say anything and my need for her silent presence. [I needed her to] just hug me, hold me."

The foundation of these gestures was empathy, an attempt by each parent to connect with a child's emotional experience. Your daughter is hungry for empathy when she is struggling socially. Remember that girls live in a peer culture that often denies or invalidates feelings: *you're being too sensitive, I didn't do that, you took it the wrong way, I was just kidding.* With so many voices saying her feelings are unfounded, she needs you to help authorize her experience. Empathy may feel like a meager contribution, but it's immeasurably important.

Yet empathy can be the first thing to go in a moment of panic or anxiety. Parents struggle for two reasons. First, when the alarm bells go off, we want to put out the fire. We assume—understandably—that we can make a child feel better by making the problem go away. Parents are habituated to this from the moment of a child's birth: feed when they are hungry, sleep when they are tired, hold when they cry. Yet as your child grows more independent, and her peer culture becomes more influential, it will become almost impossible to make her problems "go away." (In my experience, most girls come to accept that long before their parents do.) The overwhelming desire to solve the problem short-circuits the empathy muscle.

Second, empathy is painful. It involves slowing down to acknowledge and think about your child's feelings of hurt, rejection, or sadness. This can be an anguishing experience for parents. Connecting with these emotions can make you feel powerless and overwhelmed, so it's understandable why so many parents would prefer to spring into action. Linda recalled her response to her daughter with some regret. In hindsight, she said, "I wouldn't have pushed so hard [for her to fight back]... Otherwise it becomes about what I want instead of what she wants, and sometimes I think I made that mistake because it was so painful to watch."

An empathic response to a girl being targeted might sound like the following:

"I'm so sorry this happened."

"That sounds awful."

"If I were you, I would also feel really _____."

"It sounds like you're feeling pretty_____. That makes a lot of sense."

Empathy is not the same thing as expressing emotions. This moment is not about you sharing your feelings. It can be extremely uncomfortable for a child if her parent weeps or loses strength at the moment when her daughter needs it most. The message sent is that you need to be taken care of, not the other way around. And your response might influence your daughter's willingness to keep confiding in you. She may believe it's in your best interests not to know the messiest feelings she has, that on some level it is not acceptable for her to share them with you.

Suzanne Cohen had always struggled to separate her feelings from her daughter's, but when Hannah's torment began, her sense of helplessness nearly broke her. "I didn't know where [my feelings] left off and hers began and vice versa," she told me. With the help of a therapist, she learned that she could not live vicariously through her daughter, and that her behavior suggested to Hannah a need to be parented by her. "I wanted to be able to make it right," she said, but "at a certain point I kind of realized that it's not about anyone doing anything other than just listening. [I had to] give her the shoulder, let her vent, let her get it out of her system, because I am a mother, and then not respond to that in anything but a loving way, and not make it my battle." Eventually Suzanne learned how to play a role in her daughter's experience that would both honor her child's circumstances and give herself a sense of agency. It was harder than you think, she said, to do it.

Have your emotions, it has been said, or they will have you. To avoid losing yourself in your daughter's feelings, reflect on your own. Like the mothers in chapter nine, most parents bring as much to the bullying situation as their daughters. Your response to your daughter will bear the imprint of your priorities, your fears, your childhood. Ask yourself some of the following questions:

- What was the hardest part about my experiences with peers growing up? How might that influence the way I am responding right now?
- What am I most afraid of in this situation? How reasonable is my fear? How might this fear be guiding my response? Is operating from this place allowing me to parent effectively?
- If my best friend was parenting through this experience, what advice would I give him or her?

Knowing how you feel will anchor you. If you know you are angry, or scared, you will be more in control and reflective about your impulses—and less likely to act on the more destructive ones without thinking clearly. If you know where your feelings come from, you will be more thoughtful about your decisions.

To help you achieve the right balance in how you respond to your daughter, think back to when she was learning to walk. If you showed fear and panic when she slipped and fell, she'd usually sense it and wail. If you chortled, "Oops! You're okay! Up you go!" and plucked her up calmly, she probably kept on trucking. It was a combination of concern and reassurance that motivated her to continue. This is what she needs from you now. Kim Kaminski, a veteran school counselor, urges parents to rise above their alarm and be the rock for their daughters. "The parent has to be the parent and say, 'I am here for you, I am going to help you, and I know you can do this. We will find a way together.'" When a girl does not believe in herself, or think that a situation can improve, a parent's strength is hugely reassuring. Your courage will sustain her when she cannot access any on her own.

It takes spiritual brawn to carry someone through a time of pain and suffering. You need to take care of yourself, too. Call on the resources around you to be good to yourself, whether it's with exercise, friends, counseling, meditation, or cheesecake. Your success as a parent is not measured by how little you need to survive. You cannot care for others when you are diminished.

Keep in mind that empathy is conveyed through actions as well as words. Ask yourself and your child how you can make her life easier at school and home. Cover all the bases of your child's day and see where you can lighten her load. Find out what she's doing at lunch and recess: If she's alone, where is she? Would it be possible to arrange for her to go to the library or art room or gym twice a week? It's not a permanent solution, nor should she make a habit of escaping every single day, but if she is truly suffering, perhaps you can find her some space to breathe.

Are there any other friends she can play with during the day? Encourage her to join their lunch table or group at recess. If you have good friends with children your daughter can play with, talk with them about it. Be careful: avoid the appearance of trying to force your daughter into friendship with another girl. Be sure to communicate with the parent about the potential for a good fit with her child. Never assume it's another child's responsibility to help your daughter, no matter how dire your child's straits. To encourage the other child to exercise compassion at the expense of her own social needs would be to reinforce the message that care and self-sacrifice are her priority. At the end of the day, the decision should lie with the two children.

why girls don't tell their parents

Ten minutes before the last bell, and I was winding up my discussion with ninth-grade girls at Linden. Papers were rustling like leaves, bodies were starting to wriggle and fidget. "Okay!" I said, a little louder than I meant to. "One more question." I asked them if they talk to their parents about bullying, or when a girl is mean to them.

A ripple of "No way!" and "Yeah, right" crested through the room, followed by snorts, muttering, and one girl spitting up her soda.

"Right," I said coolly, trying to look unfazed. "Why? Really," I said cheerfully. "Come on, you guys."

Mollie piped up, "You can disappoint your parents if you're not friends with everyone."

"You don't want your parents to think badly of your friend because you'd get over it," Lydia added. "You want to stand up for your friend because they reflect you."

"Oh yeah!" Reena cackled. "My mother will go, 'I never liked that friend of yours anyway!'"

"Totally," murmured a voice in the corner.

"My mom's a dork. She says, 'Oh, I'll be your friend,'" Lauren said.

"I don't want to tell her if she thinks I'm wrong. If she's not on my side, it's like I failed and it's terrible because your parents are supposed to be on your side."

"I don't want my friends *and* my parents against me."

And on and on.

Most girls don't tell their parents what's going on in a bullying situation. That's not a sex difference, either; bullying is a deeply humiliating experience for every child. Since alternative aggressions lack a public identity, however, the burden of silence may be heavier. Some girls may not be able to identify what they're experiencing as wrong or punishable. Instead, they may internalize the problem as their fault and never speak of it.

A child might also feel that since there are no rules prohibiting the behavior, and so much of it slips beneath the radar of teachers, that it's somehow not worth mentioning or pursuing. Faith, an eighth-grade teacher in Ridgewood who as a student attempted suicide when her friends abandoned her, was too embarrassed to tell her mother what was happening. "I didn't think my mama had went through all this because she never told me about any of it. I didn't want her to know all this because it was really embarrassing telling your mom that a girl was picking on you and bullying you and stuff."

Talking with your children about alternative aggressions is absolutely critical. If you indicate to your child in a nonjudgmental way that you know what goes on at school—that on some level you "get" the hidden culture of girls' aggression—she will feel safe showing you its darkest corners. Be casual: Do it in the car on the way home, in the kitchen before a meal, or during a commercial while watching television. Asking leading questions can help:

- When girls are mean in your class, what kinds of things do they do?
- Does the teacher see it when it's happening? Why or why not? How does she react?
- Are some girls more secretive about their meanness? How?
- Can friends be mean to each other? How?

It helps to introduce your questions in the third person. It will give your child the chance to acclimate to talking with you about it.

Girls are socialized to care for others, so they often hold their feelings in to shield others from the weight of their pain—hence the spike in depression, self-mutilation, and anorexia that can accompany the loss of self-esteem around adolescence. Stephanie, whose silence left an ulcer in her stomach, explained, "I didn't want [my parents] to worry more. I didn't want them to think that I was a freak who couldn't, like, make the grade."

Once I got them going, the over three hundred girls I met individually and in groups spoke passionately about what their parents did wrong when it came to helping them. Here are some of the most common responses of parents to their daughters' ordeals, followed by what many girls say they'd prefer (with my own two cents thrown in for good measure).

fault lines: what not to say

WRONG: *"It's a phase"* or *"It happens to everyone, honey."*

This remark is meant to soothe, but it ends up trivializing your daughter's pain. It says, "You're a dime a dozen," when she feels just the opposite—that her pain is the worst she's ever felt, that she is surely the first to feel it this intensely, that she is the only one who's ever endured something so horrible. It may indeed be a phase, but she doesn't know that. This comment only underscores for her how little you get what she's dealing with.

A lot of parent-child communication surrounding bullying is like the children's game of Operator. What sounds like "It happens to everyone" out of your mouth might sound like "It happens to losers like you" in her ears. One of the most common reasons girls don't tell is because of the shame they feel for failing to perform socially. If girls' social identities are built on their relational skills, isolation is a disaster. The feeling of failure is only increased by comments that trivialize what they're going through.

BETTER: *"Oh, honey. That is so terrible. I'm sorry."*

Honor your child's pain as though she were the first to experience it. At the same time, tell her about alternative aggressions. As many parents are well aware, you can tell your child something and she'll turn up her nose, and when she hears it from someone else, she'll nod effusively. Explain what researchers have found. Explain that she is not alone.

ADD: *"It happened to me."*

Did it? Can you remember? If you can connect to the feelings you had as an adolescent, your daughter is far more likely to keep listening and believe you. But don't overdo it: some kids told me they hated it when their mothers insisted they knew exactly how they were feeling. "My mother says, 'I know how you feel,' but she doesn't," they said. "Things are different now." This is especially true in the age of cyberbullying. If you did not grow up in a world where aggression was unleashed at the speed of a text or e-mail, there is indeed a gulf between you and your daughter's childhood experiences.

WRONG: *"I never liked that friend of yours anyway."* Also known as *"Why are you hanging out with her/them to begin with?"* and *"How many times do I have to tell you [fill in the blank]?"*

Ever date someone your friends didn't like? Remember when they told you how wrong the person was for you? Did you say, "Oh, that's *right*! Thank you *so* much!" and dump him? The same is true for your daughter. Sure, she's hanging out with girls you may think are terrible, but she's not going to figure it out until she's ready, and you may have little to do with it when she does. At this point, it's wise to remember girls' fear of relational loss and that your child is probably looking for a way to heal the relationship, not to end it.

On-again, off-again friendships can drive parents insane, and rightly so. Depending on the day, your daughter is either thrilled or tortured, and you are a mostly helpless passenger on her roller coaster ride. Become too angry or frustrated, and your daughter may begin hiding what's happening. If she disconnects, she is that much more vulnerable.

BETTER: *Take a deep breath, and try to walk the line between responding as a parent and as a friend: as a parent, you have the right to convey your unhappiness about the way your daughter is being treated, and to weigh in about what a healthy friendship looks like. At the same time, to avoid alienating your daughter, exercise caution with your judgment as a friend might. At a certain point, girls may choose toxic friends over their disapproving parents. Remember: you want her to stay connected to you.*

Sometimes, the most you can do is ask questions that push her to reflect on her toxic relationship. Try some of these:

- What are you looking for in a good friend? Does this person give you that?
- Why do you think you are staying friends with someone who makes you feel this way?
- When you allow her to [refer to a specific act], what message are you sending her about yourself?
- When she [refer to a specific act], what message is she sending you about the kind of friend she is?

Keep in mind that at some point, your daughter will outgrow this friendship, or the other girl will simply move on. As with all painful relationships, your daughter will come away with a powerful life lesson about friendship and intimacy. This is not much consolation right now, I know, but trust me that it will not be this way forever.

WRONG: *"What could you be doing to cause this?"*

If your daughter is being bullied or cast out of her social group, it is highly unlikely that anything she does or changes about herself is going to make a difference. There's often no rhyme or reason to the moment a girl or clique finally decides to get angry or even. If there is, it's usually not traceable to any one person's fault. Moreover, your daughter is probably already cataloging her faults with the efficiency of a computer. No matter what your intention, we have the Operator problem again. You say, "What can you change about yourself?" She hears, "My mother thinks it's my fault and there's something wrong with me."

Naomi believes her mother's interpretation of her problem as a social-skills issue left a second scar. "I wanted her to be a mother lion and protect me, to treat me as endangered and not as a kid with problems. I wanted her to see a greater, more immediate danger." She needed her mother to defend her, not question her. It's okay to ask for your daughter's contribution to a situation, but tread lightly.

It should not rank in the first five of the questions you ask her when she tells you about the problem.

BETTER: *"Do you want to brainstorm together about how we got here?"*

The problem may not always be developmental. Remember Erin: all her friends repressed their problems with her, letting their anger simmer quietly for years until finally it exploded. Remembering the dynamics between herself and her friends helped Erin understand why their anger felt so disproportionate. Erin could see where she inspired anger, competition, and jealousy, and where her friends might have been afraid to talk about it or express anger. Working backward with your child by walking her through memories of tension may be similarly effective.

ALSO: *Ask the school counselor or teacher.*

Perhaps your daughter *could* improve her social skills; perhaps she's not responding to cues the right way and is drawing the ire of her peers. She may be too young or unaware to tell you that herself. Visit her guidance counselor or teacher for an evaluation. Research the resources that are available to help your family. Helping your daughter improve her social skills is another way to engage her in bettering her own situation. Asking how she may be triggering the behavior is not an inappropriate question, but as my mother always says, "It's not what you say, it's how you say it." Your approach should be balanced, respectful, and tender, one that reflects a mix of empathy for your child's pain and support for her social success.

WRONG: *"This is the way girls are. You may as well get used to it."*

Mothers who were once targets of girls' aggression often voice this sentiment. This is another instance in which the parent's experience may overwhelm the child's. No matter whom you're talking about, generalizing about a group of people never sets a positive example for your daughter. Teaching her to fear and hate other females is, of course, a mistake. There will always be challenging people in our lives. To suggest she give up the joys and comfort of female friendship will only hurt her more. Moreover, if you implicate all females in her situation, you imply that the relationship itself wasn't the problem, which is actually what your daughter needs to learn so she can find a healthier friendship the next time around.

BETTER: *"Did you know that there is research about why some girls act in these ways when they get angry?"*

Teach your daughter about how girls are socialized. Explain how many girls are denied permission to express anger, jealousy, and competitiveness openly, and how that affects the ways girls express themselves. This doesn't mean apologizing for aggressive behavior; it's about understanding where it comes from so she can feel less isolated or singled out in the experience.

Guide her to understand how conflict avoidance appears in all kinds of relationships, not just the bad ones. Help her identify her own fears of conflict, even her own acts of alternative aggression.

This is a good time to wax philosophical about love, loss, and relationship. Conflict is an inevitable and vital part of relationship. It is also the price of having intense connections: "'Tis better to have loved and lost than never to have loved at all."

WRONG: *"She's just jealous."*

This is one of parents' favorite things to say, but it doesn't connect with girls in middle school and up. It's often the case that the girl who bullies or hurts your daughter appears quite self-satisfied, attractive, powerful, or otherwise well-off. Jealousy is the last thing your daughter believes this girl would feel. She thinks, Why would someone who appears that strong and satisfied be jealous of *me*?

BETTER: *"Why do you think she's doing this?"*

If you ask this question of an adolescent, you might well get some version of "Um, if I knew that, I would have told you already" or

"Because she hates me." That's okay. Keep pushing your daughter to consider why the girl is acting this way. Little by little, as she reflects, your daughter may realize it has less to do with her and more to do with the other girl. Or she may begin to see that the friendship is fundamentally broken. This kind of clarity can actually be a comfort.

WRONG: *"Maybe you're being a little sensitive?"* or *"But you two are such good friends!"*

As my grandmother would say, "Oy vey." It would be hard to overstate the resentment adult women still feel about this particular pearl of wisdom. You may think you're toughening up your daughter, teaching her to roll with the punches, but she experiences these remarks as a blatant denial of her feelings.

Naomi grew up in the kind of home where if she fell, her grandmother would laugh and say, "I hope you didn't break the floor!" When she told her parents how the others were whittling her down, they advised her to act as though it weren't happening. She recalled,

> I couldn't cry about it. I couldn't ask for help. I couldn't fight back. I didn't have a right to defend myself. You couldn't show your pain. You couldn't react as if someone had done a really bad thing. There was this silence, this you can't speak. And I feel as though I have a right to nothing more than I have a right to my own feelings ... You have a right to do whatever you need to do to defend yourself and you have the right to feel dignity. I think that was the greatest thing that I feel was ever taken from me. And only now am I getting it back.

Remember that appearances can be deceiving. Girls easily tuck aggression into the folds of friendship, making it almost invisible. Your child's brief or casual disclosure may be the only warning you get. Faith explained how her bully's sweet exterior masked the girl's nastiness. "Nobody knew because Liz was like a straight A student, and they thought she was friends with all these people. Nobody knew what she'd do to some of her friends." If you find yourself arguing with your daughter, it wouldn't hurt to ask yourself why. After all, we see what we want to see. What do you have to gain or lose if your daughter is no longer friends with this person?

At the end of the day, if you weren't present for the episode your daughter is describing, calling her hypersensitive is unfair and judgmental. It's one of the clearest ways to signal you don't understand her or her life. It also perpetuates the silencing and invalidation of girls' aggression.

BETTER: *"How can you tell they're not joking? Are you sure they really mean to make you feel this bad?"*

If your child is recalling a situation her friends insisted was a "joke," beware. As I show in chapter three, girls use humor as a vehicle to convey negative feelings indirectly. It is also extremely common for a girl to do something hurtful, then deny it happened at all. This can make your daughter second-guess herself and even feel a bit crazy. As she lets the other girl define what is true in the relationship, she surrenders the confidence and authority she needs to stand up for herself.

In a culture that denies the anger and meanness girls visit upon one another, it is incumbent upon you as a parent to validate your child's version of events. You may be the only one who ever will. That's not to say you should overreact and overidentify with your child's painful disclosures. But you do have to take her word for it. If you don't, you may risk never hearing from her again.

beyond empathy: raising a resilient daughter

As much as the parental instinct blares to protect your child from pain, her healthy development is dependent on learning to handle life's challenges. The stresses of friendship help her learn vital coping skills she will use across a range of contexts and throughout her life. Depriving girls of these experiences, and of the opportunity to wrestle with them, does not eliminate stress; it delays its arrival, dangerously. As psychologist Madeline Levine has shown in her book *The Price of Privilege,* adolescents whose parents deprived them of opportunities to be self-reliant were unable to handle the challenges of adolescence. These teenagers had high levels of anxiety and depression. They were more likely to engage in self-destructive behaviors like substance abuse and self-mutilation.[80]

Relationships are the fourth "R"—or should be, anyway. Just like math or spelling, successful friendships involve learning and practicing a set of skills that become more sophisticated over time. If we do not expect girls to arrive at kindergarten capable of adding fractions, we should not expect them to have flawless friendships from a young age. Girls have to learn, and we have to help them. This process takes time, not to mention some stumbles and missteps along the way. It also means giving girls the space to learn on their own. For just as we know that doing her math homework for her will stunt her learning potential, doing her "relationship homework" will be equally harmful.

Best-friend heartbreaks (or "friend divorces," as I call them) confer hard-won wisdom about what we're seeking and deserve in our most important relationships. Think back to the times you have had your heart broken, either by a friend or romantic partner. It is probably true that the experiences made you stronger and taught you things that improved your later relationships. Remembering the invaluable lessons of those dark days may help as you watch your daughter endure her own.

You are not a bad parent if she gets hurt or hurts someone else. Nor, of course, is she a troubled or unusual child. Think about it this way: when girls begin dating, most realize they won't end up marrying their first crush. They accept that they will probably get dumped and will do the same to others. Why not embrace this idea when it comes to female friendship? What if we could parent girls with the expectation that friend problems will inevitably crop up, and that these are formative obstacles on the road to adulthood? This doesn't mean excusing bullying or severe aggression. It does mean approaching the situation as an opportunity to learn, and not an instant crisis or the sign of a parenting failure.

Giving your daughter an opportunity to flex her coping muscles on her own will help her become more resilient. Resilience is defined as the ability to overcome stress, challenge, or adversity. I believe a socially resilient girl can size up a challenging friend situation, think about her options, and choose a strategy whose outcome has been carefully considered.

You can build these muscles in your daughter by asking her to take responsibility for her own decisions in a relationship. After empathizing with her, you can ask, "What do you want to do about this?" She will most likely say, "I don't know." Gently push her. You can say, "I know it feels overwhelming, but what's one thing you think you could do?" Allow her to generate a few choices (doing nothing, by the way, is a choice).

Go even further and try the four-step GIRL protocol with her, which your daughter can apply to any social challenge. It works like this:

G—Gather Your Choices. (List all the choices you might make in response to the situation.)

I—I Choose ... (Make a choice. Pick one of the strategies you just listed above.)

R—Reasons Are ... (Justify your choice. List the reasons you will choose this strategy.)

L—List the Outcomes. (Think ahead: what might happen if you make this choice?)

Below is a GIRL completed by Esther, an eighth grader, whose friend ignored her when another girl was around. When Esther asked her friend why she was doing it, the girl denied it and said Esther was being too sensitive.

The first step is G, Gather Your Choices. Esther listed her options: *stop speaking to her, talk about her behind her back, ask her about it online, tell her how I feel, talk to an adult, hang out with other people,* and *ask someone else if she knows why my friend is ignoring me.*

The second step is I, or I Choose. Esther decided to talk to her friend about it online.

The third step is R, or Reasons Are. Esther said she wanted to do it online because it was easier than asking in person and she could keep it more casual that way.

The fourth step is L, or List the Outcomes. Esther predicted that her friend might deny it again, or she might feel more comfortable communicating via Facebook.

Would I advise Esther to share her feelings with a friend on Facebook? No way. But it's important to let girls realistically explore their options during the "G" step, even if you don't agree with them. I could challenge Esther, of course, but it might be useful to let her follow through so she can fully own her choice and its consequences. I have found that when girls pick strategies that will hurt themselves or others, they have second thoughts once they get to the step where they list outcomes. They often backpedal and decide to do something else.

The GIRL protocol helps a girl become more resilient by sharpening several key skills she needs to be sturdy in the face of friend drama: First, it gives her a systematic method for laying out all the possible strategies to deal with a problem. Second, it asks her to make a choice. This gives her a sense of agency and control in situations where she would otherwise feel helpless or overwhelmed—or where choices are often made for her by other adults. Third, GIRL expects her to justify and own her decision, asking her to reflect on her personal values. Finally, GIRL asks her to think long term about the consequences of her choices. This practical way of thinking is especially important for girls who trend toward aggressive, indirect, or retaliatory responses. For example, you may choose to talk about someone behind her back, but if you think about the potential for retaliation, you are likely to reconsider.

You can use GIRL verbally, by asking your daughter to reflect on the questions informally. Better yet, write G-I-R-L on a page and ask her to fill it out with you the next time she comes home with a problem. Ultimately, the questions you ask your daughter should become the questions she learns to ask herself. In other words, the GIRL protocol should become part of how she thinks about life's challenges. The point is to build the internal muscles your daughter needs to think for herself in the face of stress.

coaching your daughter as she confronts a peer

If your daughter is considering confronting a peer—or if you want her to—you can guide her with some of these ideas. To learn more about the skills girls need to navigate difficult conversations, check out my latest book, *The Curse of the Good Girl: Raising Authentic Girls with Courage and Confidence.*

Conflict is an opportunity to get what you want. As we have seen throughout this book, many girls view conflict as catastrophic to relationship. However, conflict can be an opportunity to create change in a relationship that matters to you. You talk with someone because you need something from her: you need her to stop doing something, or to start. As you consult with your daughter about her options, share instances of successfully resolved conflicts that you have had: moments when you have spoken your truth respectfully and been rewarded for it. Try, as much as you can, to loosen her negative associations with conflict.

If it doesn't go your way, it's not necessarily a loss. Your daughter may do her very best to confront a peer in a way that is sincere and thoughtful. If the other girl reacts poorly, it does not mean your daughter did something wrong. It is vital to convey to girls that they can be responsible for only how they act, not how others respond. There are too many girls who, because of their lack of comfort with conflict, associate any kind of challenging conversation with disaster (these are often the same girls who, if you say anything negative in a mild tone of voice, report that "She yelled at me!"). These girls will not under any circumstances be able to hear the truth your daughter needs to convey.

Just as a strong feeling like anger can be a sign that something is wrong within ourselves, a friend's failure to listen or respond with compassion is an important signal that a relationship may not be healthy. As painful as this kind of disappointment may be, it does offer three benefits: one, an avenue opens to leave the relationship; two, you strengthen your sense of what healthy intimacy looks like; and three, you discover what you are seeking in your closest relationships.

Resist the urge to advise your daughter to end a friendship over a single mistake. Remember that girls are still learning how to be in relationship with each other. They are also more tolerant of their friends than you are. That is a good thing: Girls need opportunities to work through issues together and without adults. This will feel uncomfortable for you, and it should. It is not natural to enjoy watching your child wrestle with something painful. But it is what she needs to develop skills and standards for healthy friendships. Obviously, tolerance should have its limits. Still, remain mindful of how your own alarm may be different from your daughter's.

Practice always helps. No one wakes up one day a "grownup" who is effortlessly able to speak her mind and heart. It takes courage, skills, and practice. The ability to have a difficult conversation gracefully does not simply happen to us. Learning to communicate is an ongoing process.

Practicing your toughest conversations first, as a role-play, is a terrific thing to do with your daughter. If you suggest it and her eyes start to roll, let her know this isn't a "kid" suggestion. Explain that adults rehearse difficult conversations all the time, with good reason: just as practicing piano or soccer makes you a better player, practicing how you communicate makes you more effective in your relationships.

In times of crisis, Ellen, a psychotherapist, found role-playing extremely effective in helping her daughter, Roma. She asked Roma and her ally to act out different scenarios of confrontation with their tormentor, Jane. "I was encouraging them to speak their truths," Ellen explained, "and to not be afraid of what [Jane] was going to say to other kids, and not let that control them. I would get very, very specific wading through with them—'Yeah, but if I say that, she'll say this!'—and I would help them figure out what they would say next. It was how to handle a situation."

Too often we dispense advice to children in a vertical way: "Tell her this!" or "Have you just tried walking away?" Role-playing is more horizontal and interactive. It makes the strategy three-dimensional and real for your daughter, while at the same time giving you a presence in her social world that will comfort both of you. Having a friend or sibling participate can shore up your child's sense of moral support and decrease the terror of isolation.

You can role-play in the car or the kitchen. Have your daughter coach you to act the way she thinks the other person would in an actual conversation. Perhaps your daughter thinks her peer will deny the problem, burst into tears, begin yelling, or just walk away. Play the part, and don't be quick to give in or give up. It doesn't help to hand your daughter an instant happy ending. By role-playing different outcomes, you indirectly affirm that people are unpredictable and, as mentioned earlier, you can be responsible for only your own reaction. Your daughter is also more invested in the outcome because she owns her plan of action.

Nerves are a big reason why girls avoid confrontation. Remind your daughter that being nervous means you care. The nerves that flare before a soccer game are driven by your investment in the match; if you didn't care, it wouldn't bother you.

interventions

So you've empathized. You've allowed your daughter to wrestle with her choices and try out a few. It wasn't enough. Now it's time to reach out and get help. If you are planning to call the school, read on. In talking with administrators, counselors, and classroom teachers, I have heard stories about parents that both horrify and inspire. Below are the wisdom and strategies I've accrued from these conversations. Use this section as a kind of "insider information" on what school professionals respond to and recoil from.

A quick note: If the only time your child's school hears from you is when you have a problem, you disadvantage yourself significantly. Teachers should get to know you in multiple contexts: normal every-day chitchat (you would be surprised how happy it can make a teacher when a parent simply takes the time to say, "How are you?"), messages of praise or simple recognition, and at events or activities where you contribute to the classroom. Short of this, staff may link conversations with you to feelings of inadequacy; that is, they will automatically associate you with an unhappy experience in which they may have come up short for your family.

Do your homework. Before you do anything, stop and think. Do you have all the information you need? It is understandable to want to contact the school immediately. However, the most effective parent will be able to derail a school's attempt to hand the problem back to the family. This means knowing, to the fullest extent possible, the status of your child's development. Get the facts from your daughter as a journalist would: find out who's doing it, how long it's been happening, what is happening, and if the teacher knows.

Do some more recon. What are her social relationships like outside the classroom? Have you spoken recently with her coaches and other instructors? What kind of disposition is your daughter perceived by others as having? Be open to the answers you may get. If you hear something that surprises or disappoints you, stay grounded. Although no child ever deserves to be bullied, stories are always more complicated than they first appear, especially with girls. You are much better off going in with that knowledge than being ambushed by it.

Reach out to other parents who have experienced similar situations. It is easy to get lost in an echo chamber of your own thoughts and feelings. Your peers can contribute strategies you haven't thought of, contacts at the school and elsewhere, and the comfort of knowing you are not alone.

Do not hesitate to contact a psychologist, social worker, or other professional counselor to help you or your daughter. This is not a failure on your part. If your daughter struggles to confide in you or someone at the school, time with an objective outsider may be exactly what you both need.

Respect her wishes. Before you pick up the phone to call the school, consider your daughter. Does *she* want you to call? Unless your child's life is endangered, exploiting parental authority to override your child's desire is unfair. She may have little left but her autonomy, and anyway, you're not the one who's going to spend seven hours a day in that classroom. Naomi remembered her parents' panicked response to her distraught behavior: "It was like I really broke down. The stress was too much, and they wanted to take me out of school. They wanted to call the school. I was like, don't, I'll die, I'll get killed, you don't understand, do not make a case out of it. I thought there was no limit. I can't—how can I emphasize enough that this was *real* to me. These were kids; adults didn't have power. I witnessed every day adults being out of the loop and kids having the power."

Even if you swear the teacher to secrecy, you can't predict what might happen. One teacher promised a girl that she would not mention the bullying in class, then pulled the perpetrating clique into the hallway and made them promise to be nice to her. The girls made a game out of pretending to be sugary sweet for the rest of the year, an agonizing fate.

Obviously there are exceptions. If your child's welfare is seriously endangered, you have to make an executive decision in her best interests. If you do this, proceed with the utmost sensitivity and caution.

Respect school protocol. Schools, like all organizations, are inherently political. At the end of the day, school leaders are mandated to keep both your child and their staff safe. Invariably and to some degree, the agitated parent will be on the "other side." Keep in mind that an organization's relationships and personalities matter as much as the business it does. This is never more true than when you contact your child's school about bullying. How you represent yourself is as important as what you say, and how you manage your relationships will affect an incident's outcome. As a parent, you have to protect your child and do it in a way you can both be proud of.

Avoid going from zero to sixty: do not begin your contact with the school by calling the principal, superintendent, or other senior officials. Call the school counselor or assistant principal first. If your child is in elementary school, speak to the classroom teacher before anyone else. Teachers understandably bristle when parents go over their heads; it makes them feel condescended to or ignored. Worse, when teachers spot parents in an administrator's office without prior notice, most assume they are going to be reprimanded. Demanding the highest authority and ignoring existing protocols lay the foundation for a potentially adversarial relationship between you and the staff at your child's school. These are people you need on your side.

Understand that most schools have a system in place for situations like yours (not necessarily an effective system, but a system nonetheless). "There are steps that the school has to follow when they get a bullying complaint," Julia Taylor, a North Carolina high-school counselor, told me. "We cannot just charge the alleged offender without investigation. There are always two sides to every story."

Set a goal. What are you seeking from this interaction with the school? Determine your goal before you begin. Be as specific as you can: do you want the school to investigate the problem, move your child's seat, give her a place to eat when she is alone at lunch, mediate among her friends? Write down notes you can use for a phone call or a meeting. Have the notes with you when it's time to speak so you stick to your talking points.

Be open to what others have to say. As upset as you are, you still need to have a conversation. Avoid the path of the middle-school parent who walked into a principal's office, pulled out a legal pad, and read for fifteen minutes, allowing no interruption. The most effective parents are upset but able to have a dialogue. John Magner, a Virginia school counselor, said, "I appreciate when a parent is open to listening and determining *with* the counselor what did actually happen with their child."

In order to investigate the problem, the school official you speak with may want to explore your daughter's contribution to the situation. Being willing to consider the possibilities is not a betrayal of your daughter, nor does it justify what has happened to her. It reflects your grip on the reality that information must be gathered, kids' conflicts are complex, and situations take time to fully understand.

School professionals are most emphatic on this point. "The parents who are least effective can't understand that their daughter, no matter how minor it may be, plays a role in the situation that is occurring. They see a black knight, white knight situation," said Brian Gatens, a New Jersey school administrator. Instant defensiveness and outrage about the role your child may have played in an incident is unproductive in the extreme. Saying "my daughter would never do that" virtually always leaves the listener thinking you don't get your kid. Taylor, the school counselor, said, "Girls are capable of doing everything you raised them not to do. I have yet to hear of a girl getting in the car or running through the front door [of] her house and announcing, 'Guess what, Mom, I was, like, totally aggressive all day! First, I spread a rumor about a girl, then I called her a bitch to her face, next, I skipped Algebra, and then I texted my friends all fourth period.'"

At a functionally responsive school, a target's contribution does not erase the accountability of the aggressor. However, be open to the possibility that as you learn more details from the school, the punishment you imagined may no longer be appropriate. Consider that the intent and impact of an incident may diverge; it is not always the case that a child set out to hurt your daughter. In these instances, the proposed solution may do little to relieve your anger and distress.

Lose your mind, then find it again. According to Gatens, it is always easier to work with parents who understand that their child is experiencing behavior that is "age appropriate, but inappropriate." These parents recognize that situations like theirs are not uncommon, and that the problem will be addressed.

Unless you just cut a fat check to your school's PTA or endowment fund, the I'll-huff-and-I'll-puff approach is generally ineffective. School officials are used to upset parents—that's part of the job—but unhappiness is never an excuse for rudeness. What pains teachers and counselors most in their interactions with parents is the loss of civility. Parents who drop by offices for intense conversations without making an appointment, who call excessively without leaving a message (yes, most schools have caller ID), who send lengthy e-mails and are outraged when there is no instant response, create discomfort and resentment in the very people whose help they need. Some parents go further, becoming verbally abusive and threatening.

Although parents who act this way comprise a small percentage of a community, they can absorb a disproportionate amount of a school or teacher's time. They can also bruise a teacher's self-esteem and professional confidence. When teachers become skittish about difficult parents, they play it safe, avoiding situations where they may encounter an aggressive parent—and possibly hanging back when certain children act out.

When a child is in any kind of danger, it is easy to let anxiety and fear overwhelm you. This comes through in how you communicate, interpret information, and react to others. Emotion can be an asset or a weapon; as the latter, Gatens says, "While it may get a lot of attention, it isn't that good in getting a lot of results because it automatically creates an adversarial relationship." For this reason, remaining as calm and respectful as you can is crucial.

There is no easy way to say it: getting labeled your school's "crazy parent" can complicate the path to a solution. Be prepared to offer clear, factual details about the situation. Using the information you gathered from your daughter and conversations with other adults in her life, share the evidence. Describe behaviors and incidents. Steer clear of personal judgments about children or adults.

That doesn't mean being a robot. Gatens explains, "The parents who are the most effective lose their minds, but then they find them again." Before you call, take your emotional temperature. Can you control yourself if the conversation does not go your way? If you feel a need to call that is so urgent you can't do or think about anything else, it may not be the right time.

There are two things to avoid: First, try not to wait until the moment you're boiling over to act. Some parents watch from the sidelines and catalogue aggressive incidents, only to explode when the situation becomes untenable. Waiting too long usually means that you are overwhelmed by the time you approach the school.

Second, do not begin a conversation from a place of anger. Accusing the school, from the first moment, of doing nothing and allowing your child to be bullied will obviously make it difficult to work together to address your problem.

"I respond much better to a parent who calls and tells me on the phone or asks to come in, thanks me, and trusts that I will do everything in my power to help her and her daughter," Julia Taylor told me. "Also," she added, "sometimes parents just need to vent, and that's okay, too."

Avoid attacking the other child. When you report what has happened, stay focused on the behavior, not the character, of the aggressive child. Do not label her or question the way she was parented; any professional worth her salt will refuse to engage on that level anyway. Stick with what is happening to your child and how you and the school can help her.

Be strong for your child. Your child goes to school every day because she knows you believe it is a safe place where she is recognized and nurtured. If you question or challenge the school excessively in your daughter's presence, her confidence in the school will falter, and along with it her faith in herself. Unless you are pulling her out of the school tomorrow, no matter what you really think, show your child that you are working in partnership with the school. If you go to a meeting with her at school, give her the space to communicate on her own behalf. Do not mirror her emotions or editorialize about the incident at length. Where possible, echo the concerns or suggestions of the professional. When you do this, Gatens said, "it strengthens the ability of the school to resolve the matter in the eyes of the child." Do not confuse criticizing the school with advocating for your child. Save your strongest feelings to be conveyed when she is not present.

Ditch incompetent adults. As in all other places of business, schools will have their share of incompetent employees. Having your complaints dismissed, your response questioned ("Perhaps you're overreacting a bit..."), or the incident ascribed to "girls being girls" is a sign you may be dealing with one. Move on to another person at the school who can help you. That said, it is easy to mistake a disappointing response for a sign of incompetence. It's okay to express dissatisfaction, but be careful when you accuse an otherwise well-regarded professional of incompetence. It can ultimately affect your reputation at the school.

calling another parent

This is potentially dangerous territory, but it doesn't have to be. Caution, however, should be exercised. These conversations can go swiftly and woefully awry. It's rarely easy for the approaching parent to conceal her discomfort and anger. Parents on the receiving end often see comments about their children as a personal affront to their parenting skills, or worse, to themselves. Their responses can be angry and defensive as a result. It's also not unusual for the parent to deny the problem altogether. Rosalind Wiseman, coauthor of *Queen Bee Moms and Kingpin Dads,*[81] tells a great story about a boy throwing sand at her son in the sandbox. She is indignant and outraged. When her son, moments later, does the same thing, she defends him by saying he is tired. You have a blind spot for your child. Every parent, even one as accountable as Wiseman, will struggle to see the rougher edges of her child's behavior. It comes with the territory.

In the area of dealing with other parents, there are some absolute, 100 percent no-no's. As I said earlier, the example you set as the parent is key. Never confront the other child directly, no matter how close you are to the other family. Do not ignore or give dirty looks to the other child when you encounter her in hallways, carpool lanes, and cafeterias. Do not confront a parent publicly without warning, or slander the other parent or child in front of your daughter.

When you call another parent (and you should call; this is rarely a conversation for e-mail or, God forbid, texting), make sure it is a good time for the other person to talk (avoid calling at dinnertime or late at night), or e-mail to set up a time to talk. Explain that you want to discuss a problem involving your children, and acknowledge up front that you know you have only one part of the story. Jot down some notes ahead of time so you can take extra care with your words.

As dispassionately as possible, describe the facts. Stick closely to the behaviors that were observed or experienced, and name the emotions your child felt as a result. Do not discuss the other person's parenting style and try not to label her child's behaviors ("rude," "unfair," "hurtful"). Allow the parent to respond, and invite him to work with you on a solution together.

Be prepared to hear a response like, "I think you might be over-reacting here. Shouldn't we just let the kids work it out for themselves?" Another: "Hey, isn't this just girls being girls? Not much you can really do. They'll figure it out!" When that happens, take a deep breath, watch your tone, and continue:

"I appreciate that, and I agree it's important to let the kids work things out when they can. I also think we have given them some chances to work it out already. [Your child's name] has done what she can [give an example if you can] and she is still having a hard time. I am asking for your help in resolving this. Can we talk about what we can do to resolve this together?"

You might also say, *"I'm letting you know because I would have wanted another parent to tell me something like this. I know how involved you are with your child, and I figured you would want to know this was happening. If my daughter is involved, please let me know."*

If you are told the situation is simply a matter of "girls being girls," try this response: *"It's true. This does seem to be how some girls act. But just because it happens to a lot of girls doesn't mean they don't need our help, or that the behavior is okay to begin with. If they've done everything they can to deal with it on their own, and they still need us, I think we need to step in."*

Wiseman's *Queen Bee Moms and Kingpin Dads* is an excellent resource guide for navigating conflict with the adults in your child's life.

switching schools, changing relationships

Does she want to switch schools? Several girls and women I met transferred to make a fresh start and never looked back. The change may seem disruptive, but it can make a huge difference. Like a storm, girl bullying is often little more than different social elements swirling together in a particular climate. There's a reason why tornadoes touch down in Kansas more often than in California, and social chemistry among girls is often the same way. Unless a girl is consistently controversial and has struggled across different contexts, changing schools may be the right answer. The stories I heard confirm that girls who are whittled down in one environment can thrive in the next.

If changing schools is a financial burden, there are other options. Elizabeth entered a weeklong youth program at the low point of her suffering in eighth grade. Angry, suspicious, and defensive at the time, she was practically dragged in by her parents. To her great surprise, Elizabeth recalled, "These perfect stranger kids would walk up and give me a hug and say, 'It's nice to meet you. I'm so-and-so.' And I was like, 'Oh my God. Are you for real? Are you serious?' But by the end of the week I skipped out of there . . . They wanted to know me and there was no catch. They weren't going to stab me in the back."

That experience, she remembered, "turned my perspective around totally." When Elizabeth went to high school that fall, she was "high on acceptance, totally high on [the fact that] it doesn't matter because, whatever, these people [from the youth program] love me for who I am." For Elizabeth, the scars may not have disappeared, but her wounds did begin to heal.

Reparative relationships can make a world of difference to girls. I will never forget the day I realized this. I co-founded and ran the Girls Leadership Institute summer camp for many years. Every day, I taught middle- and high-school girls workshops about assertiveness and healthy friendships. I am not embarrassed to admit that I believed the workshops were what brought girls back year after year. They weren't. It was the friendships. The girls were emboldened by the trusting, honest, and unselfconscious relationships we had given them a space to create. It was these connections that gave them permission to make new leaps in their development.[82]

There is no question that a new activity can mean the world to an ostracized child. Ideally, you should choose activities where kids are valued more for the contribution they make than for what they're wearing, saying, or watching. The shift in scrutiny, away from what makes a girl popular and on to what makes her a good player or writer or horseback rider or babysitter, can make the difference. So get your daughter on a team or in a club, on the school newspaper or in an afterschool writing workshop. Get her singing, dancing, throwing pottery, tumbling, volunteering: get her with other people who are disconnected from her social misfortune.

Be thoughtful: don't put your kid on the soccer team if she's got two left feet or in a gymnastics class with a razor-sharp power clique. Take the social temperature before you enroll her by talking to the adult in charge or to other parents. Set your child up to succeed, or at least blend in and enjoy herself.

Activities are exciting gateways to finding a childhood passion, and like falling in love, passion often makes the rest of life bearable. I know that no matter how bad my day was, once I got on the basketball court, it was pure focus and meditation. Nothing could touch me.

speaking truth to power: raising a courageous bystander

Your daughter lives in a peer culture with its own rules and rituals. As a parent, you can still communicate your family's values relative to that culture, regardless of your ability to change it. Your voice and perspective matter, even as your daughter may roll her eyes or inform you that you are clueless. It's her job to do that, just as it's yours to persist in telling her what's right. By questioning the terms of her social world, you introduce her to the possibility that its rules are neither right nor permanent. You give her words and permission to question it herself.

Ask your daughter if she has ever watched her friends do something that she felt guilty about, but did not challenge. Why didn't she? Let her speak and try not to judge. If you listen, she will likely say that she feared the consequences. It can be social suicide to question a peer with power. As a result, most kids don't stop bullying or aggression. They fear for themselves.

You can be sensitive to this. You should be. Would you, back in the day, have stood up to bullies in your social network? Hindsight may be 20/20, but it's not fair to relive those moments in childhood with what you know today. Keeping in mind how torn she may feel, speak with your daughter about what it means to resist silence and defend someone with less power. There are many examples in history and even today's headlines where men and women fight injustice against all odds. Point out that bystanders are everywhere: every day, moments crop up where individuals stand up and protect others.

If you can remember your own experiences as a child, share them. Can you remember a time when you wish you had intervened, but didn't? Talk about your regrets and what you wish you had done. Today, if you have an opportunity to model bystander behavior for your child, take it. Remind your daughter that even walking away from a bad situation takes a lot of skill and courage. But as hard as it may be to stand up and fight back, the bottom line is that no one is invisible in the face of cruelty. Remaining silent in the face of bullying, as justified as it may feel, still means playing a role.

Silence is not the only option when your daughter witnesses something that makes her uncomfortable. If she feels helpless or confused, she can change the subject, make a joke, or walk away. She might say, "You might not mean to be hurting this person, but you are." If she wants to, practice these strategies by role-playing. Remind her of the power of two; explain that if she can find one other person in her group to stand with her, the bully is likely to stop.[83]

Telling an adult is also a way to support a target without having to take the heat yourself. Make sure your daughter knows the difference between "telling" and "tattling." Tattling is about trying to get someone in trouble. Telling, on the other hand, is about getting someone help. Reporting a situation where someone is unsafe means you're following the rules of your school and community. It is also your ethical obligation as a human being.

When it comes to talking with girls about standing up for others, there is one exception: ganging up, or alliance building. Conflicts among girls are often settled according to loyalties; "hating who she hates" can be interpreted by a girl as standing up for someone. In fact, this kind of behavior makes conflicts much harder to resolve and thrusts girls into drama that has nothing to do with them. It cloaks aggressive behavior in the mantle of loyalty, suggesting a true friend sticks up for you by going after someone else.

dads

Each year I address thousands of parents in cities and towns all over America. Not surprisingly, most of the auditorium seats are filled by women. Some dads come, sure, but most of them defer to moms when it comes to "girl stuff."

This is a mistake. A dad's unique perspective can be exactly what a girl needs. It is precisely a man's distance from the ins and outs of a girl's social universe that make him the perfect wingman in the jungle. As I have shown, many mothers are triggered by their daughters' experiences because of their own histories. The emotional response can, at times, be limiting. Some fathers, on the other hand, may find girls' social universe unfamiliar and somewhat less threatening. Their perspective can be refreshingly different.

Many fathers question girls' avoidance of conflict, the tendency to hold a grudge, and taking problems too personally. As frustrating as these insights may sometimes be for girls ("Daaaaad! You so don't get it!"), it's a respected voice with a different perspective. Whether or not your daughter agrees with or buys into your opinions, especially during the eye-rolling years, should never be a reason to remain silent.

what if my daughter is the bully?

There is a small group of parents who attend my presentations, whose hands creep up gingerly toward the end of my Q & A. Their voices are halting and sheepish. "What if," they ask me, "your daughter is the mean one?" I can see the other heads swivel, craning to see who these brave souls are.

Everyone has a daughter who has been the "mean one"—yes, even you. As I showed in chapter six, we all have the capacity for aggression. And I have yet to meet a girl who has not done something she is sorry about. You are not a bad parent if your daughter is a bully or aggressor. In fact, the courage to admit your daughter's capacity for aggression is exactly what you need to parent well through this period. Give yourself a pat on the back for even owning up to this.

A parent's insistence that her daughter would never be rude or mean to another child may actually end up making her rude or mean to another child. Research shows that when parents ignore alternative aggression, their children are more likely to engage in it. It makes perfect sense: when parents do not discourage the behavior, girls are free to act that way to get what they want.

For example, many preschool girls use relational aggression constantly. They disinvite their parents from birthday parties or say they "won't love you anymore" when they are upset. When girls threaten to withdraw friendship, even at the age of three, it is the equivalent of biting or kicking. When the behavior is not disciplined, the child learns it is an acceptable strategy to get what she wants or express negative feelings.[84]

Parents may not take alternative aggressions seriously because, like their daughters, they live in a culture that has defined the behavior as a rite of passage or "girls being girls." Others simply do not want to see anything "wrong" in their children.

Many parents are stumped by how to deal with their daughters' psychological aggression at home. The answers are closer than you think. Begin by taking stock of how you respond to more obvious or conventional acts of aggression, like hitting or name-calling. Without being conscious of it, you probably use a protocol for disciplining your daughter: perhaps you tell her to stop, explain why she shouldn't do it, foster empathy for the target, and name some consequences. You'll need a similar intervention plan for the behavior that challenges you now.

When you observe your daughter engaging in alternative aggressions, activate your protocol. As an example, imagine a girl who rolls her eyes at her sister and ignores her at dinner. Here's how you could handle it:

"Jennifer, it is not okay for you to ignore your sister." (Stop the behavior.)

"Ignoring someone is not an appropriate way to express yourself when you are upset. And when you roll your eyes, you're sending a nasty message, even if you're not speaking." (Name the behavior.)

"How do you think your sister feels when she tries to speak to you and you pretend she's not there?" (Foster empathy for the target.)

"You need to find another way to express yourself. Even if you're angry, I expect you to be respectful toward your sister and acknowledge her." (Suggest an alternative.)

"If you can't change the way you're acting right now, you
   will have to eat dinner later or in your room." (Create a
   consequence.)

"I know you're capable of more than this." (Communicate
   positive expectations.)

If the phone rings and it's your daughter's school calling with news
that she has been involved in bullying, get all the information you
can. Do not inform the caller that your daughter "would never do"
what they are calling to inform you she did. Do not downplay or interpret the incident as "kids being kids"; if the school took the time
to call you, it's likely more than that. Instead, apologize and thank
the school for calling.

Ask your daughter, who may have beaten the school to the punch
with her own story, to respond to the school's description of her behavior. If she patently denies it, let her know that you will follow up
either way. If there is evidence of her guilt, tell her she will be punished more severely for lying to you. Give her another chance to revise her story. Ask her what the other person would say if she was
asked to tell her side of the story. Refusing to "let it go" is not about
signaling distrust of your daughter. It sends a larger message to her
that you are vigilant about her behavior toward others. It also affirms
your respect for her school's authority.

Call the school for an appointment if possible. It is always better
to speak face to face about these issues than by phone. Do not begin
e-mail correspondence on the subject. Electronic conversation about
any sensitive matter can be easily misinterpreted.

Perhaps you are not sure if your daughter is acting aggressively at
all. It's not easy, but there are ways to find out. First, just ask: talk to
her school counselor, teachers, coaches, and other adults who see her
in different contexts. Let them know you are sincerely open to their
feedback. Second, start hanging around your daughter when she's
with her friends. If they are in the kitchen, do the dishes quietly. If
they are watching TV, straighten up the room. Drive carpool: kids
have this weird ability to forget an adult is driving them, and they

will say all kinds of things in the back seat. I once met a mother who asked me if it was okay to slam on the brakes when she heard her daughter and her friends sniping about their peers. I said it was at least a start.

Joking aside, you are entitled to let the girls who sit in your car or eat in your home know how you feel about gossip and other aggressive behavior. Be sparing, though: your daughter's embarrassment could derail the teachable moment. Save your strongest feelings for a private time with her.

when it isn't bullying

Is every time a child feels socially rejected a moment of victimization? What makes a girl the "odd girl out"?

In a world without bullying, there will always be exclusion. Exclusion will happen naturally as relationships grow more intimate. Exclusion does not necessarily constitute bullying, even when we account for alternative aggressions. It would be wrong to read this book as an argument against exclusion.

Every case of exclusion is as unique as the child in question and must be evaluated on its own terms. If a child is being left out here and there, or from a certain group, then she is being left out here and there, or from a certain group—nothing more and nothing less. If she is failing to forge close relationships with others, it bears further investigation before deciding she's been bullied. If her exclusion bothers her or her parents, interrogate the disappointment. The desire to see a child become popular can color the way we view her social universe, can make the everyday rise and fall of friendship look like something else. If the child needs help with social skills, she should get it, but it's not other children's responsibility to compensate for what another girl lacks.

That girls sometimes use relationship as a weapon does not mean that every time a relationship is not offered, the girl is behaving aggressively. We must distinguish between intentional acts of meanness and the reality of children's social order. Like exclusion, popularity will outlast us all, and to cry foul at it will only make a parent appear overinvested and ignorant.

To expect girls to play nice with everyone, despite what they may really want, is to enforce upon them precisely what we are trying to stop: a "tyranny of the nice and kind"[85] that will stifle girls' voices, shuttle them into idealized, alienating relationships, and impress upon them the belief that their own needs should be subverted to others' at any cost. A common situation is one girl who silently trails after another, copying her behavior and appearance as though to absorb by osmosis what she is unable to take independently for herself. The followed girl is annoyed and embarrassed. Is she obligated to spend time with the follower, who has done nothing but hover quietly? I don't think so.

Only when a child has been shunned by most of her peers or suddenly dropped by the friends she once had does exclusion look less like social ordering and more like relational aggression. And even then, discipline may not be appropriate. This isn't to say that when one child lets go of a friendship with another to get popular, she isn't being mean. She is. But could someone have "made" me talk to Anne? Probably not. There will always be cases where we have to let girls negotiate their own social lives. What we can do is provide them with as much emotional support as possible, and let them know that life will get easier.

"I'd love to hear my daughter come up with some really strong responses," one mother told me. "I don't want to see her be weak. We want our children to be stronger than we were." In spite of this, most parents find themselves at the doorstep of the age-old question, At what point do we let our children fight their own battles, and when is it time to intervene? I always tell parents to trust their gut. If after a few days of unrest your daughter's behavior begins to change—if her eating and sleeping patterns shift, if she grows quiet, if the phone stops ringing or vibrating—something is wrong and she needs you. When parents ask me what the right thing is to do, I ask them to imagine doing nothing at all: Is the school aware of what is happening? Will someone there step in when things go too far? Does the school take these behaviors seriously?

The hidden culture of girls' aggression subsists on silence and isolation. As Mary Pipher has written, "We need to politicize, not pathologize, families." Part of this means that in order to fight the forces that prey on children outside our homes, we must first step forward to publicly acknowledge our questions and fears within them. For it is not just the girls who think they are suffering alone when they are bullied. So do parents. When families don't talk, parents can't learn from one another and it becomes easier to blame themselves for their children's problems. Blaming parents means we focus less on our daughters' peer cultures. It prevents us from realizing collectively as a society that there are systemic and social patterns to be resisted and corrected.

for girls especially (but not only): everyday truth telling and conflict

Girls have a critical role to play in changing the culture of their cliques and friendships. After all, most of us hate this way of life. I can't count the number of girls who told me they'd rather be beaten up than ignored or cut down spiritually by their peers. We need to abandon the belief that doing this is natural or unavoidable. It isn't. We can change.

It's like riding in the passenger seat of a car when you're young. You hardly ever pay attention to what the driver's doing. You don't have to. But one day, you get your learner's permit and switch seats. You're going all the same routes, only this time you have to relearn each part of the way. All the turns someone made for you, you now have to make yourself. You have to make sure the wheels don't jump the curb, that you come to a complete stop, that you check your blind spot.

It's the same thing with our relationships: we have to get in the driver's seats and relearn healthier ways of taking the twists and turns. We don't have to give in to the autopilot urge to tell someone else we're angry instead of the person who made us angry in the first place.

The biggest reason we don't talk to each other is because we're afraid we'll lose the friendship with the person we're confronting, or worse, that the person we're talking to will turn everyone against us. The fear throws up a wall that prevents us from speaking our hearts and minds to each other. As we also know, it also leads to a ton of gossip, rumor spreading, and resentment that mushroom into other kinds of nastiness.

AN EXERCISE FOR GIRLS:
THROW THE GEARS OF
OUR CULTURE INTO REVERSE

"I hate the fact that you have to go through all this stuff," Shelley said to me at Starbucks one afternoon. "You can't tell someone you're mad at them, you have no idea what's going on, you're kind of like lost. Or you end up having problems with six people when you're mad at only one person."

It doesn't have to be this way. If we talk openly with our friends about our fears of losing each other, we often discover they share the same feelings. One thing I noticed in my many conversations with groups of girls was the mixture of relief and surprise on their faces when they found their friends felt the same way. Over the three years I researched and wrote this book, I went through some pretty dramatic changes as a person. I suddenly became conscious of how often I avoided being directly angry with people, how much I held things in and acted cold or quiet while my resentment grew. When I had my fight with Jenny, I discovered what can happen when you share hidden feelings of jealousy and competition with a friend. I'm no expert, but for what it's worth, why not try this:

1. Get your closest friends together, or just one friend, and make time to talk. Get comfortable in a quiet space, however you choose to do that.

2. Talk about your fears of conflict. Ask each other, "When I make you angry or upset, do you tell me about it?" If not, talk about what you do instead of talking about it.

3. Talk about what happens when you hold your feelings inside or hide them. Is the buildup of emotion better than dealing immediately with what's happened? Explore specific situations. They can be resolved or ongoing, but think of a time when you feared speaking up. Was it when Joanna made that comment about your shorts, then said she was joking, but you felt pretty sure she wasn't? Was it when Leigh ignored you in front of the guy she liked? Try talking about it to each other and keeping the promise to respect each other's anger, to own the anger as a part of your friendship.

4. Look yourself in the eye and see the face of your own aggression. Talk about times you have felt angry, mean, competitive, or jealous. They can include feelings you've felt in your life or toward each other. Like my roommate Jenny and I, put it out on the table. Show your cards. Stop hiding and start owning your feelings, and see just how little damage they will wreak on your life once you do. See what a relief it is not to be perfect.

5. If some or all of your friends say they're afraid of losing each other or being ganged up on, make some promises. Say you won't do that. Say you won't use phones and computers as a substitute for real conversations. Say you'll be there no matter what. Say you'll work it out somehow. Say that you feel that way, too, if you do. This is nothing more than a commitment of friendship, something we're all used to making with each other. It's not that different from promising to keep a secret, or be best friends, or save a seat. We're *good* at this.

If you want to, talk about how girls are socialized to *not* be angry and aggressive and to not tell each other the truth. If you're into girl power, this is ground zero. This is taking your voices and your relationships back from the forces that would divide you from each other. When girls shut each other down, they seal the fate of their own socialization. They tell each other that anger is indeed wrong, that they do not deserve to feel it.

6. Comfort each other. Reassure your friends that their feelings are important, that conflicts bring you closer together, that you *want* each other to talk about stuff, because all of you know just how much it sucks when you have to keep it in and feel resentful and angry.

In a healthy immune system, the body can tell the difference between the cells it needs to survive and the foreign ones that threaten it. When our immune systems malfunction, our bodies mistake healthy cells for dangerous ones and start to attack. As a result, we actually weaken ourselves. Sadly, this is how many of us are taught to approach conflict: as a foreign event that threatens our very constitution. But that fear, so absurdly false, ends up breaking us down from the inside. It turns us against each other. It makes our fights much, much worse than they really have to be. To strengthen ourselves, we have to learn to recognize aggression as a healthy part of our relationships and lives, something that makes us stronger and more honest individuals.

After spending weeks talking about fears of confrontation with one group of girls, one student began speaking about anger that had been brewing toward a friend. "I decided to go up to that person and I really had to have a lot of courage to do that, and when I told the person, I was like, 'Oh, what if she's not going to be my friend anymore, and she's going to hate me? I'll lose one of my best friends.' And after I told her, she told me some of the things that I was kind of doing that were mean and annoying her. And we solved our problems and then we're like still best friends. It's not always what you think is going to happen."

BULLYING: WHEN YOU'RE IN REAL TROUBLE

"If you could go back in time and talk to yourself at the moment when you were most upset, what would you say?" This was the question I asked every woman and girl I spoke with who was bullied. I wouldn't have written this book if a small piece of me wasn't still eight years old, standing in the darkened community center theater listening to the fading giggles and footsteps running away from me. I guess I wanted to know what I could have done, what someone might have told me. So I asked.

1. get help.

Try not to do this alone. Find someone who can support you. Eleven-year-old Dina advised, "If something goes wrong and you can't stand up for yourself, then you should make friends with someone you can trust [who can] be on your side. If you don't have a friend, then go to your parent because parents should know what's going on. Maybe they've been through it so they'll know. They can call the school and say what's going on. You shouldn't just stand in the corner and try to deal with it by yourself."

Susie Johnston, also eleven, said she regrets not telling her parents how bad it was for her. "I was afraid to tell my parents because I was afraid they'd call the kids' parents and that would make things worse. I didn't tell them everything," she said. "And I just wish I had sometimes, because if I had maybe I could have gotten out of the school earlier." Once she switched to her new school, she made more friends than she'd ever thought possible.

Talk to a teacher. There may be someone who gets it, who understands how bad this is. Perhaps she'll talk with you after school or at lunchtime. Can she arrange for you to go to the art room or the library at lunch?

Haley said, "You should talk to friends who've either been through this or who are your very true friends, and that's very helpful." One of the worst things about getting bullied is that you feel so alone. Sometimes you feel like you're the only person in the world who's been through it. If you've read any part of this book, you know that's not true. But it does help to see someone in the flesh who gets it, who *knows,* and that, according to many girls, can make you feel a lot better.

2. *lose them.*

If you're miserable because you're trying to get popular, or it's your friend who's doing this to you, give it up. If you think being popular is going to make you happy, you're wrong. "The only way to get through it," said Stephanie from chapter five, "is to find the people you like because you like them, not because of their position at school, not because they're the prettiest or the most popular or all the boys want to date [them]. Find someone that you have fun with, that you share interests with." If the other girls are ignoring you, aren't inviting you out, are giving you the worst seat, aren't telling you the secrets—if they're using you as a tool to make themselves feel cooler—take the hint. You are putting yourself in emotional danger every minute you spend with them.

3. *get it out.*

Get a diary or journal and write about your feelings. Paint, dance, kickbox, run in the rain, punch a bag, write a song, bang on drums. Don't keep it inside. Don't kick the dog. The culture raises us to swallow our pain until we choke. The way to fight back is to release.

"It helps a lot to get your problems out," eleven-year-old Jill said. "Most of the time it's good to write down who's being mean to you or how they're being mean to you. And write down an equals sign next to it [and] what you can do to solve the problem." Remember: Whatever you write should remain private. Don't use social media to tell the world how you're feeling about other people.

4. *do something.*

Join the newspaper, take a workshop, join a team, take an art class, volunteer, get a job. Join an online group. Try not to curl into a ball under your blanket, or at least not all day, every day. Finding a different community of people can make the difference. Find what you love to do.

It doesn't necessarily have to be with others. When you find what you love, you come closer to finding yourself. You start putting out a vibe to others, an energy of sorts. It happened to Alizah, and it had a profound impact on her life in high school. She said, "Explore what you like to do by yourself because I really think that's where your strength lies, within yourself. People will come to you because of who you are, and I think we all have gifts."

5. *it* will *end*.

Ever try to tell a screaming three-year-old that her mother will be back in five minutes? She could sooner tell you who the forty-three presidents are than what five minutes from now is. We can get like that when someone's making it her goal in life to ruin ours. But— and you can trust me on this—one day you won't have to wake up and go to school with these people.

"You have no reason to believe me," said Naomi, "but take a leap and trust that this is not the real world. This is school. This structure will never exist again, it will never be possible again.... Things are going to get better because I'll never be defined by just one group of people's opinion of who I am."

The world may feel like it's ending. It isn't. Roma said, "It gets better. These people are the people you're with now and whose opinion matters the most now, but it's not going to be the opinion that lasts. Try and listen to what is most important to you. Try and isolate the fact that you have a whole world of possibilities and things you're going to be interested in and that you'll want to do for you. Try really hard to get in touch with those things. And when you do, hold on to those things that are most important because nobody outside of you is more important."

CHAPTER *eleven*

raising girls in a digital age

I once met a woman who slept with her teenage daughter's laptop under her pillow. "It's the only way I know she won't steal it in the middle of the night," she told me, rolling her eyes. We laughed, but she was dead serious. Parenting girls in the digital age is, all at once, mysterious, confusing, frustrating, overwhelming, and terrifying. A girl with a gadget seems to disappear like Alice down the rabbit hole, into a world that feels utterly foreign to her parents. Where kids go online, what they do, and who they do it with are questions that can become moving targets as girls click and switch from computer to phone to iPod.

As ever more gadgetry accessorizes youth, setting limits can feel impossible. This chapter is about how to parent effectively through BFF 2.0, or the virtual world girls and their friends inhabit. As confusing as social media may seem, unplugging is not an option. Your daughter needs your active involvement in her online life. She is vulnerable to saying and doing things online that she would never do in real life—and many girls will take any chance they can to avoid difficult real-life situations with friends. Social media exacerbates her normal adolescent states, like insecurity, self-consciousness, and jealousy, as well as anxiety and competitiveness. She is also likely addicted to social media because she is addicted to relationship and connection; therefore, she cannot moderate her own use.

The intensity of your daughter's demand for social media is often related to how susceptible she is to its dangers. A girl who is insistent that she must have as much access as you can give her is likely hooked on the endless, unfulfilling race to be constantly connected, in the know, and—worst of all—part of the drama. This world can make a girl volatile, self-conscious, and unhealthily invested in what others think of her.

But here's the good news. Many girls feel downright fatigued by the relentless onslaught of social media. Your child may *look* like she would prefer to sit, concave and quiet, with a laptop cracked and cell phone cocked, for hours on end. And she may do it. Yet she may also feel utterly overwhelmed by the constant stream of information she feels pressured to respond to and make sense of. Many girls go through their days with the pervasive anxiety that they must know, at all times, what is being texted and posted, lest they fall out of favor or lose status. They begin to equate the quality of a relationship with the frequency of contact. They also become hamsters on a wheel, caught in an unsatisfying, endless cycle of information consumption. A surprising number of girls have told me their friendships would be better off without social media at all. As one middle-school student told a blogger in 2010, "If everyone else stopped using it, I would, too." Said another: "I just don't want to be left out."

There are three guiding principles you can use to parent through this time. First, you are the parent. You are entitled to say no and set limits. Your daughter is not an equal partner in this conversation, and you can negotiate as much or as little as you want. Nor is her access to technology some kind of twenty-first-century entitlement. Just because your child lives in your home does not automatically qualify her for a free smart phone or Facebook account.

Second, your job as a parent is to not only protect her from others, but also to guide and monitor her behavior. Do you remember when your parents would rationalize rules you hated by saying, "It's not that I don't trust you. I just don't trust other people"? I am recommending something different here: that you don't entirely trust your daughter. That doesn't mean you approach her as some kind of criminal, just that you are realistic enough to know that the temptations of social media can bring out the worst in all of us, adults included. With frontal lobes still developing, young people are simply less reflective and more impulsive. They are also coming of age in a celebrity- and media-obsessed culture where little is considered private and "anything goes." We are doing girls a favor when we assume they will make a few mistakes. As I showed in chapter four, they are far from the "digital natives" they are made out to be.

Third, it is a myth that effective parenting in this area requires new, mysterious knowledge that only "techie" types possess. The same values you have been teaching your child—moderation, safety, responsibility, respect, good manners, and so on—apply to her online experiences. Remembering this point is vital to remaining grounded and sane while you parent through BFF 2.0. Giving up is not an option. Think about it this way: if you did not fully understand something your child was dealing with in the real world, you would not surrender to your own confusion.

Of course, not everything is the same in the virtual world, and some knowledge of social media will always be useful. But parenting is fundamentally about socializing a child: modeling and promoting healthy habits that help her thrive in the world outside your home. In this section, I outline how basic parental values carry over to the virtual world, and I also offer strategies to help your daughter navigate the dangers of cyberbullying and aggression. Please note that I do not explore the issues raised by predators, pornography, or other challenges posed by technology.

Set the example. Children learn to say please and thank you because we tell them to and because we do it ourselves. Likewise, they learn to check their phones at meals and in the middle of conversations because we do it, too. I once taught a class where fifth-grade girls practiced asking a friend to put down her phone and pay attention. One girl raised her hand to suggest a strategy. "When my mom is too busy on her phone," she told the class, "this is what I do." The evidence is everywhere: sporting events where parents sit enraptured with their gadgets, parents who overdisclose on Facebook or who cannot resist texting while they drive. Clearly, kids are not the only ones who need to upgrade their technology etiquette. Your influence as a role model continues in the virtual realm. It is hard, not to mention hypocritical, to ask your children to adopt healthy technology habits at home if you have not embraced them yourself.

Be the parent. There is no easy time to be a parent, but the twenty-first century has ushered in unique dilemmas. The onslaught of new media and gadgetry has confounded many. On top of this, with parents working harder than ever, there is less and less time to talk about the challenges of raising children. Kids exploit this isolation shrewdly. They tell their parents they will be losers, left out or worse, if they do not keep up with the latest technology privilege or gadget. Parents, fearful that their children's predictions are real, or simply wanting to avoid World War Three during precious family time, oblige. They go against their gut desire to protect their kids in favor of keeping the peace and helping their kids keep up.

When I travel around the country, I am taken aside by women who identify themselves to me as "mean moms," or parents who say "no." This is a troubling sign of the times. If using your authority is equated with meanness, then being a limit-setting parent is seen as marginal or deviant. I will not waste time in telling you that being "mean" is exactly what you need to be. In fact, if your daughter approves of your technology policy, you're probably doing something wrong. A sweeping statement, yes, but kids need limits on technology use, period.

I ask parents who struggle with not wanting to be "mean" two questions. First, can you remember the most permissive parents you knew growing up? How did you feel about them when you were a kid? What do you think about them today, as a parent? The permissive parents were probably heaven to your kid brain, but dangerous in the more evolved one you have as a parent.

Here's the second question: What is one thing your parents made you do, or forbade you from doing, that drove you nuts at the time but which you now see was exactly what you needed? Perhaps it was a family dinner on a certain night, or making you stick with playing an instrument. The point of these questions is to show that kids can't be behind the wheel on these issues. A girl's knowledge of technology does not mean she has the authority to define the terms of use. What she thinks is right—eating cupcakes for dinner, staying up all night, wearing a skirt that is more like a headband—is not necessarily going to be right for her. That is the challenge of parenting: setting limits and saying no, not because you will be thanked for it, but because it is what they need in the long term. The payoff comes later.

Getting told "no" and "not yet" is part of growing up, and some things are simply not negotiable. Anything plugged in or networked is included in this constellation of letdowns. Conflict—and there is plenty on this subject—is itself a form of connection, a way you communicate your love for your child. You hold the line because you care.

Define the use of technology as a privilege. Like being able to stay up late, drive a car, or go out alone with friends, the use of technology is a privilege that must be earned—and one that can be taken away when it is abused. The award of a privilege is usually based on a contract you have with your child. For example, in order to stay up late, she needs to maintain her GPA. To drive a car, she must obey the speed limit and special laws for minors. To go out alone with friends, she must call you and let you know where she is going, or if her location changes.

To use social media, your daughter must also abide by a contract to be safe, responsible, and ethical online.[86] It is up to you to communicate it. Rosalind Wiseman has a fantastic script for this:

Technology can be really fun to use and it gives us incredible access to the world. But it is a privilege, not a right. And because it is a privilege, you have a responsibility to use it ethically. What using technology ethically looks like to me is that you never use it to humiliate, embarrass, send personal information, misrepresent yourself or someone else, use passwords without the person's permission, share embarrassing information or pictures of other people, put someone down (elementary school), or compromise yourself by sending pictures of you naked, half naked, in your bra (junior high/high school). Remember that it is so easy for things to get out of control. You know it. I know it. So I reserve the right to check your online life, from texting to your Facebook page. If I see that you are violating the terms of our agreement, I will take all of your technology away until you can earn my trust back. This is my unbreakable, unshakeable law.[87]

Some parents elect to have their children sign a written contract outlining their obligations. Samples of ethical-use contracts are widely available online. However you decide to do it, the conversation is essential. If you have not had it with your own kids yet, it is perfectly fine to apologize for not doing it sooner, and even to acknowledge that you are still figuring out how to do the right thing as a parent. The bottom line is that you should never assume your child just "knows" how to act online, and she should know that her access depends on how she handles it.

Give age-appropriate access. Most parents award privileges gradually, as a child is able to handle them. This is never more appropriate than in the realm of technology. Giving a fifth grader an iPhone is not a sign of your affection as a parent. Her first cell phone should be able to call her family or 911. It should neither text nor take photographs. You can roll out more privileges as she demonstrates her ability to use her phone safely and responsibly.

Keep in mind that a cell phone is a computer, not a cell phone.[88] Most girls use their telephones to text far more often than speak.

They also use phones to take and send photographs, and log on to the Internet. Parents who give their children cell phones often do not appreciate the range of options they give kids to interact. Make sure you understand what your child's phone can do, and talk to your phone company about how to supervise her use and activate age-appropriate restrictions.

Elementary-school girls do not need computers (or televisions, for that matter) in their bedrooms, nor should they, or middle-school girls, ever be on Facebook. I recognize that it is now considered "normal" for middle-school girls to have a Facebook account, but that certainly does not mean it's appropriate. It is no coincidence that bullying peaks between the ages of ten and thirteen; self-consciousness, insecurity, and an inexorable desire to fit in (along with the crippling fear that you might not) are pervasive. As I show in chapter four, sites like Facebook can make girls feel they fit in, but they also inspire intense feelings of anxiety and insecurity, not to mention online conflicts that quickly spin out of control.

If your elementary- or middle-school girl is already on Facebook, increased supervision is essential. You should have her password, be her Facebook friend, and check her page once a week. If she appears inactive, she may have a private page she is hiding from you. Keep in mind that middle school (and early high school, for that matter) is a period where extra parental vigilance around social media is crucial.

Set limits. When young people have carte blanche access to electronic devices, they are more likely to get involved in drama and look at content they shouldn't see. Saying no to tech use is one of the biggest wars you may have as a parent. While it's true you have to pick your battles, this is one fight worth having.

Parents who do not permit their children to watch, eat, or wear anything they want need only extend this healthy sense of moderation to technology use. It may help to stop thinking about this world as "technology," which can seem intimidating and foreign. Instead, call what girls are doing online and with their phones "social media." In fact, social media is no different from the other media in your daughter's life that you have long regulated: you have overseen her gradual access to certain books, television shows, movies, and magazines. The same incremental approach applies with social media. Access to social media and its toys must be given gradually. It must be *earned*. And if it is not used appropriately, there must be consequences.

Of course, there is one major difference between social media and, say, watching a television show. Unlike the one-sided act of watching something, a child uses social media to connect with other people. In some ways, it is the difference between playing soccer and riding a horse. You can kick a soccer ball as many times as you want without regard for the ball. When you ride a horse, you must always be sensitive to the creature you are sitting on and working with. It is a relationship. The same is true of social media. Being allowed to use a device or website can never be a simple "yes" or "no." As a child gets access to new privileges, it is not just to push buttons but to interact with others. There is a higher obligation to this sort of recreation, and a different measure of responsibility that must be met.

Explain your choices. The expectation of safe, responsible, and ethical social media use should come with a clear explanation of why. It is rarely effective to set limits or say no "because I say so." Engaged parents explain to their children *why* they are saying no, in a way that respects the child as an individual who deserves to know the reasons why decisions are being made. Knowing why also gives your daughter real reasons to care about following the rules. That said, explaining your reasons for a rule does not mean it is open to negotiation. Once you have explained, you need not have the same conversation again and again. Yes, you may be the only parent who is setting these particular limits. That's okay. Your family is yours and no one else's—and this is where, finally, "because I say so" may be the last word.

To explain limits, you might say, "Too much of anything is never good. Healthy living is about balance. That's why we eat dessert occasionally, not at every meal. We try not to work all the time so we can make time for rest, or hang out with friends all the time so we have no time for ourselves. The same thing is true for our lives online. We're going to do that, too, in moderation, as part of a balanced life."

To explain your commitment to online civility, you might say, "We embrace respect as a core value in this family. Respect is the foundation of a safe, humane community—in this house, at school, at my workplace, and online. Without respect, people cannot learn, grow, or be themselves. Online, you are also a member of a community, and I expect you to be the same principled person I see you being in the real world. Every person's behavior in a community counts."

The dangers of social media are another reason to set limits on use, and these are also important to explain to girls. Internet safety expert Lori Getz is only half kidding when she advises parents to explain to teens that their brains' frontal lobes are not fully developed, rendering adolescents incapable of mature reason, logic, and impulse control.

Ongoing conversation will affirm your commitment to the limits and make them an organic part of how you parent. Use one of the many embarrassing electronic situations celebrities fall prey to as an opportunity to talk about the perils of social media. You can also start a conversation with your daughter about the way people act online, and don't forget to talk about what she loves about social media! Ask her how fast she can text or finger type. Have fun with it. Here are some excellent conversation starters:

- "What is your favorite thing about [choose a form of social media you know she loves]?"
- "Do you think people act online the same way they act in real life?"
- "Why are people more inclined to be mean or rude online?"
- "Technology can bring friends closer together. Can it also make you more insecure in your friendships?"

- "Does technology cause misunderstandings?"
- "Would your friendships be better or worse without technology?"

Once you have had these conversations, it is easier to introduce restrictions. Below are some ideas for keeping technology use moderate in your home.

Keep the computer in a public place. This practice creates natural limits on use. It allows for some degree of privacy while making sure you are close enough to know what's going on. Although it becomes more challenging as kids get older, no elementary-school child needs a laptop in her room. If you approach your child while she is online and she minimizes the screen, she may be doing something inappropriate. You are absolutely entitled to ask her to show you the screen.

There are additional benefits to having the computer in a public part of your home: you get to see your kids. "When we start putting computers and TVs in their rooms," says Lori Getz, the Internet safety expert, "that's where they go and we lose them."

Create a cell phone parking area. Establish a place in your home where all cell phones are parked and charged (and, if possible, silenced) during preset times. It might be for a prescribed homework period, during dinner, or both. Although this practice can feel difficult at first, most people find it a relief to let go of their phones for certain periods. With fewer external stimuli, family members are free to focus on each other and on important tasks.

Prohibit sleeping with phones. There is no good reason why a girl should be sleeping with her phone. Girls rest their phones under the pillows or on their chests so they can wake up if someone texts. If drama is afoot, late-night texts quickly become irrational and explosive. Plus, girls lose valuable hours of sleep. Let your daughter know her phone gets parked before she goes to bed (if she can't bear the idea of her phone sleeping alone downstairs, you may need to snuggle with it under your pillow, as some parents have done). If you are not sure what your daughter does with her phone at night, the answer is only as far away as your latest phone bill. A record of each number she texts and the time it was sent is easily accessible. There is one exception to this: New applications exist that allow users to text without owning a phone. There is no record of these texts. If your daughter has a device that can download "apps," you will need to check if she owns one with this new texting capability.

Limit gadgets at meals. It is a common sight at restaurants: adults talking while two children sit lost in their gadgets. Waiting for your meal can be boring, but it can also be a time for families to catch up and connect. The ability to "turn off" reality and seek refuge in a device prohibits kids from developing the ability to manage impatience, discomfort, or other difficult emotions. Being able to make small talk is also a vital skill that is stunted in children who are not expected to do it. If families give kids permission to log out of conversations, it becomes part of a child's repertoire of manners and etiquette in the world.

Make family meals, at home or out, a sacred time uninterrupted by technology. Do not respond to phones or computers. As an alternative to using gadgets at the table, try going around the table and asking each family member to name their highs and lows for the day. That is, each person should briefly describe the best and worst part of his or her day. You can do it as a nightly ritual.

Limit social media during homework. In 2010 a Kaiser Family Foundation study found that half of students ages eight to eighteen use the Internet, watch TV, or use some other form of media either most or some of the time while they do homework.[89] With the constant disruption of a vibrating phone or blinking chat window, kids do not develop habits to help them sustain longer periods of work, focus, and thought. Scientists call this study time "rich learning," the kind of knowledge required for higher-order thinking tasks like math or reading. With social media at play during homework, kids end up multitasking, or switching rapidly between different tasks.

The problem is that multitasking does not allow for rich learning, and it also results in epic amounts of distraction. Allison Miller, a high-school freshman who sends and receives twenty-seven thousand texts every month, told the *New York Times* about her struggle to balance her social and academic lives. "I'll be reading a book for homework and I'll get a text message and pause my reading and put down the book, pick up the phone to reply to the text message, and then twenty minutes later realize, 'Oh, I forgot to do my homework.'"

Researchers at Duke found that when adults do not supervise computer use, children choose playing over homework. In 2010 only three out of ten young people had rules limiting technology use. They used media about three hours less than peers with no rules.[90] Kids need parents to set these limits. Although teens may rely more on the Internet to do some homework, there are no assignments, as far as I know, that require a text message. During homework hours, have your kids park the phone with prescribed times for use (a fifteen-minute texting break every forty-five minutes, for example). This practice will allow your child to work with much less distraction.

Lori Getz suggests asking kids to try homework one night while using social media, then the next night without it. After the two nights, talk with your daughter about the difference in learning, efficiency, and effectiveness she experienced. As you consider implementing these changes in your home, keep in mind that habits take time to change. There will almost always be resistance ("I won't know what's going on," "I can concentrate better if I can text"). After the initial storm of indignation, many girls actually find the permission to unplug a relief. Alternatively, the solitude and quiet of homework time may be one of those things they thank you for when they are adults.

keeping her safe online: what to do

Just as your child needs to know how to be safe when she goes somewhere without your supervision, she needs guidance to protect herself in the digital world. There are two kinds of situations to prepare her for: cyberbullying, or sustained harassment by a peer, and cyberdrama, the day-to-day dust-ups that can occur between friends.

In this section, I will list safety precautions you can take, as well as strategies to talk about with your daughter so she stays safe online.

Know the passwords. At the moment you give your daughter access to new technology, whether it is a device, software, or Web page, know her passwords. Be there when she sets them. Establish, from the beginning, that you will play a supervisory role in her digital life. Let her know you will do random checks, in her presence, on her phone, social networking page, or computer. Do not abuse your monitoring privileges, or your daughter may seek other avenues for privacy that you never discover.

If you allow your daughter to be on Facebook, insist that you are her "friend." Alternatively, ask another adult trusted by your family to friend her.

Read the phone bill. It bears repeating: know who she's texting, how many she's sending, and what time the texts go out. Wireless phone companies have safety controls for kids' phones; call, find out what they are, and talk with your daughter if you're considering using them.

Check in and ask questions. Lori Getz advises parents to inquire about kids' virtual lives in the same way they would about their physical world. "You always want to know who they're with, where they're going, how long have they been there and what are they doing," she says. To do this in the virtual world, ask your daughter about the applications on her phone: which ones does she use the most? Have her show you the photos she has posted or that others have posted of her. Ask to see her friend list and who she has been texting with lately. Are they people she knows personally? You may not get the answer to every question, but you are owed a reply. If you get the silent treatment, it may be time to monitor her remotely.

If you spy, do it openly. A cottage industry of spyware has sprung up to help parents remotely monitor everything from texts and websites to keystrokes. It is understandably tempting to know what she's typing and where she's going. How closely you monitor your child's life online should not diverge dramatically from your real-world parenting style. "If you are the type of parent that would ask a whole bunch of questions but not necessarily pick up the phone and listen to a child's conversation, then you should be the kind of parent who asks a lot of questions but doesn't pick up the phone and read text messages," Getz says.

If you spy without telling your daughter and end up letting her know later, she will feel betrayed—and rightly so. No matter your intent, spying sends the message that, on some level, you do not trust her. The lines from earlier in the chapter—"It's not that I don't trust you. I just don't trust other people"—don't hold up here. Consider that there are other steps you can take before going to this extreme.

In other words, don't make spyware your first intervention as a parent. Give your daughter a chance to make you proud and prove to you that she can use social media responsibly. You can let her know that is exactly what you are doing by *not* using spyware! Instead, as a first step, try random checks of your daughter's phone, social networking page, and computer (while she is on it). If you still feel nervous or unsure, that's when you take the next step. Remember, while you are entitled to monitor, she is also entitled to know she is being watched.

High school does not mean total privacy. No matter how hard she tries to convince you otherwise, your daughter's increasing independence does not entitle her to freedom from parental oversight online. In the "real world," more freedom is cause for more questions: as she begins to drive on her own or with others, you ask where she is going and who she is with. You expect she will encounter challenges to her values, so you talk about the issues and let her know she can call you, no matter what. The same is true online. No matter what she tells you—and teens are especially gifted at pressuring parents to give up or give in on the subject of online supervision—you do not "graduate" from parenting in the digital realm.

Keep her off websites with anonymous commenters. Prohibit your daughter from visiting websites where people can post anonymously. As I show in chapter four, destructive websites like Formspring.me are heavily trafficked by middle- and high-school girls. Formspring allows girls to open an account and receive a personal page on the site. Anonymous or known commenters can then ask the girls random questions on their pages, and girls usually answer.

Formspring pages have become free-for-alls of cruelty, fueled by the anonymity the site affords. They are online venues where girls sign up and are demeaned and harassed by people they know but can never identify. Here is what I tell girls about using these sites:

- When people post anonymously, there are no consequences or costs to what they do. People write things they would never say. They also lie, just because they can. They say things to get a rise out of other people visiting your page. You can't trust anonymous posters because you don't know their motive, or even who they are. Anonymity doesn't give people courage to say what they really think; it lets people say anything, true or false, which is why you can't trust it.
- By inviting people to say harmful things to you, and then reading and responding, you give them credit. No matter how clever a comeback you come up with, you make it seem like their words are worth responding to when you reply.
- You will never be someone who is 100 percent liked by everyone, so stop thinking you're going to be. This is why so many girls sign up for sites where people can comment on them; they believe they might be that person who everyone loves. This is a useless waste of time. Focus on the relationships that bring you happiness and security, not people who tear you down. If you are worried about what other people think of you, ask the people you trust and who know you, not cowards who hide behind a cloak of anonymity to hurt you.

keeping her safe online: what to say

Here are the most important things to tell your daughter about online safety and digital citizenship.

There is no such thing as privacy online. It doesn't matter if you only wrote it in an e-mail, or the person promised not to share it. Once something is electronic, it can be forwarded and shared endlessly. Imagine you are holding a pillowcase filled with feathers at the top of the Empire State Building. If you cut open the pillow, empty the feathers out, take the elevator down, and run along the street, you could collect some of the feathers, but never all. Carried along by the wind, cars, and shuffling feet, they will disappear to places unknown. The same is true when your words or image are put online. Once something begins to get forwarded, it becomes like those feathers. It's gone.

Ask your daughter what the difference is between making a funny face at you and taking a photo of her face and sending it to a friend. One of these images is in her control, and one isn't. The face she made at you can be re-created by only her; what she sent, if a friend forwarded it, could be re-created over and over again, as new people encounter it in their phones and in boxes. It could be digitally altered and re-sent as an entirely new image. The same is true of her e-mails, chats, and texts.

A good rule of thumb is for her to ask herself a question before posting or sending: If this showed up on the front page of our local newspaper, would I be okay with that? If the answer is no, she is taking a risk by putting the content out there. Remember, too, that when online content lives forever, it can besmirch a girl's reputation among college admissions officers or employers.

Stop, Block, and Report.[91] Internet safety experts recommend three steps for responding to a cyberbully. First, stop. Do not engage with the cyberbully by retaliating or, in the event of an anonymous attack, attempt to track the bully down. This is not a battle a child can ever "win," and responding usually only provokes the cyberbully. Second, block the cyberbully. This can be done for texting, e-mail, and chat (if you don't know how, Google "how to block a user on [type in the website name, phone, or software]." If necessary, delete old accounts and create new ones for your child. Third, report the cyberbully. Encourage your child to save or print the offending material, and then discuss it with you. No matter how upset you are, encouraging your child to retaliate teaches your child that aggression is appropriate self-defense and exposes her to more danger.

You are there no matter what. The only thing worse than getting cyberbullied is having to go through it alone. The kids who don't disclose when they are targets fear that parents will overreact without consulting them or take their technology away. Staying calm is key. An alarmist response—shouting, crying, making threats against the school—will upset your daughter further and probably silence her the next time something happens. For more on how to handle this moment, read chapter ten. Make sure your child knows she won't lose her devices if she is targeted (though a temporary hiatus may be called for in order to cool off), and that she can come to you for any reason and under any circumstance. Let her know you will work with her on the right response. You do not have to promise that you won't have feelings about it, and you can say there may be times when you need to make a tough decision as a parent. The most important thing is that you want her to feel comfortable coming to you.

Do not share your password under any circumstances. Many girls share a password to bond with a friend, but it's precisely these friends who may abuse it. It is all too common for girls to break into each other's accounts and send out e-mails, photos, or texts pretending to be someone else. Advise your daughter to treat her password like a credit card; in other words, there are some valuable things we do not share with our closest friends, no matter how much we love them. If your daughter resists, tell her to blame her secrecy on you the next time she is asked for her password. You can also tell her it's okay to let you know she gave out her password so you can change it together. In general this is a good opportunity for girls to learn how to set healthy boundaries with friends.

Help others in need. You have likely taught your daughter to look out for others as well as herself. In the virtual realm, the same civic obligations exist. Forwarding a hurtful message is an active way of participating in cyberbullying. When you share a hurtful e-mail or image with ten people, it's the same thing as writing ten separate notes and passing on that information to each person, one by one. Online, you can actually stand up for someone by doing nothing—that is, by refusing to forward an embarrassing message.

Remind her of times she stood up for a friend or peer in "real life." Draw the analogy online: if she sees harassing messages, embarrassing photos, or other wrongdoing, you expect her to exercise the same kindness. Her role as a witness is a vital part of her contract with you.

"Walk away" from a bad situation online. Anyone—your daughter, you, the president of the United States—who is typing while crying, seething, panicking, or exhibiting any other intense feeling should not be typing. We will all invariably say something we do not mean.

If your daughter is upset and holding an electronic device, take away the device. Expect a fight, of course, along with fervent insistence that typing is the only way to resolve the conflict. You have two choices: The first is to take the device away, let her calm down for a while, and invite her to call the person in question. You can offer to take her to the person's house or encourage her to make a time to meet him or her at school the next day. The second choice is to allow her to finish her conversation and talk with her later about the perils of typing while distraught. Either way, do not let the moment pass.

Other toxic typing temptations include alliance building, or ganging up. Girls constantly pressure each other to get involved in conflicts that are not their own. The same is true online, and it can be even easier to get sucked in with just a few typed words. Work together to brainstorm strategies to deal with the pressure. Here's what I suggest girls type in the face of a request to get involved in someone else's conflict: "I'm really sorry this is happening to you. I don't think I should get involved. I promise I won't talk to [the other person], either. No matter what happens between you guys, things between us will stay the same." Some lower-intensity responses include, "I don't feel comfortable doing this (or "I'm not cool with this"). Let's talk later." If she can, she should simply change the subject.

If someone is directly confronting your daughter, encourage her to type something like this: "I really don't want to talk about this online. Can I call you right now?" Another option: "Can we talk tomorrow at school at [suggested time]?"

If you wouldn't say it, don't send it. When they are upset, girls constantly type things they would never say to someone's face. Conflict is the unavoidable result. Surges of panic, insecurity, anger, jealousy, or fear lead to impulsive messages that leave smoldering holes in relationships. It is unrealistic to think we can monitor girls' every conversation. That said, talk with your daughter about the temptation to be someone online that you are not in real life, and the consequences that may follow.

I give girls two tips to avoid making this mistake. First, if you are obsessed with the need to send a message, and it is a need so powerful that your house could be burning down, but you would want to keep texting (or chatting, or whatever), you should not be typing. You are too upset and likely to say something you don't mean. Put down the phone or walk away from the computer.

Second, if you suspect a conflict is brewing with someone via text or online, slow yourself down. Before you post or send your message, read aloud to yourself what you have written. Ask yourself: Would you actually say these words to the person? If the answer is yes, press send. If the answer is no or maybe, go back and edit it. Say it out loud again: Does it sound like something you would say? Are you using capital letters to "yell" online when you probably wouldn't raise your voice in real life? Do not press send until what you have written matches what you might say.

Do not fight with your friends online. If you want to parent effectively, respect what appeals to girls about online conflict. First, you don't have to look the person in the eye or hear her voice. Second, you have all the time you need to come up with just the right reply. Go ahead and acknowledge these perks to your daughter—then pick them apart.

When you're not looking at someone, you stop thinking about her feelings. When we do not make eye contact, we are less sensitive to hurting the other person and more focused on venting our own emotions. We are likely to say things we don't mean. We get puffed up with false confidence that quickly evaporates and leaves us with a mess.

When we can't hear someone's voice, it's hard to know what tone the other person is using. Take the sentence, "I never said she stole your boyfriend." Repeat the sentence several times, each time placing emphasis on a different word. The sentence can sound angry, defensive, confused—you get the picture.[92] Misunderstandings happen constantly: All we see are words, but we might decide the person is angry without actually knowing the truth. Unnecessary drama often results.

Tell your daughter that fighting online can seem like a good idea when you think about it, but when you actually try it, it gets messy quickly. Technology is never a substitute for honest, real relationships. As hard as it feels to talk to someone face to face or voice to voice, this is the best and only way to settle conflicts with respect and maturity. E-mail can be an exception, if it is used with care. When e-mail becomes a gateway for angry texts or chats, it is no longer productive.

Do not use social media to vent about your relationships. Social media allows users to post status updates, quick public statements that usually say where or how they are. Unfortunately, as I show in chapter four, many girls use status updates to vent about people, inviting their entire social network to observe, weigh in, or, worse, become involved. To wit, an update posted by a middle-school student, available to several hundred of her closest "friends": "So glad ur nt in my life anymore! Im beta off without you!" These are almost guaranteed drama starters because the subject of the update feels embarrassed, angry, or otherwise compelled to retaliate. Talk to your daughter about what is appropriate to share in an update, and what is best left between individuals.

Talk about sexting. While sending sexual photos or text does not obviously fall into the area of bullying or aggression, embarrassing photos in the wrong hands can become a powerful weapon used by boys and girls alike. As I show in chapter four, boys may ask girls to send a revealing photograph as a way to flirt. Unfortunately, many also do it so they can show it to their friends. Being in possession of a naked or half-naked photo of a peer is a source of status for boys and a way to affirm their masculinity. Many girls fear if they do not send a photo, the guy will lose interest. To maintain the relationship, they comply.

Speak frankly with your daughter about what to do if she is asked to send a photograph. You will have more credibility with her if you can critique sexting as a practice without making it seem like you oppose flirting or (if you are comfortable saying so) dating. Rosalind Wiseman wisely writes, "A reasonable fifteen-year-old girl in real life would never stand in front of a guy she liked, take off all her clothes and ask, 'Now do you like me?' Nor would she think it was acceptable for that boy to bring all his friends over to weigh in on the decision . . ."[93] The issue is not her attraction to a boy, but the power she gives him when she presses send. Even if the boy promises not to share the photo, there are countless stories of said trusted boys having their phones wrestled away by eager peers who forward the photo to their own devices.

If she does sext, and an image or message gets out of control, she must be able to turn to you for support. If she is being humiliated electronically, focus on getting through the crisis and helping her face going back to school. When the consequences of her behavior die down, you can step in and introduce your own.

I speak with parents all over the country about the challenges of parenting in the digital age. At the end of my workshops, I leave time for parents to share homespun strategies and struggles. Like the first kernels of popcorn popping slowly in a microwave, the voices begin tentatively. One parent talks about finding her daughter texting in the middle of the night, while another confides he can't stop checking his BlackBerry. Heads nod in recognition, and they laugh. They share their own rules (or lack thereof) at home. The parents leave with the confidence to try something different with their kids.

No matter how advanced technologies become, our very human habits and instincts remain. When people talk, they learn from each other. They create communities that provide affirmation and comfort. Do not underestimate the power of your peers to help you reclaim the authority your gadget-obsessed daughter may be working hard to take away. Most important, remember what you stand for as a parent. When families commit to the core values that have guided their parenting from day one, technology becomes a lot less daunting. There is nothing that happens online that you cannot help your child through. No gadget, no website, no application will ever change the fact that you are the parent. The most important manual you will need is the one that guides your own heart.

CHAPTER twelve

the road ahead for educators and administrators

When I first wrote *Odd Girl Out,* I had no experience in the classroom other than as an observer. All that changed when the book was published. I began working with schools to develop strategies to reduce bullying. I went into the trenches, serving as a classroom teacher with girls in elementary, middle, and high schools. I cofounded the Girls Leadership Institute and wrote curricula to develop girls' social-emotional learning skills. Today, I am a teacher myself.

One of our best hopes for changing the hidden culture of girls' aggression is educators. An educator can create a classroom culture that understands the range of girls' aggressions, refuses to tolerate them, invites girls' private and public discussion of them, and seeks solutions wherever possible. It is in the classroom that a girl can learn that alternative aggressions are nonassertive acts. Educators can teach girls that indirection and manipulation are unsatisfactory ways to express negative feelings.

Beginning in preschool, along with how to stand in line, how to be quiet when the teacher asks, how to take care of the pet guinea pig, and how to wait their turn, girls and boys can learn that alternative aggressions are not acceptable. Just as they are taught that punching to get what you want is a kind of violence, students must learn that threatening to not be someone's friend is, too. The lessons must begin early and continue year after year. Just because alternative aggressors sigh instead of shout, snort instead of tease, roll their eyes instead of taunt, or turn their backs instead of hit, they shouldn't be let off the hook. Banning these behaviors and socializing girls *away* from them should become as important as any other lesson in character education.

Yet educators alone cannot be expected to carry this load. If this is a culture that blames parents for everything wrong at home, it's also a culture that blames educators for everything wrong at school. Educators cannot be the architects of lasting change without the support of colleagues, principals, and superintendents. On a day-to-day level, educators must feel that time spent on these issues is neither wasted nor stolen but instead important to their students' education and development. This chapter examines girl bullying from an educator's perspective. I explore the obstacles professionals face, along with strategies they can use right now to create a safer learning environment for students.

barriers to intervention

Pursuing alternative aggressions in and out of the classroom can be as treacherous for educators as it is for girls and parents. Pushed and pulled by parents and administrators, working under vague or nonexistent anti-bullying policies, faced with impossibly high standards and shrinking budgets, and exhausted and undercompensated, educators may be less inclined to discipline behavior that is often invisible. It is not uncommon for public school classrooms to be crowded with as many as thirty-five students. As Peggy Orenstein points out in *Schoolgirls,* educators sometimes have only girls to thank for the few moments of order in class. Girls have long played the straight man to the boys' class clown; the American Association of University Women has documented the dwarfing of girls' voices in schools by more rambunctious boys. It is precisely girls' reputation for civility that provides the perfect cover for covert aggressors, giving them unrestricted movement beneath the radar.[94]

To complicate matters, girl fights lack the boldly drawn lines of battles between boys. Girls' conflicts run deep under the ground like the roots of an old tree. The lack of awareness of these behaviors only reinforces the anxiety many adults feel toward girls' relational conflicts. "Girls' relationships make me nervous," one veteran teacher confided, "and I'm not qualified to recommend psychological help."

Many educators who would otherwise be willing to lend a hand are adrift without a disciplinary infrastructure or public language to describe girls' behavior. Marilyn, who has taught elementary school for over twenty years, explained, "I mean, how do you say to a parent, 'Your child is a consummate liar'? They don't want to hear that from me!" A new vocabulary shared by a school community would report on children's behavior in less inflammatory terms. Parents could refer to acts of relational, indirect, or social aggression such as rumor spreading, alliance building, or nonverbal gesturing. In turn, educators might feel less fearful about approaching parents.

It is in part the invisibility of girls' aggression that puts educators on such shaky ground. Many refuse to discipline behavior they did not themselves see. Marilyn explained, "It's easier to stop the physical because it's visual, and if you come across it, if you see one child stick his foot out, or see somebody hit somebody, or move a chair out from behind someone, that's very easy to confront because it's right there. The innuendo or slight—you have to be present, and you have to be right on top of it."

Barring cameras in the classroom, educators aren't going to get instant replay; behavior that is open to question may remain so. "I don't hesitate to confront a child if I know I have ground to stand on. But you don't want to put yourself in jeopardy or a situation where you're not quite sure what's going on," Marilyn said. Later, she added, "Parents are always watching you. They can be your best ally and worst enemy."

Indeed. Even a note in a message box from a parent can be enough to make a teacher panic. An elementary-school teacher described the intense anxiety she feels when confronting a parent over a child's problem. "You get a note and you go home [anxious], and you stay up all night talking to your husband. Educators walk out of the building crying over things like this." Marilyn has concluded it's generally useless to inform parents about the misbehavior of their children. "There's no rationale. It's not an intellectual reaction. It's like the lioness and her cubs. They're going to protect them no matter what. As a teacher," she said, "you don't want to touch that. I'm not the enemy," she noted, "but at some point, you just back off and don't go there anymore."

These days educators have their noses to the grindstone to keep their students working at a demanding academic pace. A teacher in a top-rated public school district explained, "Girls bullying each other is the farthest thing from our minds. I'm sorry, but I wasn't looking for it. It doesn't happen in that fifty-minute [class period]. I'm not noticing it. I'm not focused on it. I'm too focused on instruction. I don't have time for that.

"We're not trained to look for that," she added. "We are trained to make sure they are doing their books." The idea that educators should be attuned to students' body language exasperates her. "It's so hard to be up all the time. You have to be on top of everything and you're bombarded constantly. And now, on top of everything, you have to be aware of the situation they're going through, aware of body language—all of it!"

Not surprisingly, educators are apt to misinterpret problems at school. Maryann, also a twenty-year veteran of the classroom, told me that sometimes girls "misunderstand" other girls. "There's two girls who have a secret together," she explained to me. "It could be a good secret or a bad secret, just something that the two of them want to keep for themselves." She told me the story of a third grader who became "hysterical" when her best friends stopped talking every time she approached. She was devastated that her two best friends had left her out.

"I don't know how they could have voiced [the need to exclude her] without hurting her feelings. Even if they had said, 'Look, this is something we need to keep private between us,' she would have still felt left out." Maryann took the three girls outside and tried to help the excluded girl understand that some people needed to keep secrets.

When I press Maryann about why she permitted the girls to do this, she admits she didn't know what the secret was, just that she respected their right to keep it. "They said it was private," she explains. Yet there is a difference between keeping information private between two people and flaunting the privacy itself. Making distinctions like this one is critical to understanding how subtle the aggression between girls can be.

There is a darker misunderstanding between educators and students to explore. Educators do not have access to a neutral language to name girls' aggression, and many are unaware of the social and psychological impact of stifling anger. As a result, it becomes easier to resent girls' behavior and give in to cruel stereotypes. One of my old teachers put it simply, echoing a remark I've heard more times than I care to count: "I'd much rather deal with men. They are generally straightforward and honest with you. With men, you know where you stand." The impact of such attitudes on educators' work in the classroom is unknown.

None of this is to say educators prefer ignorance. When I called Lynn, the same school counselor I wept to when Abby took me on in the third grade, she was thrilled to hear from me. A slight woman with a globe of brown curls, a freckled face, and the presence of a center forward, she hugged me, asked me about my brother (himself no stranger to this office), then settled back into her chair. "The biggest difficulty I encounter, the hardest thing to work through, is this awful thing that girls do to each other," she said, crossing her legs and frowning. "I have been waiting twenty-five years for someone that would explain this to me."

Like Lynn, some educators have chosen to confront alternative aggressions despite the shroud of silence that surrounds the topic. For Amber it is the memory of her own victimization that moves her. An elementary-school teacher in Mississippi, she sat with me one day in her classroom and told me about it: "I was short, had buck teeth and glasses. I know how it feels, and it's not gone away, and it's been twenty years. It's never gone away. I'm the most insecure person in the whole world. No one in my classroom would probably know that because I'm always telling them that we can do anything. I still, you know, I still can hear those kids calling me names and not accepting me because of my looks, my physical appearance."

Amber hawkishly forbids verbal cruelty in her classroom. She recalled escorting a boy and girl into the hall after they traded insults and speaking to them frankly about her own life. "It hurts, doesn't it?" she said. "I've been there. I had buck teeth. They may not be now, but [the teasing] hurt me." When she takes girls outside, she often gives them equal time to tell their stories.

In schools where physical violence is common, psychological aggression can take a back seat. School professionals triage student battles, focusing on the most violent altercations. Unfortunately, this is like waiting until a fire has fully consumed a house to call the fire department. As I show in chapter eight, girls' brawls are virtually always the endgame of a drama that began beneath the radar, using weapons like relational aggression, gossip, negative body language, and so on. The aggression may become visible with a shove or yank, but it almost never began there.

creating a safe school culture

A classroom sensitive to alternative aggressions is managed by an educator who openly discusses its different forms. An educator may use lessons with stories of children who experience alternative aggressions. She may openly discuss her own history with bullying. He may use instruction time to talk about the social dynamics of the class. She may work with colleagues to share effective discipline strategies and discuss the social climate of the grade. He may take time out to praise acts of truth telling and assertiveness in the classroom.

None of this can occur sustainably without the support and authority of an administrator. The decision to create a safe school culture must be made at the top and integrated into every part of a community. In the next section, I outline the structural changes needed to reduce bullying in schools. Much of my thinking in this area has been guided by the work of Dan Olweus and the Olweus Bullying Prevention Program, a rigorously researched and evaluated anti-bullying initiative for schools. From where educators should stand in the hallways to how lunchtimes can be made safe for all, the wide-ranging program works with every level of a school community and attempts to redefine the norms associated with bullying itself.

Develop an anti-bullying policy. There is no excuse for a school to lack an anti-bullying policy. It's like not having a fire safety plan. Although many states now require public schools to develop an anti-bullying policy, several states still do not; private schools are under no obligation at all.

The purpose of a policy is both symbolic and practical. Its existence sends a clear signal to the community about the school's core values and priorities. Knowing a policy is in place authorizes educators to use their judgment with confidence as they manage their classrooms. A good policy also stipulates protocol—that is, a systematic way of doing things—which lets the community know that cases will be handled on their merits and rules applied consistently, without regard to family, class, race, or gender.

School anti-bullying policies and handbooks must be revised to reflect the new research on alternative aggressions. Schools need to define clearly what constitutes aggressive behavior among *all* students such as rumor spreading, alliance building, and severe episodes of nonverbal aggression. For example, it might acknowledge that intentionally damaging another child's relationships is a form of actionable aggression.

Policy development should occur among individuals who represent different constituencies in the school: students, parents, staff, faculty, and administrators. A robust policy will not only designate unacceptable behaviors but affirm the school's values and desired behavior across its entire community.

The best school policies attend to electronic aggression. In the twenty-first century, it is impossible to keep students safe at school without holding them responsible for cyberbullying. The vast majority of schools decline to intervene in these episodes because they occur off school grounds. Yet anyone who has spent five minutes in a school knows that what happens off campus comes back into the school the next day, disrupting the community. Conflicts intensify, students can't focus, and school counselors and administrators are brought in to clean up the mess. Without the ability to hold students responsible for their actions, a vacuum is created where students can act out against each other without deterrent.

While there are important legal issues of free speech to consider here, it is no longer acceptable to argue that anti-bullying policy remain squarely within the school's gates. Cyberbullying is a game changer; it literally shatters the walls between school and home. There is no escape. As Wired Safety founder Parry Aftab has said, cyberbullying follows you everywhere: home, to summer camp, to Grandma's house.

Increasingly, schools are arguing that students must be held accountable for what happens off campus because of the school resources required to manage the aftereffects of cyberbullying. This is the right direction for schools to be heading.

Develop a consistent intervention protocol for educators. When a community has not come to agreement about what bullying means and how it should be addressed, enforcement can be wildly erratic. Consistent intervention with girls—indeed, with any student—is crucial to creating a safe school climate. As Dan Olweus and Susan

Limber have written, "Students need to experience that adults in your school will address bullying in roughly the same way, using the same rules and similar guidelines for use of positive and negative consequences. This... assures students who are bullied that adults will take action to stop bullying."[95]

When only certain students get in trouble, it sends the message that some students live above the law. At a public high school in the South, a cheerleader was caught with marijuana in her bag on a school trip. The squad's sponsor, who was also a teacher at the school, asked the assistant principal to remove the girl from the squad. Legal charges were pending, but the administrator refused. The girl's father was a prominent community figure and booster club donor, and her brother was the quarterback on the football team.

Intermittent enforcement erodes a student's sense that she is safe at school. This invariably adds to student anxiety, makes kids think they can break the rules with certain adults, and leads to a pervasive loss of faith in adults at the school. Administrators cannot be people pleasers. The most effective school leaders are willing to risk losing a prominent family in order to keep their communities safe.

Enforcement may be inconsistent because educators do not know how to respond to peer aggression. Graduate schools of education rarely train teachers in this area, so administrators should never assume that a teacher simply "knows" how to reprimand and discipline a student.[96] It is simply unfair to assume educators are ignorant or unwilling to address bullying. Staff need training to know what to say and how to say it. When they do not feel empowered to intervene, staff send the message that bullying is acceptable and will not be disciplined by authority figures at the school.

When I visit schools, educators ask me all the time for scripts and strategies to deal with an aggressive girl. Many of them seem to think extraordinary or unusual tricks are required to intervene effectively. This is a myth. In fact, dealing with girls is not all that different from how many staff already address more conventional forms of aggression or rule breaking.

Imagine witnessing an act of aggression you have seen several times before—say, a nasty remark or one student shoving another. What would you do? Most likely, you would follow a set of steps you have grown accustomed to in similar situations. Perhaps you would stop the behavior, make sure the student is okay, send the offending student to the assistant principal, and so on.

To respond to visible alternative aggressions, I recommend educators adopt some combination of these steps:

1. *Stop the behavior and ensure the target is safe.* As I have said elsewhere in this book, some of the most aggressive girls are downright angelic around adults. When confronted, many girls (and plenty of boys) will revert to denial, or the claim they were "just kidding." The Olweus program advises staff to avoid giving students an opportunity to reject their interpretation of events. Instead of asking, "What are you doing?" or "What did you just say?" don't hesitate: "I saw what you were doing and that is unacceptable behavior at this school." If girls reply that it was a joke—even if the target seems to agree—hold your ground: "It doesn't matter how you meant it. What you said is not okay."

2. *Define the violation.* When it comes to alternative aggressions, you may need to explain why the behavior is considered wrong in the first place. For example, some students may not understand that threatening not to be someone's friend, or convincing others not to sit with a peer, is a form of aggression. It can be useful to compare the behavior to one they already take seriously. "When you roll your eyes at her every time she raises her hand, it's hurtful. It's like calling her a mean name."

When dealing with a group of girls, do not talk to them together. Instead, speak to each one in quick succession,[97] and do not allow the girls to congregate outside an office while they wait (otherwise, they may "get their stories straight").

3. *Outline the consequences, if any;* OR *refer the student to a disciplinary official.* Every situation is different, so consequences will vary depending on the circumstances. In addition, consequences do not always have to be punitive. Students can be asked to complete writ-

ten reflection assignments that ask them to explain their action, its impact, and their feelings about their behavior. Alternatively, you can ask students to write a letter of apology to the target. The point is to not let the behavior go. Students should know that aggression comes at a cost.

Since so much of girls' aggression occurs without detection, denial of bad behavior is rampant. Yet a she-said, she-said situation does not necessarily mean you have to back down. Let's say a student has been implicated in using a nasty code name to describe another girl. There is no proof, yet you feel pretty sure it happened. You can tell the student you are not blaming her but still weigh in on the behavior itself: "Using a code name to talk about someone is really hurtful, and it's the kind of thing we don't tolerate at this school. Can you imagine how embarrassed and put down that girl would feel if she found out?"

Then, you can talk about the "hypothetical" consequences for engaging in the behavior, in the event someone is caught doing it: "I just want you to know that if someone did do that, and I found out, that person would definitely get a detention and phone call home."

New Jersey school counselor Kim Kaminski asks a clever question when a girl denies wrongdoing or seems to withhold incriminating information: "When I ask the other person about this, what do you think she's going to say?" The question, Kaminski says, can have a fairly magical effect on quiet or stubborn girls.

If educators are uncertain about the limits of their permission to intervene, they should be advised to ask the administrator responsible for discipline. Students can read the hesitation of staff. Adolescent girls are exquisitely gifted at talking their way out of trouble, and staff may back down as a result. Educators' confidence will increase with the knowledge that they are fully authorized to step in.

4. *Communicate expectations for future positive behavior.* Discipline is rarely effective when its recipient is left feeling hopeless or shamed. It is always important to give a student an opportunity to

redeem herself. This can be done by emphasizing a student's prior displays of good character, or by suggesting a specific action the student can take to correct the impression that has been left by her negative behavior.

This moment has the potential to become the point where a girl is told to "be nice" to the other girl. Better, instead, to emphasize the need for respect. "Nice" is a loaded word for girls. For adults, "nice" means polite and respectful. To girls, "nice" means being friends with that person. This is usually not feasible (or fair). Moreover, it is in part the pressure girls get to be "nice" that drives their behavior underground in the first place. This is an opportunity to talk with a girl about what respect means and looks like in practice. Girls do not have to be friends with every student, but they do owe their peers respect.

5. *Report or record the incident.* Research shows that when educators report bullying incidents, the situation is more likely to be addressed. If you are not already mandated by law to do so, require staff to report aggressive incidents to the school counselor or assistant principal. It is vitally important for incidents of bullying and aggression to be flagged and moved to the top of an administrator's list. If too much time passes between a report and an intervention, it may be too late to make an impact.

Each week a summary incident report can be circulated in writing to staff or reviewed in a staff meeting. Reports do not always have to lead to action; they can also serve as an information-sharing device that activates support for a struggling student. For example, if an art teacher reads a report that one of her students is being bullied, she may reach out to the student, take care to recognize her work, or offer to let her collaborate on a special project.

Every staff or team meeting should make time to review "red flag" or struggling students. This evaluation needs to cover both bullies and targets. When more educators are aware of who needs help, they can work together and provide the necessary support or discipline.

Train the entire school staff. All individuals employed by a school, whether they work in the cafeteria, drive a bus, or clean the building, should be trained to understand what bullying looks like and what to do when they see it. Most bullying and aggression occurs in places with the least adult supervision, which is everywhere a teacher may *not* be. This includes bathrooms, carpool lanes, cafeterias, buses, and hallways. Making a school safe is an effort that must be undertaken by every adult in the community.

Make sure students know the rules. Every student at your school should know what bullying is, what to do when bullying is observed, and what the consequences are for engaging in it. The rules should be conveyed in the context of discussions, suggested later in the chapter, or accompany other learning experiences such as school assemblies. Making rules or exercising authority "because we say so" never goes very far with kids. They need to understand why the rules exist and have an opportunity to reflect on how they pertain to their own wellness and safety.

Separate the roles of counselor and disciplinarian. School counselors and clinicians working at a school cannot be tasked with both counseling students and taking disciplinary action against them. Unfortunately, in understaffed schools, this is precisely what happens. Students need to feel safe approaching a counselor, without worry that disclosures will lead to punishment. Asking a counselor to play both roles puts him in a compromised position and makes his student support services highly conditional. Under such terms, students are far less inclined to visit a counselor and get the help they need before a situation worsens.

Take social-emotional learning (SEL) seriously. The core skills of SEL include "recognizing and managing our emotions, developing caring and concern for others, establishing positive relationships, making responsible decisions, and handling challenging situations constructively and ethically. They are the skills that allow children to calm themselves when angry, make friends, resolve conflicts respectfully, and make ethical and safe choices." Some SEL-focused activities might include exercises where students practice identifying emotions, explore what it means to be a good or true friend, and devise strategies for telling a bully to back down.[98]

SEL is not about only classes or skills. It also refers to the core values and priorities of a school. When administrators take a social-emotional approach to their leadership, safety becomes a priority that is embedded in the operation and culture of the school. These school leaders do not just assign lunch periods randomly, but purposefully create lunch periods and seating arrangements that separate targets from aggressors. They oversee school counselors who place vulnerable students in nurturing teachers' classrooms. They separate the students who create more trouble when they are paired. Emotional safety is seen as a way of life, not an afterthought; steps are consistently preventative and do not come only in response to crisis.

With its evidence-based success, the SEL field is finally gaining the widespread credibility it deserves. A host of studies find that a child's SEL is directly linked to her academic and social success. Despite these findings, there is often little time available during the school day devoted to SEL. As I wrote in chapter ten, relationships are the fourth "R." The skills for safe and ethical relationships must be taught, not assumed. When students have the tools to manage their feelings and relationships, and make ethical choices, they are less likely to be involved in bullying.

Provide guidance to parents and staff about how to communicate. Bullying episodes have a lifespan; that is, the actual incident is only the beginning of a longer process. As administrators and parents become involved, the need for protocol and clear expectations about behavior does not evaporate. If anything, having a system in place becomes more important than ever. Parameters on the school-parent relationship hold all players to a standard of behavior that can be easily left behind when emotions become intense. In 2010 "vigilante parents" was a popular term, as sure a sign as any of the need for boundaries between educators and parents.

Schools can stipulate how parents should communicate with the school and, in turn, how the school will respond. One independent school introduced a "parent covenant" that parents must sign each year in order for their children to attend. The document points out that "we enroll families, not just students" and explains the "reasonable expectations we have of each other" in working as partners to fulfill the school's mission. Among the promises parents make to this school are to:

- Respect the school's responsibility to do what is best for the entire community, while recognizing the needs of the individual child . . .
- Seek to resolve problems and secure information through appropriate channels which are teacher/advisor and then if further discussion is needed, with the Assistant Headmaster and/or Headmaster . . .
- Model and exercise respect, honesty, and a professional attitude, in the face of the inevitable differing points of view and challenges with staff, faculty, administration, and other parents within the community.

The covenant further asks that parents behave in a way that reflects the school's character goals both on and off campus.

At every school, it should be standard for staff to be permitted twenty-four hours to respond to a parent's message. Parents should also be encouraged to make formal appointments with educators to discuss a problem, so that staff can be optimally prepared to respond.

Educators need to know their senior administrators are available for support when communication with a parent becomes challenging, and that it is not a failure on a teacher's part to need or ask for help. Meanwhile, at parent meetings, an administrator should never question or undermine a teacher publicly. This embarrasses the teacher, challenges her authority, and gives the appearance of incoherent school leadership. Finally, educators need scripts to respond to difficult parents and clear instruction about the boundaries they can set with parents. Do not assume a teacher knows she is permitted to set limits with parents, or even that she knows how.

classroom strategies

Of the many joys of teaching, one has always stood out to me: the privilege of presiding over a community that travels together, for better or for worse, for an entire academic year. This journey is never just intellectual. Classrooms are tight-knit groups with powerful social dynamics, and the social-emotional vibe of a class can make or break a student's learning potential. Classrooms can be dangerous places where only a few are safe, or nurturing environments where every member feels recognized. In the next section, I share strategies classroom teachers can use to foster connectedness and care among students and their families.

Set a positive tone from the beginning. Take time to e-mail or call to introduce yourself to your parents at the beginning of the year. Develop a parent-teacher relationship where parents see you as an individual who teaches their child, rather than the person who calls only when their child has or is a problem. Making a few minutes of small talk or noticing something positive about a student is money in the bank: when it's time to have a tough conversation, you'll have some equity in the relationship.

Create a class contract. At the beginning of the year, spend time with your students developing a class contract that outlines how they want to be treated in your classroom, by both you and each other. Contracts remind students of the important role they play in the smaller classroom community. The rules affirm that each of them is a member of a group, and each has an important responsibility to fulfill.

Some questions to get the ball rolling are, "What do you need, from me and each other, in order to feel safe and respected in this classroom?"[99] You might also ask, "What are some ways that people can be disrespectful toward each other during class? What about before and after class?" Put students into small groups and ask them to create their own suggestions for how the class should conduct itself. Then, bring them together as a large group to hammer out the final contract. When it's done, create a poster of the contract and have every student sign it. When rules are broken, remind students this was a contract written by them, not you.

Create a prosocial classroom culture. Develop classroom rituals that give students opportunities to be kind to each other. For example, establish a hand signal students can use to silently offer agreement or support during class discussion. Have students give "snaps" to each other when someone answers a tough question or takes a risk. This is not about making each student feel "special," a trend that has seen its rightful share of skepticism in recent years. Rather, it is a way to set a classroom tone of community and kindness, modeled by the teacher and made rewarding for students.

Maggie Bittel, a veteran elementary-school teacher, taught her students to offer each other a "put-up"[100] (as opposed to "put-down"), a way to recognize someone's good character or personality. She began by giving the group detailed put-ups when they worked together well. Then she had students give themselves put-ups by creating a collage of characteristics or skills they admired in themselves. The class talked about the difference between bragging and knowing something good about yourself, and they discussed the difference between complimenting an external or internal quality of a peer.

Bittel read aloud from books with characters who had low self-esteem, and she asked students to reflect on the feeling of being lifted by another person when you feel sad. Finally, she made each student in the class responsible for noticing a teacher or peer for a full day. At the end of the day, with permission from the observed and the observer, students shared what they noticed in a card they wrote. Sometimes the assigned person was a secret; at other times everyone knew who was observing them. Finally, Bittel created a put-up wall in her classroom, where students could (with Bittel's permission) post a put-up they wrote about peers. Bittel intervened and gently encouraged students to notice those with fewer put-ups on the wall.

In high schools, where classroom size and stress mushroom, it is especially easy to ignore student wellness. Alyssa Yff, a social studies teacher in Raleigh, North Carolina, makes it a priority. She asks each student to complete a "History of Me" project, which integrates methods and precepts of history with social-emotional learning. During each student's presentation, Yff praises student creativity and celebrates differences. She posts the projects for the rest of the semester and refers to them if students disagree or "don't all have the same opinion."

Yff believes it is vital for educators to get to know each student personally. She invites hers to lunch, attends sporting and fine arts events, encourages students to stay after school, and makes herself accessible. "When kids trust you they will come to you," she said. "You have to nurture them both socially and academically, listen and not just hear, always role-model positive behavior, and create a safe atmosphere." Yff understands that her students will not learn if they don't feel safe, and that respect is a two-way street. When a student answers a question wrong and others laugh, she will say, "Okay, I see how you got that." By creating a foundation for an emotionally safe learning environment, Yff's students can experiment with new ideas.

Develop a body language glossary. Vigilance toward aggressive body language is important for social and academic safety. Angry glares or knowing looks can make a student feel anxious and threatened when she should be focusing on the lesson. In middle and high school, getting an answer wrong or expressing a strong opinion can be met with snickering or eye rolling. When such a pattern takes shape in a classroom culture, students take fewer intellectual risks. A sense that self-expression is not safe, or is circumscribed by unwritten rules set by a few aggressive students, can diminish a classroom's effectiveness.

It is always better to address the issue before it becomes a problem. Spend twenty minutes in your classroom asking students to come up with a list of ways kids can disrespect each other without speaking. Explain that even when we stop speaking, our body still communicates; like a muted television with captions, there are captions to our gestures. Have students make a list of gestures and, alongside each, the "caption" of what each gesture means:

> Mean look—"I hate you."
>
> Eye rolling—"You are annoying." "You are stupid."
>
> Laughing—"You're an idiot." "I can't believe you just said that."
>
> Silent treatment—"You're not worth my time."
>
> Whispering and staring—"We're talking about you right now."[101]

Some of the named gestures may not be relevant to the classroom. That's okay. The point is for students to own what their bodies are saying. When you weigh in on this issue during class time, you send the message that not only are you not clueless, you take the safety of your students seriously.

Define gossip and rumors as a form of violence. In a culture that has minimized psychological aggression, students need to understand explicitly that inflicting damage on a peer's relationships is a form of violence. One of the most common ways this harm occurs is through everyday gossip and rumors. Teach your students the connection between gossip and rumors and the loss of relationship. Explain that gossip has a ripple effect, and that what may begin as something between two people spreads until the target is excluded or harassed by others as a result.

To illustrate this process, draw three concentric circles on the board. In the smallest circle, write some fictional gossip, such as "Did you hear what she did at the party?" Ask students to imagine two people having the conversation, and then ask them to consider what realistically happens next. Fill in their response in the second circle. Continue on and add larger circles if need be, until you reach the point where the target of gossip suffers a loss or damage to her relationships.

The point of this exercise is to be clear that gossip and rumors are more than words. It's not just that calling someone a slut or gay hurts them personally; it's that the words cause others to mistreat the target. Perhaps peers will look at the person strangely, whisper and stare, harass them online, stop speaking to them, or insult them directly. All of this happens because two people, in that smallest circle, begin to talk. Bullying and aggression are not always direct.

Be the teacher who "gets it." As a teacher I was taught that even when under the gun, taking five minutes to play a game that focuses stressed or tired students can make the remainder of the class more effective, even if you lose valuable teaching time. Likewise, taking time to talk with students about their social culture fosters the safety and community your class needs to thrive. There are three conversations I have found successful with students. The first explores our social obligations to each other, and the exchange allows students to talk about norms for dealing with social challenges:

> Does every girl (or student) have to be friends with every other girl here? Is that a good or bad thing?
>
> What does respect mean to you?
>
> What does respect look like in the cafeteria? How should you act if someone sits down next to you who is not your friend? How do people really act?
>
> What does respect look like in class?
>
> What should you do if you hear someone talking about your friend behind her back? Is it better to tell her?
>
> What is the best way to have a conflict with someone?
>
> What should you do if you are bullied?

The second conversation focuses on psychological aggression and the behaviors that often go unnoticed by adults:

> Are there differences between the ways girls hurt each other and the ways guys do? (List the behaviors and similarities.)

How can people be hurtful without speaking?

What percentage of the time when girls (or people) say they are just kidding do you really think they are just kidding? If your number was low, why?

When someone says "no offense, but," what kinds of statements come next? What is your opinion of the way people use that phrase?

What gives girls power and status? What do you think about that?

How can friends hurt each other? How is that different from being hurt by someone you don't know that well?

How do people hurt each other electronically?

Would your friendships be easier or harder without technology?

The third conversation measures students' insights about bullying.[102]

How often do students report bullying?

How do students feel about bullying?

How responsive are adults to bullying at school?

What are the places where bullying or aggression is most likely to occur at school?

How do students feel about the reliability of classmates intervening?

In North Carolina, a high-school teacher asks these questions via e-mail or the website Survey Monkey. She randomly surveys her students with questions such as "Is this a safe environment? How am I doing? What can I do?" Students can e-mail her privately or answer the survey anonymously.

It is still remarkable to me how many girls believe adults are clueless when it comes to girl drama. Do not underestimate the power of devoting "official" class time to these issues. In doing so, you send the message that you are a teacher who "gets it." Take the time, at the end of these discussions, to let students know you are available to talk, or direct them to the individual who is.

Some educators open the channel by asking students to e-mail their concerns, or by placing a "suggestion box" where students can anonymously report problems. E-mail is always preferable after elementary school. Julia Taylor, the high-school counselor, advises educators to introduce the option by saying, "If you do not feel emotionally safe in my classroom, or you need help, e-mail me. I promise to keep what you write confidential unless you're in danger of harming yourself. We can talk about it and come up with strategies to help you deal. Don't spend thirty-six weeks in my class feeling like you're not safe." This approach can be effective as long as students who are "nominated" as bullies or aggressors are carefully investigated. Some students go after peers by falsely claiming they were hurt or attacked. To avoid this situation, seek different perspectives on an accused student and do not jump to conclusions.

Be a sounding board. When girls are young, it is much easier to intervene successfully in their social crises. Moments of glory are far more rare for middle- and high-school educators. Adolescence brings a tangle of relationship problems and conflicts that are not easily repaired. As a teacher, being the sounding board who listens, brainstorms, and empathizes can make the most lasting and immediate impact. What most teens want is to be seen and heard for who they are. They also want to know that life is not completely out of their control.

The GIRL decision-making tool I introduced to parents in chapter ten is an excellent strategy to use with struggling adolescents. GIRL helps students sort through their options for dealing with a social problem so they can identify the most effective strategy. In some ways, GIRL can be used even more effectively by educators because they are usually more dispassionate than parents. As you work with the student, you help her take charge of finding a solution and let her know you care. These are nourishing moments for a student who is suffering.

Set limits with parents. It is not a failure on your part to ask an administrator to join you in a meeting with a parent. Know when to ask for help. Having another person in the room, especially one senior to you, will underscore your authority to the parent and provide you with support in case the conversation goes south. It also gives you a witness. Be wary of parents who try to question your version of events, and do not second-guess yourself. Although parental denial is well intentioned, and usually stems from a desire to protect kids, trust yourself and stay the course.

Know, too, when to end a conversation. If you feel disrespected, unsafe, or uncomfortable, you are entitled to say, "I think it would be best if we ended this conversation for now and talked again at another time. I'm not comfortable with the tone of this discussion and I think we should take a break. Let's reconnect tomorrow." Your job description does not include service as a punching bag.[103]

Evaluate the example you set. After my workshops for educators, I am often taken aside by a teacher or two. "You know that assembly on bullying that you just gave to the students?" they ask. "You should be giving it to the educators." We laugh a bit, but the point is serious: educators are not exempt from aggression, and their behavior can swiftly undermine a school's message of kindness and respect. Educators can form exclusive cliques, gossip about colleagues, and reject newcomers outright. Some of this behavior is easily observed and overheard by students. A colleague at a school where I once taught advised me that it was okay to break a school rule after the principal had walked by the room, because she was so uptight. We were standing in front of twenty ninth-grade girls at the time.

This is not to say every educator is supposed to be an angel. Yet it is all too easy to confine anti-bullying messages like mine to youth without taking responsibility for what we bring to a community. I have trouble agreeing with educators who say they are not there to be social workers, but only to teach. We are not only models of intellect and academic inquiry; we are equally examples of good manners and citizenship.

Very little training would be required to train educators to identify and discipline alternative aggressions. The question is whether or not we want them to. When I asked Kendra, an elementary-school teacher, how she can tell it's happening in her classroom, she said it's obvious. "[Girls become] very withdrawn, their personalities change. Their facial expressions change. It's almost like a sadness, an intimidation... Even their posture. It almost sounds silly. They just withdraw—from the teachers, their group of friends... You can just look. I like for a child to smile. Lots of times I say, "Give me a smile," and if they really cannot smile, you know something is wrong.

Of course, even the most well-intentioned educators miss some covert aggression. Kendra cautioned, "They will try to hurt without anyone seeing it. You really have to see the expressions on their faces to know who's being left out or what's happening." Even Jenny, my old roommate who is a teacher and target of bullying herself, often comes home frustrated because she cannot fathom when it is Princess manages to psychologically flatten fragile Maya. In these situations, only the child can be relied upon to come forward and explain. And if she believes that her teacher will trivialize or ignore her pain, or approach the problem insensitively, she will remain silent.

No one should have to rely on ad hoc moments of compassion or personal experience to confront an epidemic. It is only through enforceable public rules and systematic staff training that we will begin to scratch the surface of this problem. If we don't make alternative aggressions a clear responsibility of school officials, children will continue to be vulnerable to bullying and abuse.

conclusion

Writing this book brought light to the dark corners of my life. Naming the alternative aggressions allowed me to see myself and my relationships in an entirely new way. It gave me a way to talk with others, to come to peace with what I remembered and what I continue to experience today.

I believe our task now is to give every girl, every parent, and every teacher a shared, public language to address girls' conflicts and relationships. A world that acknowledges the hidden culture of girls' aggression would empower girls not only to negotiate conflict, but to define relationship in new and healthier ways. Girls would learn that relationship is an option and not a mandate. They would understand relationship as a chosen partnership in which care and conflict are comfortably exchanged.

When girls understand that relationship can be chosen and that conflict is natural, their social identities will cease to hinge on how many idealized friendships they can rack up. Conflict will no longer feel like a violation of relationship but rather will be seen as a by-product of relationship, even a worthy skill to be honed. Conflict will not be something to be kept locked out of relationship. It will not feel, as it did to Carmen Peralta, like a bomb, splintering friendship beyond repair.

Parents would show girls that conflict-free relationships do not exist. Instead of believing conflict terminates relationship, girls could learn that *no relationship can survive without conflict.* Girls would learn not to be controlled by fear, understanding that relationships ebb and flow beyond the power of one.

In a world that acknowledges the hidden culture of aggression, girls would cease to play out their own fearful prophecies of loss. Knowing that conflicts are periodic, and that relationships survive them, girls might be less inclined to engage in the repression, back-stabbing, and ganging up that so often rise up to crush friendships. Most of the behaviors mapped out in this book—nonverbal gesturing, ganging up, behind-the-back talking, rumor spreading, the *Survivor*-like exiling of cliques, note passing, the silent treatment, nice-in-private and mean-in-public friends—are fueled by the lack of face-to-face confrontations. If girls could recognize their anger and upset, the intensity and scope of their reprisals might very well subside.

In a world that acknowledges the hidden culture of aggression, girls who are victimized would know they are not alone. They would have a language to assign meaning to what happened to them. They would enjoy protection at school. They could assimilate girl bullying into their lives as a painful, but not earth-shattering, event. Schools would have the resources, research, and strategies to address the wide range of alternative aggressions. Parents would have the confidence to approach their schools and properly protect their children.

the price of alternative aggressions

In the course of writing this book, I watched alternative aggressions and conflict avoidance intersect with three areas of girls' lives: leadership, relationship violence, and the reported loss of girls' self-esteem around adolescence.

GOOD LEADERS, GOOD GIRLS

At a girls' leadership workshop for twenty middle-class teenagers, one third of whom were nonwhite, we were talking about what made us uncomfortable about leadership, what we were calling "danger zones." As the girls began discussing their fears, I was amazed that nearly every concern related to how others would react to what they say or do.

Over and over again, looking bad or stupid—in their parlance, "getting judged"—was their worst fear. Whether meeting new people, speaking in public, reciting, or debating, the girls feared being "shut down"; they worried that people would not give them a chance to explain themselves and that others would shatter their self-confidence. As a result, they worried, people would not like them, would not want to be their friends, would turn their backs on them.

"The most remarkable thing about the socialization of aggression in girls is its absence," writes sociologist Anne Campbell. "Girls do not learn the right way to express aggression; they simply learn not to express it."[104] Many girls at the workshop, for instance, perceived being agreed with or supported as a sign of personal connection and being opposed as relational loss. Intriguingly, the dread they felt toward certain leadership practices was a mirror reflection of the fears so many girls voiced about *personal* conflict. In other words, these girls felt a comparable anxiety toward the "good" aggressions (confidence, competition, assertiveness) as many did toward the "bad" ones (interpersonal confrontation, anger, overt meanness). Like the girl who will not say why she is angry because she is afraid of losing her friend, the workshop participants predicted similar relational loss if they acted as leaders.

Throughout the workshop, more parallels emerged. These girls imagined themselves at work on everything from extracurricular projects to their future ventures as adults. Among the girls' most salient fears was being seen as conceited, which they believed would make them unlikable to coworkers. Girls who would do anything to avoid being seen as "all that" about a boyfriend were similarly alarmed when they envisioned professional conduct. Instead of thinking about how much they could achieve at work, they were wondering how to appear as though they hadn't, or how to look like they didn't think they deserved to.

The same thing happened with competition and desire. Many workshop participants told me they were afraid of being called competitive or bossy at work. What they were thinking about at work was not what they wanted and how to get it, but how to appear as though they didn't care as they maneuvered their way patiently toward their goals.

Finally, the workshop participants confided a fear of "messing up" or losing control by saying the wrong thing. This anxiety would force them to think every little thing through, driving them away from the risk taking and shoot-from-the-hip thinking so critical to success in the workplace.

At the following year's workshop, thirty middle-class teenagers were scattered in a circle on cushions in a recreation room. One quarter of them were nonwhite. We were talking about what makes a good leader. I asked them to call out the words they thought described her, and I scribbled along on an easel at the front of the room. When I stepped back to look at their list, here is what I saw:

A GOOD LEADER IS . . .

Loving	**Dedicated**	Outgoing
Loud	**Sensitive**	Organized
Good listener	**Cooperative**	**Respectful**
Helpful	Creative	**Open-minded**
Optimistic	Unique	**Understanding**
Flexible	Expressive	Mature
Proud	Talented	**Caring**
Determined	**Willing**	**Patient**
Committed	Bold	Responsible

Thoughtful	Honest	Friendly	ODD
Supportive	Trustworthy	Kindhearted	*girl*
Balanced	Open	Well-mannered	OUT
Independent	Positive	Insightful	

Passive, yielding, caring words (in bold) overwhelmed the list. Only four of the words, or less than 10 percent of their "good leader" (underlined) words, suggested a person unwilling to be nice.

To these girls, a good leader was a good girl.

Taking charge, saying no, and engaging in conflict were not signs of their good leader. The girls' leader was easy to get along with. She was nice. She was caring. She was someone you'd like to have as your friend. Looking back at the "anti-girl" list the group made the day before, mentioned in chapter five (see page 166), I was shocked by what they believed was wrong in girls: "Brainy," "Opinionated," "Pushy," "Mean," "Professional," "Serious," "Strong," "Independent," "Egocentric," "Unrestrained," "Artsy." The qualities that are the ingredients for a strong leader are the qualities of a bad girl.

Unfortunately, this is not a passing phase. In *Play Like a Man, Win Like a Woman*, CNN Executive Vice President Gail Evans explores why women struggle for equality in the corporate world. After decades of watching women hit the glass ceiling, Evans concludes that a misguided focus on personal relationships is partly to blame.

Evans argues that women struggle when hearing the word no from colleagues or superiors, construing it as a sign of interpersonal conflict. Because of this, women will avoid asking questions they anticipate will end in a no, hearing it as "a sign the relationship between us and our superiors has failed." Many women also avoid risk taking because they fear situations in which they may need to act like they know more than they really do, or bluff. Like the girls who fear being seen as "all that," women workers fear coming off as a person who thinks she's better than everyone else.

Evans notes that girls who wait to be asked "to go out on a date, to get called on in class," turn into women who wait to be asked to do projects rather than get out there and do them. Girls who, like seventh-grader Lily Carter in chapter three, communicate with friends through "hints" turn into women who "assume" the boss knows their work is excellent.

Because women have not been taught to see fighting as a sport or acceptable event, Evans explains that "the concept of a fair fight is an oxymoron. A fight shouldn't take place. If it does, the rules go out the window." Where Evans has watched men buy each other a beer after a conflict at work, a woman often takes it personally. She may storm away angry, reflecting a lifetime association of conflict with relational loss. Women who, as girls, never learned to be comfortable with conflict now as adults have trouble distinguishing normal, day-to-day disagreements from personal attacks.[105]

Evans's observations are not surprising. When girls learn to assert themselves indirectly, or not at all, they claim power similarly as adults. They may become helpers instead of leaders, work behind the scenes instead of at center stage, serve as deputies and vice presidents instead of chiefs and presidents.

To be sure, corporate culture does nothing to discourage this view. Women who are confident, who brag, who are assertive, and who fight are often called "manly" or "bitchy," "frigid," "castrating," or "aggressive." Their courage is not an asset. It's considered inappropriate. The California-based Bully Broads program is singular evidence: the instructor teaches female executives how to appear less assertive, advising them to stutter and cry in public in order to "soften" their image.[106] Small wonder the very girls who feel comfortable lost in the crowd end up as working women holding the short end of the stick.

BULLYING AND RELATIONSHIP VIOLENCE

Listening to the stories of Vanessa, Natalie, and Annie in chapter two, the word "bullying" sounds hollow. These girls endured protracted emotional abuse at the hands of their closest friends. They refused to give up their friendships, struggling at any cost to remain connected to their bullies. When I spoke to these girls and others, I could not help but ask how they could stay involved with people who were so hurtful. Their responses often sounded like those of battered women.

One girl wanted to leave her friend, but she was afraid of sitting at lunch and recess alone. Another insisted that her friends would be nicer tomorrow, or next week. I was reminded of the way a battered woman refuses to leave an abusive spouse because of her fears of living alone, or because he "said he was sorry." Conventional anti-bullying strategies at school are misplaced in these situations because they are built on the assumption that the aggressor and target are not friends. The intimacy of girlfriends is a central component of relational aggression between girls, and current strategies used by relationship violence experts might be more helpful for girls trapped in these situations.

Indeed, the warning signs of relationship violence bear a powerful resemblance to bullying between best friends. Like Lucia in chapter seven, abusers "can make you feel like you are the most special person in the whole world." No matter how hard a target of relationship violence tries, she can never meet her abuser's expectations, a dynamic prominent in Reese's and Natalie's relationship. As in Annie's friendship with Samantha, an abuser can try to cut the target off from friends, family, or anyone who could help her leave the relationship. The abuser will argue these individuals are "untrustworthy or don't like the abuser."

If we care about teaching girls to choose healthy relationships of all kinds, it is vital that we promote awareness of submissive and aggressive behaviors in girls' relationships. When abusive dynamics are without a language, and when anger cannot be properly voiced, girls may not develop the ability to name what is happening or extract themselves from destructive situations. As a result, girls may be learning submissive behavior they will import, uninterrupted, into intimate adult relationships. In other words, the failure to recognize abuse may not confine itself to girls, or to girlhood. Consciousness of these behaviors is absolutely critical to stopping vulnerability to abuse at the earliest possible ages.

THE BERMUDA TRIANGLE REVISITED

The middle-school years are what many would call the epicenter of the crisis of female adolescence. By now well known, the story of the crisis is often read as a eulogy to the intrepid, authentic girl. Uncovered most famously by psychologists Mary Pipher in *Reviving Ophelia,* and Carol Gilligan and Lyn Mikel Brown in *Meeting at the Crossroads,* the event marks a moment that has by turns been described as a "Bermuda triangle" in which the "selves of girls go down in droves" and a crossroads at which girls undergo a second socialization by the culture into womanhood.

Over the course of a few years, as girls become conscious of the culture around them, they are forced into abrupt disconnection with themselves. Their truthful voices, their fearless capacity to speak their minds, their fierce appetite for food and play and truth, will no longer be tolerated. To be successful and socially accepted, girls must adopt feminine postures of sexual, social, verbal, and physical restraint. They must deny their own versions of what they see, know, and feel. To avoid rejection, they must enter whitewashed relationships, eschewing open conflict and becoming shackled to cultural rules that deny their freedom to know the truth of themselves, their bodies, and their feelings. It is here, in the growing space between what girls know to be true and what they must pretend to feel and know with others, that their self-esteem shrivels.

The crisis of female adolescence has been described mostly in individual terms, its interpersonal consequences largely ignored.[107] In fact, the loss that is taking place is not simply one of the authentic self but of the self that is able to engage with her peers. The crisis, Brown and Gilligan report, is fundamentally relational. Pressure to deny the authenticity of *themselves* robs girls of the ability to communicate sincerely with one another. After all, girls are making Faustian bargains, sacrificing their true selves for damaged, false relationships with others. Disconnecting internally, they fall apart interpersonally, suppressing conflict and anger, adopting facades of the "nice and polite," and striving toward interactions that deny the realities of human relationship. They lose the ability to "name relational violations," or assert feelings of hurt and anger toward another person. "Feelings are felt, thoughts are thought," but they are "no longer exposed to the air and the light of relationship." Instead, they are sequestered in an "underground."

If we look at the crisis as a moment where alternative aggressions intensify, the loss of girls' self-esteem may be seen in a new light. By adjusting the lens we use to examine girls' lives, the underground appears as not just an emotional end point where girls store their true feelings. It may itself be an active medium to communicate conflict, especially alternative aggressions. Further investigation of this link may offer a new portal into the kinds of help we can give girls during this difficult period. If alternative aggressions are a major symptom of girls' loss of self-esteem, perhaps we can strengthen our attack against the onset of this crisis by focusing more resources and research on girls' interpersonal relationships. We might work harder to prohibit girls from engaging in alternative aggressions and instead guide them into more assertive acts of truth telling and direct aggression.

Teach girls to be aggressive? Well, yes. I return again to a major symptom of girls' loss of self-esteem: idealized, or conflict-free, relationships. If we can guide girls into comfort with "messy" feelings such as jealousy, competition, and anger, they will be less likely to take them out of their relationships with others. They will feel free to confess strong feelings, and they will stay in touch with themselves. They will be less likely to repress the feelings that over time simmer into rageful acts of cruelty.

Events of unexplained aggression and loss mark some girls forever. The worry that there is always a hidden layer of truth beneath a facade of "niceness" can leave girls permanently unsure about what they can trust in others and in themselves. These stories in particular haunt me. These are the girls, it seems, who drift away from other girls, who cease to support one another, who mature into mistrust and even hatred toward their peers.

Marcie was one of the first adult women I interviewed. The odd girl out more often than not during elementary and middle school, she confided that her current relationships with other women today are bittersweet. Now in her late twenties, she remarked, "Quite often, I feel like it's me who doesn't fit in with the rest of them. I know it's internal, and that there's a little part of me that will never quite trust them. There's a little part of me that believes they will turn on me at any moment."

Marcie's words were echoed in the voices of many girls and women I later met. Women like Marcie, injured in childhood by their peers, are still speaking in girls' voices. They feel a raw hurt and bewilderment that belies the years that have passed. These women are asking why the people around them, sometimes their closest friends, expressed anger indirectly and at times without warning, leaving them disoriented, alone, and full of self-blame.

When we can agree that nice girls get really angry, and that good girls are sometimes quite bad, we will have plowed the social desert between "nice" and "bitch." When we have built a positive vocabulary for girls to tell each other their truths, more girls will raise their voices. They will pose and answer their own questions and solve their own mysteries of relationship.

What greater gift can we give girls than the ability to speak their truths and honor the truths of their peers? In a world prepared to value all of girls' feelings and not just some, girls will enjoy the exhilarating freedom of honesty in relationship. They will live without the crippling fear of abandonment. It is my hope that as they, and any woman who has ever been the odd girl out, collect their thoughts to speak their minds, they will whisper to themselves, "What I most regretted were my silences. Of what had I *ever* been afraid?"[108]

notes

1. Michelle Anthony, *Little Girls Can Be Mean* (New York: St. Martin's Griffin, 2010).

2. See Marion K. Underwood, *Social Aggression Among Girls* (New York: Guilford Press, 2003). Also see the publications of Nicki R. Crick at the Institute of Child Development, University of Minnesota.

3. Lyn Mikel Brown and Carol Gilligan, *Meeting at the Crossroads: Women's Psychology and Girls' Development* (Cambridge, MA: Harvard University Press, 1992).

4. Adrienne Rich, "From Women and Honor: Some Notes on Lying," in *On Lies, Secrets, and Silence: Selected Prose, 1966–1978* (New York: W. W. Norton, 1979).

5. Anne Campbell, *Men, Women, and Aggression* (New York: Basic Books, 1993).

6. Lyn Mikel Brown and Carol Gilligan, *Meeting at the Crossroads*.

7. Peggy Orenstein, *Schoolgirls: Young Women, Self-Esteem, and the Confidence Gap* (New York: Doubleday, 1994). In the first part of this quote Orenstein cites Lyn Mikel Brown and Carol Gilligan, "The Psychology of Women and the Development of Girls," paper presented at the Laurel-Harvard Conference on the Psychology of Women and the Education of Girls, Cleveland, OH, April 1990; Orenstein also advises readers to see Lyn Mikel Brown and Carol Gilligan, *Meeting at the Crossroads*.

8. For other examples, see Beverly I. Fagot and Richard Hagan, "Aggression in Toddlers: Responses to the Assertive Acts of Boys and Girls," *Sex Roles* 12 (1985): 341–51; David G. Perry, Louise C. Perry, and Robert J. Weiss, "Sex Differences in the Consequences that Children Anticipate for Aggression," *Developmental Psychology* 25 (1989): 312–19.

9. Kaj Bjoerkqvist and Pirkko Niemela, "New Trends in the Study of Female Aggression," in *Of Mice and Women: Aspects of Female Aggression,* ed. K. Bjoerkqvist and P. Niemela (San Diego: Academic Press, 1992).

10. Kaj Bjoerkqvist, Kirsti M. J. Lagerspetz, and Ari Kaukiainen, "Do Girls Manipulate and Boys Fight? Developmental Trends in Regard to Direct and Indirect Aggression," *Aggressive Behavior* 18 (1992): 117–27.

11. Lyn Mikel Brown and Carol Gilligan, *Meeting at the Crossroads.*

12. Carol Gilligan, *In a Different Voice: Psychological Theory and Women's Development* (Cambridge, MA: Harvard University Press, 1982).

13. Adrienne Rich, "Compulsory Heterosexuality and Lesbian Existence," in *Blood, Bread, and Poetry: Selected Prose, 1979–1985* (New York: W. W. Norton, 1986).

14. Anne Campbell, *Men, Women, and Aggression.*

15. For example, see Patricia A. Adler and Peter Adler, *Peer Power: Preadolescent Culture and Identity* (New Brunswick, NJ: Rutgers University Press, 1998).

16. Nicki R. Crick, Maureen A. Bigbee, and Cynthia Howes, "Gender Differences in Children's Normative Beliefs about Aggression: How Do I Hurt Thee? Let Me Count the Ways," *Child Development* 67 (1996): 1003–14.

17. For the best overview of research on relational aggression, see Nicki R. Crick, et al., "Childhood Aggression and Gender: A New Look at an Old Problem," in *Gender and Motivation,* ed. Dan Bernstein (Lincoln: University of Nebraska Press, 1999).

18. Nicki R. Crick, "The Role of Overt Aggression, Relational Aggression, and Prosocial Behavior in the Prediction of Children's Future Social Adjustment," *Child Development* 67 (1996): 2317–27; Nicki R. Crick and Jennifer K. Grotpeter, "Relational Aggression, Gender, and Social-Psychological Adjustment," *Child Development* 66 (1995): 710–22; Nicki R. Crick, Maureen A. Bigbee, and Cynthia Howes, "Gender Differences in Children's Normative Beliefs about Aggression: How Do I Hurt Thee? Let Me Count the Ways."

19. Lyn Mikel Brown and Carol Gilligan, *Meeting at the Crossroads.*

20. Ibid.

21. Ibid.

22. Lynn Smith, "Hey, Poo-Poo Head, Let's Be Friends: Childhood Teasing Needn't Be Traumatic," *Los Angeles Times,* 6 December 2000, sec. E, p. 1.

23. Alice H. Eagly and Valerie J. Steffen, "Gender and Aggressive Behavior: A Meta-Analytic Review of the Social Psychological Literature," *Psychological Bulletin* 100 (1986): 309–30; Ann Frodi, Jacqueline Macaulay, and Pauline R. Thorne, "Are Women Always Less Aggressive Than Men? A Review of the Experimental Literature," *Psychological Bulletin* 84 (1977): 634–60.

24. Don E. Merten, "The Meaning of Meanness: Popularity, Competition, and Conflict among Junior High School Girls," *Sociology of Education* 70 (1997): 175–91.

25. Erica Goode, "Scientists Find a Particularly Female Response to Stress," *New York Times,* 19 May 2000, sec. A, p. 20.

26. danah boyd, "'Bullying' Has Little Resonance with Teenagers," November 15, 2010, blog post at www.zephoria.org. See also "Victimization of Adolescent Girls" by Amanda Burgess-Proctor, Sameer Hinduja, and Justin Patchin. Cyberbullying Research Center (2010), www.cyberbullying.us. I have also noticed this in informal surveys I take when I visit schools around the country.

27. Thankfully, this is changing. Increasingly, state laws are mandating that schools include cyberbullying in their anti-bullying policy.

28. danah boyd, "Friendship," in *Hanging Out, Messing Around and Geeking Out,* eds. Mizuko Ito, et al. (Cambridge, MA: MIT Press, 2010).

29. "Popularity math" is a phrase suggested by Lilly Jay to describe this phenomenon.

30. S. Hinduja and J. W. Patchin, *School Climate and Cyber Integrity: Preventing Cyberbullying and Sexting One Classroom at a Time* (Thousand Oaks, CA: Sage Publications/Corwin Press, 2012, in press).

31. I first read this on danah boyd's blog as a single statement.

32. Jan Hoffman, "As Bullies Go Digital, Parents Play Catch Up," *New York Times,* 4 December 2010.

33. *Generation M2: Media in the Lives of 8–18 Year Olds.* Kaiser Family Foundation Study (January 2010).

34. The Nielsen Company, *US Teen Mobile Report* (October 2010). In their study, *Teens, Cell Phones and Texting,* the Pew Internet and American Life Project (2006) also found that 1 in 3 teens sent 3,000 texts per month.

35. S. Hinduja and J. W. Patchin, *School Climate and Cyber Integrity: Preventing Cyberbullying and Sexting One Classroom at a Time.* See also Pew Internet and American Life Project "Cyberbullying" (2006). Online at www.pewinternet.org.

36. Cyberbullying Research Center, *Cyberbullying: Identification, Prevention, and Response* by Sameer Hinduja and Justin Patchin (2010).

37. Racial disparity has grown significantly in recent years. According to the Kaiser Family Foundation, black and Hispanic children consume nearly

4.5 hours more media daily than white children. While the largest difference is in television viewing, there is less of a gap in computer and phone use. In 2009 white youth texted for an average of 1:22 a day, while black and Hispanic youth texted an average of 2:03 and 1:42, respectively.

38. *Teens, Cell Phones, and Texting.* Pew Internet and American Life Project (April 21, 2010).

39. Girl Scout Research Institute, *Who's That Girl* study (2010).

40. Girl Scout Research Institute, *Who's That Girl* study (2010).

41. This conversation has been published as it was delivered to me. Typos and other errors were in the original exchange.

42. National Campaign to Prevent Teen and Unplanned Pregnancy, *Sex and Tech: Results from a Survey of Teens and Young Adults* (Washington, DC: The National Campaign to Prevent Teen and Unplanned Pregnancy, 2009). Two surveys in 2009 (by MTV and Cox Communications) found only 10 percent and 9 percent of teens, respectively, had sexted.

43. See Sharon Lamb, *The Secret Lives of Girls: What Good Girls Really Do—Sex Play, Aggression, and Their Guilt* (New York: Free Press, 2002).

44. Obviously, the sample of girls who submit requests for advice is not random. Girls who are looking for advice may already be struggling with insecurity.

45. According to the report, the complete definition of sexualization is when a person's value comes only from his or her sexual appeal or behavior, to the exclusion of other characteristics; a person is held to a standard that equates physical attractiveness (narrowly defined) with being sexy; a person is sexually objectified—that is, made into a thing for others' sexual use, rather than seen as a person with the capacity for independent action and decision making; and/or sexuality is inappropriately imposed upon a person.

46. APA Study (link www.apa.org/pi/women/programs/girls/report .aspx). Report of the APA Task force on the Sexualization of Girls (Washington, DC: American Psychological Association, 2007).

47. For example, see Jean Kilbourne, *Deadly Persuasion: Why Women and Girls Must Fight the Addictive Power of Advertising* (New York: Free Press, 1999); Deborah L. Tolman and Elizabeth Debold, "Conflicts of Body and Image: Female Adolescents, Desire, and the No-Body Body," in *Feminist Perspectives on Eating Disorders,* eds. Melanie Katzman, Patricia Fallon, and S. Wooley (New York: Guilford Press, 1994).

48. Peggy Orenstein, *Schoolgirls.*

49. Patrick Welsh, "Bully-Boy Focus Overlooks Vicious Acts by Girls," *USA Today,* 12 June 2001, sec. A, p. 15.

50. Elizabeth Wurtzel, *Bitch: In Praise of Difficult Women* (New York: Doubleday, 1998).

51. A welcome exception to this rule appears to be athletics, where competition among girls is embraced and encouraged. However, the freedom to compete openly has yet to move off the field.

52. Lyn Mikel Brown, *Raising Their Voices: The Politics of Girls' Anger* (Cambridge, MA: Harvard University Press, 1998).

53. Deborah L. Tolman, "Daring to Desire," in *Sexual Cultures and the Construction of Adolescent Identities,* ed. Janice Irvine (Philadelphia: Temple University Press, 1994).

54. Mimi Nichter and Nancy Vuckovic, "Fat Talk: Body Image among Adolescent Girls," in *Many Mirrors: Body Image and Social Relations,* ed. Nicole Sault (New Brunswick, NJ: Rutgers University Press, 1994).

55. Jill McLean Taylor, Carol Gilligan, and Amy M. Sullivan, *Between Voice and Silence: Women and Girls, Race and Relationship* (Cambridge, MA: Harvard University Press, 1995).

56. Nicki R. Crick, et al., "Childhood Aggression and Gender."

57. Perhaps this is because the memory of being victimized buffered these speakers against the feelings that may have deterred others from telling their stories.

58. Adrienne Rich, "From Women and Honor: Some Notes on Lying."

59. Wiseman's Empower Program group in Washington, DC, works to end violence of all kinds between teenagers, and her "Owning Up" curriculum can be found at *www.empowered.org.*

60. Lyn Mikel Brown and Carol Gilligan, *Meeting at the Crossroads.*

61. Patricia A. Adler and Peter Adler, *Peer Power.*

62. Carolyn G. Heilbrun, *Writing a Woman's Life* (New York: Ballantine, 1988).

63. Lyn Mikel Brown and Carol Gilligan, *Meeting at the Crossroads.*

64. Ibid.

65. American Association of University Women, *Shortchanging Girls, Shortchanging America: A Call to Action* (Washington, DC: American Association of University Women, 1991).

66. Niobe Way, "Between Experiences of Betrayal and Desire," in *Urban Girls: Resisting Stereotypes, Creating Identities,* ed. Bonnie J. Ross Leadbeater and Niobe Way (New York: New York University Press, 1996).

67. bell hooks, *Bone Black: Memories of Girlhood* (New York: Henry Holt & Co., 1996).

68. Dorothy Allison, *Two or Three Things I Know for Sure* (New York: Dutton, 1995).

69. Lyn Mikel Brown, *Raising Their Voices.*

70. Jill McLean Taylor, Carol Gilligan, and Amy M. Sullivan, *Between Voice and Silence.*

71. Janie Victoria Ward, "Raising Resisters: The Role of Truth Telling in the Psychological Development of African-American Girls," in *Urban Girls: Resisting Stereotypes, Creating Identities,* ed. Bonnie J. Ross Leadbeater and Niobe Way (New York: New York University Press, 1996).

72. Ibid.

73. Patricia Hill Collins, "The Meaning of Motherhood in Black Culture and Black Mother-Daughter Relationships," in *Double Stitch: Black Women Write about Mothers and Daughters,* ed. Patricia Bell-Scott, et al. (Boston: Beacon Press, 1991).

74. Lyn Mikel Brown and Carol Gilligan, *Meeting at the Crossroads.*

75. Jill McLean Taylor, Carol Gilligan, and Amy M. Sullivan, *Between Voice and Silence.*

76. Tracy Robinson and Janie Victoria Ward, "'A Belief in Self Far Greater Than Anyone's Disbelief': Cultivating Resistance among African American Female Adolescents," in *Women, Girls, and Psychotherapy: Reframing Resistance,* ed. Carol Gilligan, Annie Rogers, and Deborah Tolman (New York: Harrington Park Press, 1991).

77. Ena Vazquez-Nuttall, Zoila Avila-Vivas, and Gisela Morales-Barreto, "Working with Latin American Families," in *Family Therapy with School Related Problems,* ed. James Hansen and Barbara Okun (Rockville, MD: Aspen Systems Corp., 1984).

78. Janie Victoria Ward, "Raising Resisters: The Role of Truth Telling in the Psychological Development of African-American Girls."

79. Jill McLean Taylor, Carol Gilligan, and Amy M. Sullivan, *Between Voice and Silence.*

80. Madeline Levine, *The Price of Privilege: How Parental Pressure and Material Advantage Are Creating a Generation of Disconnected and Unhappy Kids* (New York: HarperCollins, 2006).

81. Rosalind Wiseman and Elizabeth Rapoport, *Queen Bee Moms and Kingpin Dads: Dealing with the Difficult Parents in Your Child's Life* (New York: Three Rivers Press, 2007).

82. An article by Judith Jordan was particularly helpful to me on this point. J. V. Jordan, "Relational Resilience," No. 57. Stone Center for Developmental Services and Studies, Wellesley, MA, 1992.

83. Consult the work of Stan Davis for more information on how to empower your child as a bystander, especially *Empowering Bystanders in Bullying Prevention* (Champaign, IL: Research Press, 2007).

84. N. E. Werner, S. Senich, and K. Przepyszny, "Mothers' responses to preschoolers' relational and physical aggression," *Journal of Applied Developmental Psychology* 27 (2006): 193–208.

85. Lyn Mikel Brown and Carol Gilligan, *Meeting at the Crossroads.*

86. Internet safety expert Lori Getz uses this phrase to describe the three most important values of digital citizenship.

87. Rosalind Wiseman, *Queen Bees and Wannabes* (New York: Three Rivers Press, 2009).

88. Ibid.

89. Kaiser Family Foundation, "Generation M2: Media in the Lives of 8–18 Year Olds" (January 2010).

90. Ibid.

91. Internet safety experts widely recommend this protocol.

92. I got this exercise from materials distributed by the Girl Scouts of Nassau County, New York.

93. Rosalind Wiseman, *Queen Bees and Wannabes.*

94. Peggy Orenstein, *Schoolgirls.*

95. Dan Olweus and Susan Limber, *Olweus Bullying Prevention Program, Schoolwide Guide* (Center City, MN: Hazelden, 2007).

96. Ibid., 59.

97. Ibid., 70.

98. Website of the Collaborative for Academic, Social and Emotional Learning (CASEL), www.casel.org. In addition, there are several excellent curricula that specialize in developing girls' skills in these areas. "Girl Meets World," the curriculum of the Girls Leadership Institute; "Full of Ourselves" by Lisa Sjostrom and Catherine Steiner-Adair; and GIRLS by Julia Taylor and Shannon Trice-Black (Champaign, IL: Research Press, 2007).

99. I learned about class contracts from Rosalind Wiseman, *Owning Up: Empowering Adolescents to Confront Social Cruelty, Bullying and Injustice* (Champaign, IL: Research Press, 2009).

100. Maggie Bittel is not credited with creating the term "put-up."

101. I created this exercise following a conversation with Maggie Bittel about her use of a similar glossary in her classroom.

102. Olweus and Limber, *Olweus Bullying Prevention Program, School-wide Guide,* pp. 34 and 37.

103. For more insight on how to talk with challenging parents, see Michael Thompson and Alison Fox Mazzola's *Understanding Independent School Parents: An NAIS Guide to Successful Family-School Relationships* (Washington, DC: National Association of Independent Schools, 2005), or *Dealing with Difficult Parents* by Todd Whitaker and Douglas Fiore (Larchmont, NY: Eye on Education, 2001).

104. Anne Campbell, *Men, Women, and Aggression.*

105. Gail Evans, *Play Like a Man, Win Like a Woman* (New York: Broadway Books, 2000).

106. Neela Banerjee, "Some 'Bullies' Seek Ways to Soften Up; Toughness

Has Risks for Women Executives," *New York Times,* 10 August 2001, sec. C, p. 1.

107. For example, see Lyn Mikel Brown and Carol Gilligan, *Meeting at the Crossroads;* Mary Pipher, *Reviving Ophelia.*

108. Audre Lorde, "The Transformation of Silence into Language and Action," in *Sister Outsider: Essays and Speeches* (Trumansburg, NY: Crossing Press, 1984).

Adler, Patricia A., and Peter Adler. *Peer Power: Preadolescent Culture and Identity.* New Brunswick, NJ: Rutgers University Press, 1998.

———. "Dynamics of Inclusion and Exclusion in Preadolescent Cliques," *Social Psychology Quarterly* 58, no. 3 (1995): 145–62.

Allen, LaRue, et al. "Acculturation and Depression among Latina Urban Girls." In *Urban Girls: Resisting Stereotypes, Creating Identities,* edited by Bonnie J. Ross Leadbeater and Niobe Way. New York: New York University Press, 1996.

Allison, Dorothy. *Two or Three Things I Know for Sure.* New York: Dutton, 1995.

American Association of University Women. *Shortchanging Girls, Shortchanging America: A Call to Action.* Washington, DC: American Association of University Women, 1991.

Angier, Natalie. *Woman: An Intimate Geography.* New York: Houghton-Mifflin, 1999.

Anzaldúa, Gloria. *Borderlands—La Frontera: The New Mestiza.* San Francisco: Aunt Lute Books, 1987.

Atwood, Margaret. *Cat's Eye.* New York: Doubleday, 1988.

Banerjee, Neela. "Some 'Bullies' Seek Ways to Soften Up: Toughness Has Risks for Women Executives." *New York Times,* 10 August 2001, sec. C, p. 1.

Bell-Scott, Patricia, et al., eds. *Double Stitch: Black Women Write about Mothers and Daughters.* Boston: Beacon Press, 1991.

Bjoerkqvist, Kaj, Kirsti M. Lagerspetz, and Ari Kaukiainen. "Do Girls Manipulate and Boys Fight? Developmental Trends in Regard to Direct and Indirect Aggression." *Aggressive Behavior* 18 (1992): 117–27.

Bjorkqvist, Kaj, and Pirkko Niemela, eds. *Of Mice and Women: Aspects of Female Aggression*. San Diego: Academic Press, 1992.

Borg, Mark G. "The Emotional Reaction of School Bullies and Their Victims." *Educational Psychology* 18, no. 4 (1998): 433–44.

Bosworth, Kris, Dorothy L. Espelage, and Thomas R. Simon. "Factors Associated With Bullying Behavior in Middle School Students." *Journal of Early Adolescence* 19, no. 3 (1999): 341–62.

Brook, Judith S., Martin M. Whiteman, and Steven Finch. "Childhood Aggression, Adolescent Delinquency, and Drug Use: A Longitudinal Study." *Journal of Genetic Psychology* 153, no. 4 (1992): 369–83.

Brown, Lyn Mikel. *Raising Their Voices: The Politics of Girls' Anger*. Cambridge, MA: Harvard University Press, 1998.

Brown, Lyn Mikel, and Carol Gilligan. *Meeting at the Crossroads: Women's Psychology and Girls' Development*. Cambridge, MA: Harvard University Press, 1992.

Brown, Lyn Mikel, Niobe Way, and Julia L. Duff. "The Others in My I: Adolescent Girls' Friendships and Peer Relations." In *Beyond Appearance: A New Look at Adolescent Girls,* edited by Novine G. Johnson, Michael C. Roberts, and Judith Worell. Washington, DC: American Psychological Association, 1999.

Brumberg, Joan Jacobs. *The Body Project: An Intimate History of American Girls*. New York: Vintage, 1997.

Campbell, Anne. *Men, Women, and Aggression*. New York: Basic Books, 1993.

Chodorow, Nancy J. *The Reproduction of Mothering: Psychoanalysis and the Sociology of Gender*. Berkeley: University of California Press, 1978.

Claiborne, Liz, Inc. "What You Need to Know about Dating Violence: A Teen's Handbook." New York: Liz Claiborne, Inc., 2000.

Coie, John D., John E. Lochman, Robert Terry, and Clarine Hyman. "Predicting Early Adolescent Disorder from Childhood Aggression and Peer Rejection." *Journal of Consulting and Clinical Psychology* 60, no. 5 (1992): 783–92.

Corsaro, William A., and Donna Eder. "Children's Peer Cultures." *Annual Review of Sociology* 16 (1990): 197–220.

Cott, Nancy F. *The Bonds of Womanhood: "Woman's Sphere" in New England, 1780–1835*. New Haven: Yale University Press, 1977.

Craig, Wendy M., and Debra J. Pepler. "Observations of Bullying and Victimization in the School Yard." *Canadian Journal of School Psychology* 13, no. 2 (1997): 41–59.

Crick, Nicki R. "Engagement in Gender Normative Versus Nonnormative Forms of Aggression: Links to Social-Psychological Adjustment." *Developmental Psychology* 33, no. 4 (1997): 610–17.

———. "The Role of Overt Aggression, Relational Aggression, and Prosocial Behavior in the Prediction of Children's Future Social Adjustment." *Child Development* 67, no. 5 (1996): 2317–27.

———. "Relational Aggression: The Role of Intent Attributions, Feelings of Distress, and Provocation Type." *Development & Psychopathology* 7, no. 2 (1995): 313–22.

Crick, Nicki R., et al. "Childhood Aggression and Gender: A New Look at an Old Problem." In *Gender and Motivation,* edited by Dan Bernstein. Lincoln: University of Nebraska Press, 1999.

Crick, Nicki R., and Maureen A. Bigbee. "Relational and Overt Forms of Peer Victimization: A Multiinformant Approach." *Journal of Consulting & Clinical Psychology* 66, no. 2 (1998): 337–47.

Crick, Nicki R., Maureen A. Bigbee, and Cynthia Howes. "Gender Differences in Children's Normative Beliefs about Aggression: How Do I Hurt Thee? Let Me Count the Ways." *Child Development* 67, no. 3 (1996): 1003–14.

Crick, Nicki R., Juan F. Casas, and Monique Mosher. "Relational and Overt Aggression in Preschool." *Developmental Psychology* 33, no. 4 (1997): 579–88.

Crick, Nicki R., and Jennifer K. Grotpeter. "Relational Aggression, Gender, and Social-Psychological Adjustment." *Child Development* 66, no. 3 (1995): 710–22.

Crick, Nicki R., and Nicole E. Werner. "Response Decision Processes in Relational and Overt Aggression." *Child Development* 69, no. 6 (1998): 1630–39.

Davis, Angela Y. *Women, Race, and Class.* New York: Vintage, 1981.

Debold, Elizabeth, Marie Wilson, and Idelisse Malave. *Mother Daughter Revolution: From Betrayal to Power.* Reading, MA: Addison-Wesley, 1993.

Dolan, Deirdre. "How to Be Popular." *New York Times Magazine,* 8 April 2001, sec. 6, pp. 44–46.

Eagly, Alice H., and Valerie J. Steffen. "Gender and Aggressive Behavior: A Meta-Analytic Review of the Social Psychological Literature." *Psychological Bulletin* 100, no. 3 (1986): 309–30.

Eder, Donna. "Serious and Playful Disputes: Variation in Conflict Talk among Female Adolescents." In *Conflict Talk: Sociolinguistic Investigations of Arguments in Conversations,* edited by Allen D. Grimshaw. Cambridge, UK: Cambridge University Press, 1990.

Eder, Donna, and Janet Lynne Enke. "The Structure of Gossip: Opportunities and Constraints on Collective Expression among Adolescents." *American Sociological Review* 56, no. 4 (1991): 494–508.

Eder, Donna, and David A. Kinney. "The Effect of Middle School Extracurricular Activities on Adolescents' Popularity and Peer Status." *Youth & Society* 26, no. 3 (1995): 298–324.

Evans, Cathy, and Donna Eder. "No Exit: Processes of Social Isolation in the Middle School." *Journal of Contemporary Ethnography* 22, no. 2 (1993): 139–70.

Evans, Gail. *Play Like a Man, Win Like a Woman: What Men Know about Success That Women Need to Learn.* New York: Broadway Books, 2000.

Fagot, Beverly I., and Richard Hagan. "Aggression in Toddlers: Responses to the Assertive Acts of Boys and Girls." *Sex Roles* 12, nos. 3/4 (1985): 341–51.

Fagot, Beverly I., Mary D. Leinbach, and Richard Hagan. "Gender Labeling and Adoption of Sex-Typed Behaviors." *Developmental Psychology* 22, no. 4 (1986): 440–43.

Fein, Ellen, and Sherrie Schneider. *The Rules: Time-Tested Secrets for Capturing the Heart of Mr. Right.* New York: Warner Books, 1995.

Fine, Michelle. "Sexuality, Schooling, and Adolescent Females: The Missing Discourse of Desire." *Harvard Educational Review* 58, no. 1 (1988): 29–53.

Friedan, Betty. *The Feminine Mystique.* New York: W. W. Norton, 1983.

Frodi, Ann, Jacqueline Macaulay, and Pauline R. Thorne. "Are Women Always Less Aggressive Than Men? A Review of the Experimental Literature." *Psychological Bulletin* 84, no. 4 (1977): 634–60.

Galen, Britt Rachelle, and Marion K. Underwood. "A Developmental Investigation of Social Aggression Among Children." *Developmental Psychology* 33, no. 4 (1997): 589–600.

George, Thomas P., and Donald P. Hartmann. "Friendship Networks of Unpopular, Average, and Popular Children." *Child Development* 67, no. 5 (1996): 2301–16.

Gilligan, Carol. *In a Different Voice: Psychological Theory and Women's Development.* Cambridge, MA: Harvard University Press, 1982.

Gilligan, Carol, Nona P. Lyons, and Trudy J. Hanmer, eds. *Making Connections: The Relational Worlds of Adolescent Girls at Emma Willard School.* Cambridge, MA: Harvard University Press, 1990.

Goode, Erica. "Scientists Find a Particularly Female Response to Stress." *New York Times,* 19 May 2000, sec. A, p. 20.

Green, Laura R., Deborah R. Richardson, and Tania Lago. "How Do Friendship, Indirect, and Direct Aggression Relate?" *Aggressive Behavior* 22, no. 2 (1996): 81–86.

Groneman, Carol. *Nymphomania: A History.* New York: W. W. Norton, 2000.

Grotpeter, Jennifer K., and Nicki R. Crick. "Relational Aggression, Overt Aggression, and Friendship." *Child Development* 67, no. 5 (1996): 2328–38.

Hanley, Robert. "Girl in Shooting Was Seen as Dejected." *New York Times,*
9 March 2001, sec. A, p. 16.

Harris, Judith Rich. *The Nurture Assumption: Why Children Turn Out the
Way They Do.* New York: Touchstone, 1998.

Heilbrun, Carolyn G. *Writing a Woman's Life.* New York: Ballantine, 1988.

Henington, Carlen, Jan N. Hughes, Timothy A. Cavell, and Bruce Thompson. "The Role of Relational Aggression in Identifying Aggressive Boys
and Girls." *Journal of School Psychology* 36, no. 4 (1998): 457–77.

Hey, Valerie. *The Company She Keeps: An Ethnography of Girls' Friendship.*
Bristol, PA: Open University Press, 1997.

hooks, bell. *Bone Black: Memories of Girlhood.* New York: Henry Holt &
Co., 1996.

Hudson, Barbara. "Femininity and Adolescence." In *Gender and Generation,* edited by Angela McRobbie and Mica Nava. London: MacMillan,
1984.

Hughes, Linda A. "'But That's Not Really Mean': Competing in a Cooper-
ative Mode." *Sex Roles* 19, nos. 11/12 (1988): 669–87.

Ialongo, Nicholas S., Nancy Vaden-Kiernan, and Sheppard Kellam. "Early
Peer Rejection and Aggression: Longitudinal Relations with Adolescent
Behavior." *Journal of Development & Physical Disabilities* 10, no. 2 (1998):
199–213.

Irvine, Janice M., ed. *Sexual Cultures and the Construction of Adolescent
Identities.* Philadelphia: Temple University Press, 1994.

Jarrell, Anne. "The Face of Teenage Sex Grows Younger." *New York Times,*
2 April 2000, sec. 9, p. 1.

Jones, Jacqueline. *Labor of Love, Labor of Sorrow: Black Women, Work and
the Family from Slavery to the Present.* New York: Vintage, 1985.

Kantrowitz, Barbara, and Pat Wingert. "The Truth About Tweens."
Newsweek, 18 October 1999, 62–72.

Kaukiainen, Ari, et al. "The Relationships Between Social Intelligence, Empathy, and Three Types of Aggression." *Aggressive Behavior* 25, no. 2
(1999): 81–89.

Kerber, Linda K., et al., "On *In a Different Voice:* An Interdisciplinary
Forum: Some Cautionary Words for Historians." *Signs: Journal of
Women in Culture and Society* 11, no. 2 (1986): 304–10.

Kerns, Kathryn A., Lisa Klepac, and AmyKay Cole. "Peer Relationships and
Preadolescents' Perceptions of Security in the Child-Mother Relationship." *Developmental Psychology* 32, no. 3 (1996): 457–66.

Kilbourne, Jean. *Deadly Persuasion: Why Women and Girls Must Fight the
Addictive Power of Advertising.* New York: Free Press, 1999.

Kindlon, Daniel, and Michael Thompson. *Raising Cain: Protecting the Emotional Life of Boys.* New York: Ballantine, 1999.

Kumpulainen, Kirsti, Eila Racsacncn, and Imeli Henttonen. "Children Involved in Bullying: Psychological Disturbance and the Persistence of the Involvement." *Child Abuse & Neglect* 23, no. 12 (1999): 1253–62.

Lagerspetz, Kirsti M., Kaj Bjoerkqvist, and Tarja Peltonen. "Is Indirect Aggression Typical of Females? Gender Differences in Aggressiveness in 11-to 12-Year-Old Children." *Aggressive Behavior* 14, no. 6 (1988): 403–14.

Laurence, Patricia. "Women's Silence as a Ritual of Truth: A Study of Literary Expressions in Austen, Brontë, and Woolf." In *Listening to Silences: New Essays in Feminist Criticism,* edited by Elaine Hedges and Shelley Fisher Fishkin. New York: Oxford University Press, 1994.

Lees, Sue. *Losing Out: Sexuality and Adolescent Girls.* London: Hutchinson, 1986.

Lever, Janet. "Sex Differences in the Complexity of Children's Play and Games." *American Sociological Review* 43, no. 4 (1978): 471–83.

Lorde, Audre. *Sister Outsider: Essays and Speeches.* Trumansburg, NY: Crossing Press, 1984.

Maccoby, Eleanor Emmons. "Gender and Relationships: A Developmental Account." *American Psychologist* 45, no. 4 (1990): 513–20.

Maccoby, Eleanor Emmons, and Carol Nagy Jacklin. *The Psychology of Sex Differences.* Vol. 1. Stanford, CA: Stanford University Press, 1974.

Magner, Carolyn. "When They Were Bad." Salon.com., 9 October 2000 (http://www.salon.com/mwt/feature/2000/10/09/freeze_out).

McMillan, Carol. *Women, Reason, and Nature: Some Philosophical Problems with Feminism.* Princeton, NJ: Princeton University Press, 1982.

Menesini, Ersilia, et al. "Cross-National Comparison of Children's Attitudes towards Bully/Victim Problems in Schools." *Aggressive Behavior* 23, no. 4 (1997): 245–57.

Merten, Don E. "Enculturation into Secrecy among Junior High School Girls." *Journal of Contemporary Ethnography* 28, no. 2 (1999): 107–37.

———. "The Meaning of Meanness: Popularity, Competition, and Conflict among Junior High School Girls." *Sociology of Education* 70, no. 3 (1997): 175–91.

———. "The Cultural Context of Aggression: The Transition to Junior High School." *Anthropology & Education Quarterly* 25, no. 1 (1994): 29–43.

Miller, Jean Baker. *Toward a New Psychology of Women.* 2nd ed. Boston: Beacon Press, 1986.

Neary, Ann, and Stephen Joseph. "Peer Victimization and Its Relationship to Self-Concept and Depression among Schoolgirls." *Personality & Individual Differences* 16, no. 1 (1994): 183–86.

Nichter, Mimi, and Nancy Vuckovic. "Fat Talk: Body Image among Adolescent Girls." In *Many Mirrors: Body Image and Social Relations,* edited by Nicole Sault. New Brunswick, NJ: Rutgers University Press, 1994.

Oesterman, Karin, Kaj Bjoerkqvist, Kirsti M. J. Lagerspetz, Ari Kaukiainen, et al. "Peer and Self-Estimated Aggression and Victimization in 8-Year-Old Children from Five Ethnic Groups." *Aggressive Behavior* 20, no. 6 (1994): 411–28.

———. "Cross-Cultural Evidence of Female Indirect Aggression." *Aggressive Behavior* 24, no. 1 (1988): 1–8.

Okin, Susan Moller. *Women in Western Political Thought.* Princeton, NJ: Princeton University Press, 1979.

Orenstein, Peggy. *Schoolgirls: Young Women, Self-Esteem, and the Confidence Gap.* New York: Doubleday, 1994.

Paquette, Julie A., and Marion K. Underwood. "Gender Differences in Young Adolescents' Experiences of Peer Victimization: Social and Physical Aggression." *Merrill-Palmer Quarterly* 45, no. 2 (1999): 242–66.

Pateman, Carole. *The Sexual Contract.* Cambridge, England: Polity Press, 1988.

Pepler, Debra J. "Aggressive Girls: Development of Disorder and Outcomes." Report #57, La Marsh Research Centre Report. Toronto: York University, 1999.

Perry, David G., Louise C. Perry, and Robert J. Weiss. "Sex Differences in the Consequences that Children Anticipate for Aggression." *Developmental Psychology* 25, no. 2 (1989): 312–19.

Pipher, Mary. *Reviving Ophelia: Saving the Selves of Adolescent Girls.* New York: Ballantine, 1995.

Pollack, William. *Real Boys: Rescuing Our Sons from the Myths of Boyhood.* New York: Random House, 1998.

Raymond, Janice G. *A Passion for Friends: Toward a Philosophy of Female Affection.* Boston: Beacon Press, 1986.

Rhodes, Jean E., and Anita B. Davis. "Supportive Ties between Nonparent Adults and Urban Adolescent Girls." In *Urban Girls: Resisting Stereotypes, Creating Identities,* edited by Bonnie J. Ross Leadbeater and Niobe Way. New York: New York University Press, 1996.

Rich, Adrienne. *On Lies, Secrets, and Silence: Selected Prose, 1966–1978.* New York: W. W. Norton, 1979.

———. *Of Woman Born: Motherhood as Experience and Institution.* New York: W. W. Norton, 1986.

———. "Compulsory Heterosexuality and Lesbian Existence." In *Blood, Bread, and Poetry: Selected Prose, 1979–1985.* New York: W. W. Norton, 1986.

Rigby, Ken. "The Relationship between Reported Health and Involvement in Bully/Victim Problems among Male and Female Secondary Schoolchildren." *Journal of Health Psychology* 3, no. 4 (1998): 465–76.

Robinson, Tracy, and Janie Victoria Ward. "'A Belief in Self Far Greater Than Anyone's Disbelief': Cultivating Resistance among African American

Female Adolescents." In *Women, Girls, and Psychotherapy: Reframing Resistance,* edited by Carol Gilligan, Annie Rogers, and Deborah Tolman. New York: Harrington Park Press, 1991.

Rogers, Annie G. "Voice, Play, and a Practice of Ordinary Courage in Girls' Lives and Women's Lives." *Harvard Educational Review* 63, no. 3 (1993): 265–95.

Rotheram-Borus, Mary Jane, et al. "Personal and Ethnic Identity, Values, and Self-Esteem among Black and Latino Adolescent Girls." In *Urban Girls: Resisting Stereotypes, Creating Identities,* edited by Bonnie J. Ross Leadbeater and Niobe Way. New York: New York University Press, 1996.

Rys, Gail Summers. "Children's Moral Reasoning and Peer-Directed Social Behaviors: Issues of Gender and Development." Ph.D. diss., University of Delaware, 1998. Abstract in *Dissertation Abstracts International* 58 (1998): 5167B.

Rys, Gail Summers, and George G. Bear. "Relational Aggression and Peer Relations: Gender and Developmental Issues." *Merrill-Palmer Quarterly* 43, no. 1 (1997): 87–106.

Sadker, Myra, and David Sadker. *Failing at Fairness: How America's Schools Cheat Girls.* New York: Scribner's, 1994.

Salmivalli, Christina, Arja Huttunen, and Kirsti M. J. Lagerspetz. "Peer Networks and Bullying in Schools." *Scandinavian Journal of Psychology* 38, no. 4 (1997): 305–12.

Sheldon, Amy. "Conflict Talk: Sociolinguistic Challenges to Self-Assertion and How Young Girls Meet Them." *Merrill-Palmer Quarterly* 38, no. 1 (1992): 95–117.

Silver, Marc, and Joellen Perry. "Hooked on Instant Messages." *U.S. News & World Report,* 22 March 1999, 57–58.

Simon, Robin W., Donna Eder, and Cathy Evans. "The Development of Feeling Norms Underlying Romantic Love among Adolescent Females." *Social Psychology Quarterly* 55, no. 1 (1992): 29–46.

Slee, P. T. "Situational and Interpersonal Correlates of Anxiety Associated with Peer Victimization." *Child Psychology & Human Development* 25 (1994): 97–107.

Smith, Elsie J. "The Black Female Adolescent: A Review of the Educational, Career, and Psychological Literature." *Psychology of Women Quarterly* 6, no. 3 (1982): 261–88.

Smith, Lynn. "Hey, Poo-Poo Head, Let's Be Friends: Childhood Teasing Needn't Be Traumatic." *Los Angeles Times,* 6 December 2000, sec. E, p. 1.

Smith, Peter K., Helen Cowie, and Mark Blades, eds. *Understanding Children's Development.* 3rd ed. Oxford, England: Blackwell, 1998.

Smith-Rosenberg, Carroll. "The Female World of Love and Ritual: Relations between Women in Nineteenth-Century America." *Signs: Journal of Women in Culture and Society* 1 (1975): 1–29.

Spelman, Elizabeth. "Anger and Insubordination." In *Women, Knowledge, and Reality: Explorations in Feminist Philosophy,* edited by Ann Garry and Marilyn Pearsall. Boston: Unwin Hyman, 1989.

Stack, Carol B. *All Our Kin: Strategies for Survival in a Black Community.* New York: Harper, 1974.

Stanley, Lisa, and Tiny (C. M. J.) Arora. "Social Exclusion Amongst Adolescent Girls: Their Self-Esteem and Coping Strategies." *Educational Psychology in Practice* 14, no. 2 (1998): 94–100.

Sutton, Jon, and P. K. Smith. "Bullying as a Group Process: An Adaptation of the Participant Role Approach." *Aggressive Behavior* 25, no. 2 (1999): 97–111.

Sutton, Jon, P. K. Smith, and J. Swettenham. "Social Cognition and Bullying: Social Inadequacy or Skilled Manipulation?" *British Journal of Developmental Psychology* 17, no. 3 (1999): 435–50.

Tanenbaum, Leora. *Slut! Growing Up Female with a Bad Reputation.* New York: Seven Stories Press, 1999.

Taylor, Jill McLean, Carol Gilligan, and Amy M. Sullivan. *Between Voice and Silence: Women and Girls, Race and Relationship.* Cambridge, MA: Harvard University Press, 1995.

Thompson, Kevin M., Stephen A. Wonderlich, Ross D. Crosby, and James E. Mitchell. "The Neglected Link between Eating Disturbances and Aggressive Behavior in Girls." *Journal of the American Academy of Child & Adolescent Psychiatry* 38, no. 10 (1999): 1277–84.

Thompson, Michael, Lawrence J. Cohen, and Catherine O'Neill Grace. *Best Friends, Worst Enemies: Understanding the Social Lives of Children.* New York: Ballantine, 2001.

Thorne, Barrie. *Gender Play: Girls and Boys in School.* New Brunswick, NJ: Rutgers University Press, 1993.

Tolman, Deborah L. "Daring to Desire." In *Sexual Cultures and the Construction of Adolescent Identities,* edited by Janice Irvine. Philadelphia: Temple University Press, 1994.

Tolman, Deborah L., and Elizabeth Debold. "Conflicts of Body and Image: Female Adolescents, Desire, and the No-Body Body." In *Feminist Perspectives on Eating Disorders,* edited by Melanie A. Katzman, Patricia Fallon, and S. Wooley. New York: Guilford Press, 1994.

Tracy, Laura. *The Secret between Us: Competition among Women.* Boston: Little, Brown, 1991.

Tronto, Joan C. *Moral Boundaries: A Political Argument for an Ethic of Care.* New York: Routledge, 1993.

Vasquez-Nuttall, Ena, Zoila Avila-Vivas, and Gisela Morales-Barreto. "Working with Latin American Families." In *Family Therapy with School Related Problems,* edited by James Hansen and Barbara Okun. Rockville, MD: Aspen Systems Corp., 1984.

Walkerdine, Valerie. *Schoolgirl Fictions.* London: Verso, 1990.

Ward, Janie Victoria. "Raising Resisters: The Role of Truth Telling in the Psychological Development of African American Girls." In *Urban Girls: Resisting Stereotypes, Creating Identities,* edited by Bonnie J. Ross Leadbeater and Niobe Way. New York: New York University Press, 1996.

Way, Niobe. "'Can't You See the Courage, the Strength That I Have?' Listening to Urban Adolescent Girls Speak about Their Relationships." *Psychology of Women Quarterly* 19, no. 1 (1995): 107–28.

———. "Between Experiences of Betrayal and Desire: Close Friendships among Urban Adolescents." In *Urban Girls: Resisting Stereotypes, Creating Identities,* edited by Bonnie J. Ross Leadbeater and Niobe Way. New York: New York University Press, 1996.

Welsh, Patrick. "Bully-Boy Focus Overlooks Vicious Acts by Girls." *USA Today,* 12 June 2001, sec. A, p. 15.

White, Jacquelyn W., and Robin M. Kowalski. "Deconstructing the Myth of the Nonaggressive Woman: A Feminist Analysis." *Psychology of Women Quarterly* 18, no. 4 (1994): 487–508.

Wiseman, Rosalind. *Queen Bees and Wannabes.* New York: Three Rivers Press, 2009.

Wiseman, Rosalind, and Elizabeth Rapoport. *Queen Bee Moms and Kingpin Dads: Dealing with the Difficult Parents in Your Child's Life.* New York: Three Rivers Press, 2007.

Wolf, Naomi. *Promiscuities: The Secret Struggle for Womanhood.* New York: Ballantine, 1997.

———. *The Beauty Myth: How Images of Beauty Are Used Against Women.* New York: Random House, 1991.

Wurtzel, Elizabeth. *Bitch: In Praise of Difficult Women.* New York: Doubleday, 1998.

Zollo, Peter. *Wise Up to Teens: Insights into Marketing and Advertising to Teenagers.* Ithaca, NY: New Strategist Publications, 1999.

acknowledgments

It would be hard to overstate how much this book owes its life to the help of others.

From the first moment we met, R. K. had faith in me and this project. She put her reputation on the line for me, opened doors for *Odd Girl Out,* and became a supervisor, confidante, and friend. Lynn Arons, Bernice Berke, Tamika Ford, Rabbi Reuven Greenwald, Marti Herskovitz, Rudy Jordan, Eloise Pasachoff, Rebecca Prigal, Sherie Randolph, Laura Rebell, Kate Sussman-Reimer, Joan Vander Walde, Toby Weinberger, and Claire Wurtzel provided me with the critical resources and access I needed to interview girls.

Stella Connell and Andrew Mullins believed in my project and led me to Ridgewood, where I had one of the most special experiences of my life. I am especially grateful to the Superintendent's staff, C. H., S. B., and M. V.; and the teachers of Ridgewood, M. F., P. P., S. P., and G. P., gave me as authentic a Southern experience as a woman could wish to have and friendships I will cherish for a lifetime.

For reasons I will never quite understand, the wonderful people at Harcourt never blinked when my brief residence at Twenty-sixth Street turned into a six-month stay. Their companionship eased the solitude of writing, and I am deeply grateful for their hospitality. For their support and hard work, I thank Susan Amster, Jennifer Gilmore, Jennifer Holiday, David Hough, Arlene Kriv, and Jacqueline Murphy. Kent Wolf provided me with much-needed comic relief during my stay. Jennifer Aziz was a brilliant editorial assistant and friend. Rachel Myers was a superb copyeditor.

I am grateful to an extraordinary group of friends and colleagues who supported me throughout this journey. Many of them reached out to their friends on my behalf and enabled the project to go forward. I wish to thank Elaine and Lydia Amerson, Peter Antelyes, Julie Barer, Jill Erlitz, Frances Fergusson, David Gmach and Sally Friedman, Zoe Holiday Grossman, Sula Harris, Jane Hanson, Judith Holiber and Kim Warsaw, Sandra Hershberg, Kari Hong, Karen Maxwell, Rhonda Kleiner and Alizah and Elana Lowell, Ilana Marcus, Terri McCullough and Howard Wolfson, Danielle Merida, Noa Meyer, Heather Muchow, Nancy Needle, Carmen Peralta, Sid Plotkin and Marjorie Gluck, Rose Polidoro, Elana Waksal Posner, Lisa Sacks, Robert and Stacy Skitol, Freyda Spira Slavin, Leigh Silverman, Taije Silverman, Elizabeth Stanley, Linsey and Kelly Tully, Diane Tunis, Annie Weissman, Susan Wellman and the Ophelia Project, and Rosalind Wiseman and Empower.

I thank Sameer Hinduja, Jane Isay, Lilly Jay, Kim Kaminski, and Julie Mencher for their insightful comments on sections of the revised edition. Parry Aftab and Brian Gatens provided wisdom and contacts for 2010 interviews, and Jenna Johnson skillfully edited the new chapters.

Special thanks to Abdul Aziz Said and the Center for Global Peace at American University; Paulette Hurwitz, whose generous care and counsel helped me find the strength to embrace risk; Molly Shanley, a steadfast friend, colleague, and mentor who talked me down from the proverbial ledge more times than I can count; Senator Charles Schumer and Iris Weinshall for their friendship and support; Sandy Kavalier, who captured me perfectly in the photograph for this book; and Ashleigh May, Ilana Sichel, and Virginia Wharton, who provided me with excellent research assistance.

I will always be indebted to Maryana Iskander, who helped me make the hardest decision of my life and believed in me at every turn, especially when I didn't. It was over lunch in London that Jeremy Dauber became the first person to hear about a book on bullying and girls. Back in New York, on my most frantic days, he ministered carefully to my thinking and prose.

It is hard for me to put into words how much the support of my closest friends has meant. Maggie Bittel, Luke Cusack and Denis Guerin, Ellen Karsh, Astrid Koltun, Cathie Levine and Josh Isay, Lissa Skitol, and Daniella Topol are my family. The force of their faith, listening, love, and laughter guided me through every day of this challenge. I could not have survived it without them.

Odd Girl Out would not have been possible without the unflinching support of my family. My wise brother Joshua was my comic savior and the best friend I could call twenty times a day. My grandfather Bernard Simmons astonished me with his swift acceptance of the changes I made in my life, and he immediately became a devoted press secretary. My grandmother Lia Simmons peppered my computer screen with supportive instant messages and stuck bills in the mail with notes begging me to "stop eating burritos." My Bubby Frances Goldstein is a true inspiration, and my Aunt Sylvia Brodach never forgets me. Finally, my Uncle Bill Goldstein's support has been invaluable, and my inimitable cousins Sergei and Ziggy, who joined our family during the writing of this book, have made spirited additions to our family.

Finally, and most importantly, I thank the extraordinary group of women and girls who trusted me with their stories. I continue to be awed by your courageous voices. Above all, you are the ones who will show the readers of this book they are not alone. I hope your stories touch girls' lives as profoundly as you have touched mine, and that *Odd Girl Out* makes you proud to have spoken up.

When boys act out, get into fights, or become physically aggressive, we can't avoid noticing their bad behavior. But it is easy to miss the subtle signs of aggression in girls—the dirty looks, the taunting notes, or the exclusion from the group—that send girls home crying.

In *Odd Girl Out,* Rachel Simmons focuses on these interactions and provides language for the indirect aggression that runs through the lives and friendships of girls. These exchanges take place within intimate circles—the importance of friends and the fear of losing them is key. Without the cultural consent to express their anger or to resolve their conflicts, girls express their aggression in covert but damaging ways. Every generation of women can tell stories of being bullied, but *Odd Girl Out* explores and explains these experiences for the first time.

Educator Rachel Simmons sheds light on destructive patterns that need our attention. With advice for girls, parents, teachers, and even school administrators, *Odd Girl Out* is a groundbreaking work that every woman will agree is long overdue.

about the author

Rachel Simmons graduated from Vassar College, where she studied women's studies and political science. A Rhodes Scholar, she is the cofounder of the Girls Leadership Institute and develops programs for girls, young women, parents, and educators. She writes frequently for *Teen Vogue*. Rachel lives in western Massachusetts. Visit her website at www.rachelsimmons.com and follow her on Twitter @racheljsimmons.

discussion questions

1. More than once in the introduction to *Odd Girl Out*, Rachel Simmons refers to her book as a "journey." What kind(s) of journey-taking is she suggesting? And what sort of journey did you, as a reader, experience? Where did this book take you? Someplace new? Someplace familiar? Both? Explain.

2. Simmons believes that the loss of a close friend in childhood is often a girl's first experience of heartbreak, rivaling even a romantic loss. Debate this statement.

3. Near the beginning of chapter three, Simmons writes: "Girls don't have to bully [to] alienate and injure their peers... The word *bullying* couldn't be more wrong in describing what some girls do to hurt one another." Why does the author find this term inadequate? What other term(s) would you use instead? In addressing these queries, reflect on both your own experiences and the idea of "alternative aggressions" (which is explored throughout the book).

4. Consider the question Simmons poses at the end of chapter four: If girls use social media to project a particular image, or can only express certain opinions or feelings online, are girls still being "real"? How does this affect a girl's integrity? How does it affect her relationships?

5. Would your friendships be better or worse without social media? What can girls do to reduce online drama and cyberbullying? What is the responsibility of adults?

6. Simmons often looks back at her own girlhood experiences to make a point or give an example. Nowhere is this more evident than in chapter six ("The Bully in the Mirror"). How does Simmons owning her own mistakes and insecurities make this book more effective? Why is this kind of personal exploration so vital to changing the hidden culture of aggression in girls?

7. What is it about the desire for popularity that causes girls to give up their authentic selves? What is the relationship between popularity and aggression? Have you ever done something you regretted in order to be accepted by a person or group? Describe the moment and explore your feelings about it now.

8. Reread the section in chapter eight called "When Cultures Collide." Consider your own experience with girls of an ethnicity or race different from your own. Do you agree that girls' aggression can be influenced by their racial or ethnic groups? Do you think there are certain behaviors that all girls engage in?

9. Simmons tells parents that "when it's your child suffering, rational thoughts can go out the window." Do you agree? How does your own past experience with bullying affect your ability to parent, or to interact with other parents and school officials? Which advice for parents did you respond to? Why?

10. Review as a group the strategies Simmons offers to combat alternative aggression, particularly how educators can improve school climate. Point out which ones seem most realistic, helpful, and workable. What makes these particular strategies seem convincing and effective to you?

11. In her conclusion, Simmons writes: "Most of the behaviors mapped out in this book—nonverbal gesturing, ganging up, behind-the-back talking, rumor spreading, the exiling of cliques, note passing, the silent treatment, nice-in-private and mean-in-public friends—are fueled by the lack of face-to-face confrontations." Describe a key moment in your life when you stood up to someone face to face, or a time when you wish you could—or would—have stood up to someone.

tips to further enhance your reading of Odd Girl Out

1. Visit www.rachelsimmons.com and watch Simmons's "Real Girl Tip" videos. How do these tips further help your understanding of girl bullying and what you can do about it? Which were most helpful, and why?

2. For more on the changing technology landscape and how to handle it, log on to www.rachelsimmons.com and watch Simmons's video series "BFF 2.0." What did you learn? What advice or knowledge will you incorporate into your use of social media?

3. Look again, in chapter five, at the "Ideal Girl/Anti-Girl" chart that Simmons helps a group of girls at a leadership workshop compose. Try creating your own chart, with each member of your group contributing traits and qualities for each of these two archetypes. Then compare and contrast the chart you made with the one appearing in chapter five. What lessons can you draw from looking at these two charts side by side?

4. Take a fresh and creative approach to what you have learned from *Odd Girl Out* about yourself and all girls and young women. As a direct and honest response to the book, communicate your own ideas and impressions about girl bullying in a short story or poem, depict them in a drawing or painting, or set them to music. Remember to include in your creation the feelings and notions (and memories?) that came to you while reading the book.